Nursing Ethics and Professional Responsibility

IN ADVANCED PRACTICE

Second Edition

Edited by

Pamela J. Grace, PhD, RN, FAAN

Associate Professor
Ethics and Adult Health
William F. Connell School of Nursing
Boston College
Chestnut Hill, Massachusetts

JONES & BARTLETT
LEARNING

World Headquarters
Jones & Bartlett Learning
5 Wall Street
Burlington, MA 01803
978-443-5000
info@jblearning.com
www.jblearning.com

Jones & Bartlett Learning books and products are available through most bookstores and online book-sellers. To contact Jones & Bartlett Learning directly, call 800-832-0034, fax 978-443-8000, or visit our website, www.jblearning.com.

Substantial discounts on bulk quantities of Jones & Bartlett Learning publications are available to corporations, professional associations, and other qualified organizations. For details and specific discount information, contact the special sales department at Jones & Bartlett Learning via the above contact information or send an email to specialsales@jblearning.com.

Production Credits

Executive Publisher: William Brottmiller
Senior Editor: Amanda Harvey
Editorial Assistant: Rebecca Myrick
Production Editor: Amanda Clerkin
Senior Marketing Manager: Jennifer Stiles
VP, Manufacturing and Inventory Control:
Therese Connell

Composition: Cenveo Publisher Services
Cover Design: Michael O'Donnell
Rights & Permissions Coordinator: Joseph Veiga
Printing and Binding: Edwards Brothers Malloy
Cover Printing: Edwards Brothers Malloy

Library of Congress Cataloging-in-Publication Data
Nursing ethics and professional responsibility in advanced practice / [edited by] Pamela J. Grace. — 2nd ed.
   p. ; cm.
Includes bibliographical references and index.
ISBN 978-1-4496-6742-9
I. Title.
[DNLM: 1. Ethics, Nursing. WY 85]
RT85
174.2—dc23
                                        2013014339
6048

Printed in the United States of America
17 16 15 14   10 9 8 7 6 5 4 3

CONTENTS

SECTION I   FOUNDATIONS OF ADVANCED PRACTICE NURSING ETHICS   1

**Chapter 10   Nursing Ethics and Advanced Practice:
Adult-Gerontologic Health. 349**
Jane Flanagan

**Chapter 11   Nursing Ethics and Advanced Practice:
Psychiatric and Mental Health Issues 397**
Pamela J. Grace and Pamela A. Terreri

**Chapter 12   Nursing Ethics and Advanced Practice in the Anesthesia
and Perioperative Period 425**
Gregory Sheedy, John Welch, and Brian T. Sim

**Chapter 13   Nursing Ethics and Advanced Practice: Palliative
and End-of-Life Care Across the Lifespan** **483**

Vanessa Battista, Gina Santucci, Susan DeSanto-Madeya, and Pamela J. Grace

The first edition of *Nursing Ethics and Professional Responsibility in Advanced Practice* was very well received internationally. In the United States, it won the Association of Jesuit Colleges and Universities national book award in the category of Health Sciences and the Alpha Sigma Nu Honor Society national book award. Nevertheless, this second edition has been fairly extensively revised in response to the comments and suggestions of reviewers, faculty, students, and clinicians. This second edition is more inclusive of international perspectives, issues, and initiatives, and there is increased emphasis on the development of advanced practice nursing (APN) roles internationally, including the proliferation of doctor of nursing practice (DNP) programs in the United States.

The book aims to provide a consistent thread that relates advanced practice both to nursing practice and to the need for the provision of good health care via effective policies. It is unique in its application to professional issues associated with advanced practice roles. Although this book is specifically directed to the education of APNs, much of the content is applicable to allied healthcare professionals who practice in expanded roles. As with any book concerned with practice, supplementary reading materials may be needed to gain in-depth or extant knowledge of a specific problem. Additional readings are suggested throughout as appropriate. The content is accessible to anyone who is charged with the ethics education of APN students, including non-nurse philosophers or ethicists. A foundational assumption of the book is that APNs have augmented responsibilities to patients, communities, and society that derive from the nature of the role.

This assumption grounds the initial purpose of developing this book—to fill a critical knowledge and skill gap. In teaching a mandatory ethics course for advanced practice nursing students, it became obvious to me that no suitable comprehensive book existed. A resource was needed that would locate APNs' understanding of their responsibilities within the goals and perspectives of their profession while providing them with a strong background in ethical decision making, methods of problem analysis, and strategies for problem resolution. The augmented responsibilities of the APN role demand a resource that is specifically dedicated to exploring the types and complexities of issues faced by this set of nurses. It had become increasingly clear to me over time, and as a result of a variety of experiences, that this book was needed. I became an APN nearly 25 years ago. Since that time, I have taught advanced practice nursing courses, gained a doctorate in philosophy with a concentration in medical ethics, and for the past 13 years taught among other courses one entitled "Ethical Issues in Advanced Practice Nursing."

One of the foundational assumptions of the book is that the development of confidence in moral decision making is possible and that this is facilitated by practice in moral reasoning. Nurses already possess clinical knowledge and expertise, but they also need the tools to identify and articulate to others the requirements for good care in their practice settings, and they need the motivation to provide good care in the face of obstacles. Facilitators of confidence in moral decision making are exposure to contemporary ethics literature, seriously listening to the views of others with whom one would normally disagree in an attempt to understand why the person thinks the way he or she does, practice in exploring difficult cases and articulating salient aspects to others, and understanding the sources of one's own biases and prejudices. Exercises for practicing these skills are offered at the end of most chapters.

The methods I use for teaching my "Ethical Issues in Advanced Practice Nursing" course are eclectic and depend to some extent on the size and makeup of the class. However, it is usually quite interactive, so I do set ground rules and they have proved to be invaluable for getting input from all class members, whether this is in the large group discussion or in smaller group discussions. That these ground rules facilitate participation by even the most timid is evidenced both in class interactions and course evaluations. Ground rules for discussion are that persons should consider their points carefully, articulate them succinctly (this skill can take time to learn), be nonjudgmental in any challenge to the point of view of others, consider all sides of an issue carefully, and be willing to try to understand another person's perspective even when disagreement exists. In the small group case, discussion members take turns leading the group and reporting the group process.

This book is divided into three sections. The first section lays a foundation for understanding ethical advanced practice nursing. The chapters in this section build upon one another. Chapter 1 traces the development of professional ethics back to its origins in moral philosophy, that is, in the development of theories about what it is good for human beings to be or do. Chapter 2 explores the idea that nursing ethics is both an area of study about what are good nursing actions and why and is also an appraisal of nursing actions.

The second section investigates common issues in advanced practice that occur regardless of setting or in most settings and provides resources and strategies for dealing with these. Chapter 3 explores the characteristics needed for good advanced practice, decision-making issues as these relate both to patients and APNs, concerns about privacy and confidentiality, and the importance of truth telling. Chapter 4 explores the tensions for APNs between attending to the needs of individuals and the needs of the larger society. It discusses human rights and the idea of professional advocacy for ethical healthcare environments. Chapter 5 is new to this edition, and it explores the leadership obligations of APNs and DNPs. Chapter 6 discusses advanced practice roles related to the ethical treatment of persons who are human subjects of research or who are considering whether they should enroll in a research study.

The third and final section consists of seven chapters, each of which is dedicated to a separate area of specialty practice. The chapter authors each hold advanced practice qualifications in the specialty area and/or have knowledge of the ethical issues peculiar to the content area. The specialty areas are neonatal, pediatrics, women's health, adult health and gerontology, psychiatric, nurse anesthesia, and palliative care and end-of-life issues. Both the women's health chapter and the palliative care/end-of-life chapters have undergone significant revisions.

ACKNOWLEDGMENTS

This edition was made possible by the ongoing support, insight, and experiences of countless past and current patients, nurses, colleagues, students, friends, and family. Additionally, I was fortunate to be granted a sabbatical from full-time teaching responsibilities by my institution, Boston College. I owe special thanks and praise to guest authors, who each provided "true" accounts and illustrations of issues faced in their specialties and without whose contributions this book could not achieve its purpose. Additionally, the editorial and marketing staff at Jones & Bartlett Learning proved superb at keeping me on track, providing assistance, and answering questions. They quietly, diligently, and encouragingly did their work, paying attention to every detail.

Since the publication of the first edition, my mother, who was a nurse and a midwife, passed away. Her influence as my nursing role model lives on in many ways, however, and especially in this work. The late David Roberts was also a strong influence on my educational development. I would like to acknowledge several of my colleagues for their ongoing support and friendship. Nan Gaylord contributed two chapters and is a dear friend and colleague. She was instrumental in encouraging me to develop the book. Dorothy Jones, Ellen Mahoney, Sister (Sr.) Callista Roy, and Danny Willis have all continued to provide intellectual stimulation and advice. I am grateful to Anne Fleche for her careful review of Chapter 6. A current collaboration with Ellen Robinson, Martha Jurchak, and Angelika Zollfrank on a funded project to increase the confidence of nurses in their ethical decision making within the hospital setting has enriched and informed the content in various ways, and I am very grateful for these professionals' ongoing collegiality and friendship.

In addition to nursing colleagues, my thanks go to faculty in the philosophy department at the University of Tennessee–Knoxville who helped me develop and hone philosophical skills—although they didn't completely succeed in getting me to exchange my "nursing hat" for a philosopher's. Glenn Graber deserves a special mention for his steadfast support of my desire to apply the fruits of philosophical study to nursing problems. I have also benefited from the lasting friendships of my philosophy student cohort. Finally, many thanks to my husband Chris Hayford, who manages to hold on to his sense of humor as well as mine.

CONTRIBUTORS

Vanessa Battista, MS, RN, CPNP
Pediatric Nurse Practitioner
Pediatric Advanced Care Team
The Children's Hospital of
    Philadelphia
Philadelphia, Pennsylvania

**Susan DeSanto-Madeya,
    PhD, RN**
Clinical Associate Professor
William F. Connell School
    of Nursing
Boston College
Chestnut Hill, Massachusetts

Jane Flanagan, PhD, APRN, BC
Associate Professor
William F. Connell School
    of Nursing
Boston College
Chestnut Hill, Massachusetts

Nan M. Gaylord, PhD, RN, CPNP
Associate Professor
College of Nursing
University of Tennessee
Knoxville, Tennessee

**Gina Santucci, MSN, RN
    APRN-BC**
Family Nurse Practitioner
Pediatric Advanced Care Team
The Children's Hospital of
    Philadelphia
Philadelphia, Pennsylvania

Peggy Doyle Settle, PhD, RNC
Nurse Manager
Neonatal Intensive Care Unit
Massachusetts General Hospital
Boston, Massachusetts

Gregory Sheedy, MS, CRNA
Anesthesia Associates of
    Massachusetts
Clinical Instructor
William F. Connell School
    of Nursing
Boston College
Chestnut Hill, Massachusetts

Brian T. Sim, MS, CRNA
Department of Anesthesia
Brigham and Women's Faulkner
    Hospital
Boston, Massachusetts

Katharine T. Smith, MS, RN, CRNP
Doctoral Student
University of Pennsylvania School
   of Nursing
Philadelphia, Pennsylvania

Pamela A. Terreri, MS, APRN-BC
Clinical Assistant Professor
William F. Connell School of
   Nursing
Boston College
Chestnut Hill, Massachusetts

John Welch, MS, CRNA
Boston Children's Hospital
Boston, Massachusetts

SECTION I

FOUNDATIONS OF ADVANCED PRACTICE NURSING ETHICS

CHAPTER 1

Philosophical Foundations of Applied and Professional Ethics

Pamela J. Grace

Believe those who are seeking the truth. Doubt those who find it.
—ANDRE GIDE,
So Be It, or, The Chips Are Down (Ainsi Soit-Il, ou, Les Jeux Sont Faits), 1959

Introduction

For the purposes of this text, the term "APN" is used to denote any and all nurses who are working in expanded roles, regardless of their country of practice. This chapter explains that the roots and strength of advanced practice nurses' (APNs') professional responsibilities are in philosophical understandings about what constitutes good human action and why. From this foundation, it is possible to trace the development and nature of professional responsibility to the population served by the nursing profession. A clear argument is presented about why membership in a profession that provides an important service to individuals and society involves stronger obligations to further the human good than exists in civilian life. Finally, an exploration of the appropriate roles of philosophical skills, theories, and principles in decision making about good action provides a basis for examining the complex issues encountered by APNs. This is an important first step for developing and enhancing APNs' confidence in their ethical decision-making skills.

Groundwork

The Problem of Professional Responsibility

Most nurses and allied health professionals understand that the privilege of professional healthcare practice is accompanied by both moral and legal accountability for professional judgments and resulting actions. However, many are not confident that they are adequately equipped to address obstacles to good practice or the complex ethical problems that can arise in direct care or supervisory situations. Nevertheless, good patient care requires the following essential clinician characteristics: knowledgeable, skillful, and experienced; perceptive about inadequacies in the care-giving environment; willing to focus on the individual needs of the patient in question; and motivated to resolve problems at a variety of levels as necessary. Professionals also need to understand the limits of their knowledge and be willing to draw on the expertise of others. These characteristics are important for obvious reasons and are discussed in more detail in Chapter 2, but less obvious is the idea that those in need of healthcare services are often not knowledgeable about what is required to meet their current or future health needs; they are not qualified to evaluate the quality of the services offered and/or they cannot advocate effectively to receive the care they need (Newton, 1988). Unmet or even unrecognized health needs make people more than ordinarily vulnerable to the ups and downs of life. The effects of unaddressed health needs on human functioning and flourishing make it crucial that healthcare professionals can be trusted to maintain their primary focus on individual and societal healthcare needs, even when faced with economic, institutional, or time pressures.

FIDUCIARY RELATIONSHIPS

Many scholars have argued that the healthcare professional–patient relationship is fiduciary (Grace, 1998; Pellegrino, 2001; Spenceley, Reutter, & Allen, 2006; Zaner, 1991). That is, it is based on trust. People with healthcare needs are forced to rely on clinicians to understand, anticipate, and provide what is needed. Yet in questioning professionals about their responsibilities, how strong or binding these are, or about the basis for claiming that professionals are responsible for good practice, answers are varied and inconsistent; sometimes clinicians even express bewilderment that the question is being raised. Chambliss (1996), in the course of his study of nurses working in institutional settings, noted that when nurses see themselves as powerless to influence change in a setting where there are problematic practices, they can become numbed to the ethical content involved and fail to address it. Others have also documented the problems of nurses feeling powerless. In addition to ceasing to respond to unethical practices when they feel powerless, some nurses leave the setting or seek other types of employment and/or can experience lasting unease, also called *moral distress* (Corley, 2002; Corley, Minick, Elswick, & Jacobs, 2005; Gallagher, 2011; Jameton, 1984; Mohr & Mahon, 1996). Additionally, there is reason to believe that some nurses do not understand the ethical nature of daily practice (Grace, Fry, & Schultz, 2003). Thus, recognition of the fiduciary nature of practice responsibilities requires the nurse to reflect on practice in an ongoing fashion in order to avoid becoming anesthetized to recurrent problematic situations that at best fail to focus on optimal care and at worst are detrimental to patients. Throughout this text, reasoning and support are provided for the idea that professional responsibility exists to address both immediate problems and more deeply rooted systemic or societal obstacles to practice. APNs are ideally prepared and situated to see their responsibilities broadly and influence change, whether this is within their immediate environment or the social contexts of care delivery, the education and supervision of others, or empowering patients and patient populations to get their needs met.

GOOD PRACTICE

From a philosophical stance, *good practice* is equivalent to ethical practice. *Ethical practice* is the use of disciplinary knowledge, skills, experience, and personal characteristics to conceptualize what is needed either at the level of the individual or of society. Ethical professional practice uses the goals and perspectives of the given profession to direct action. Although it is true that various healthcare professions share common goals such as promotion of health, cure of disease, and relief of suffering, they nevertheless have different practice philosophies and draw on different knowledge bases to achieve these goals.

Even when professionals understand the strength of their responsibilities, many factors can interfere with accomplishing good care. This is especially true in contemporary healthcare settings, where competing interests can make it difficult to provide good patient care to individuals even when the clinician's judgment about what is needed is sound. Barriers to autonomous practice are frequently encountered and can include economic interests, institutional priorities, interpersonal communication difficulties, or provider conflicts of interest. Some obstacles to practice are recurrent and arise out of underlying contextual or societal conditions that disadvantage groups of people and thus require a broader understanding of professional responsibility as relating to individuals, institutions, and society (Ballou, 2000; Grace, 2001; Grace & Willis, 2012; Spenceley et al., 2006).

As noted, this and the next three chapters are designed to provide a firm basis for APNs, master's- or doctor of nursing practice (DNP)-nurses, and those from other countries practicing in expanded roles, to understand the origins, scope, and limits of their responsibilities to patients and society. The text provides the APN and equivalent with the knowledge, tools, and skills for ethical practice. Included in the necessary skill set is an understanding of the language of clinical ethics. This is because all nurses—but especially APNs—collaborate with others on behalf of their patients and need a common language for articulating their concerns about the ethical issues they face in practice.

Philosophy, Professional Responsibility, and Nursing Ethics: What Is the Connection?

Nursing ethics and *professional responsibility* are equivalent concepts. However, one cannot merely say this is so and expect to be met with acceptance; the assertion has to be supported by discussion and evidence. This is one of the techniques of philosophical argumentation. As a starting place, it is important to grasp that the idea and possibility of ethical practice lie in philosophical understandings about human beings and their relationship to the world in which they live.

To trace the development of the concept "professional responsibility"—or the obligations of a profession's members toward the population served—from its origins in philosophy, it is helpful to rely on an analogy commonly seen in primary care settings, that of a family tree. The tree and its branches are traced here to give an overview, and then pertinent aspects are discussed in more detail. A word of caution: The branches are made distinct for the purposes of clarity, but there are often areas of overlap or shared space.

PHILOSOPHY'S FAMILY TREE

The discipline of philosophy is the starting point where all theorizing about the nature of the world and our place in it begins. There are several branches of the parent philosophy. These branches represent particular areas of philosophical inquiry: "aesthetics, ethics, epistemology, logic, and metaphysics" (Flew, 1984, p. 267), as shown in **Figure 1-1**. They all share some common

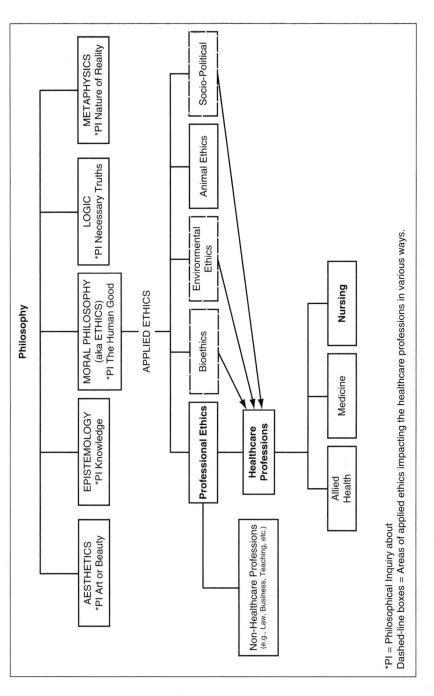

*PI = Philosophical Inquiry about
Dashed-line boxes = Areas of applied ethics impacting the healthcare professions in various ways.

■ Figure 1-1   The relationship of philosophy to nursing ethics

characteristics. They all use questioning and reasoning (the methods of philosophy) to try to understand the relationship of human beings to the world. However, their themes or focuses of inquiry are different. For example, *aesthetics* is philosophical inquiry about art or beauty. *Ethics* is philosophical inquiry about the good and is also called *moral philosophy* (everyday definitions of *ethics* differ from this, as discussed shortly). *Epistemology* is philosophical inquiry about knowledge—what it is, what we can know, who is the knower, how reliable is the knowledge, and for what purposes. *Ontology* is another branch of philosophy; it investigates the meaning of an entity's existence. Nursing's ontology, then, results from inquiry by nursing scholars—informed by practice environments and the needs of society—about what nursing is, what nurses do, and why nursing exists.

For present purposes, our interest is in Ethics viewed as philosophical inquiry about the good. Philosophical inquiry about what is good in human action branches further into areas of applied ethics. *Applied ethics* are the practical applications of theoretical ethics. Branches of applied ethics include *eco-* or *environmental ethics* (what is good human action with regard to the environment?), *animal ethics* (how should we treat animals and why?), *bioethics* (what are the implications of biological advances and how should they be used?), and *professional ethics* (what is the nature of a given profession's services, and what are the implications of this for those served?).

As noted earlier, there are areas of overlap. For example, bioethics is inquiry about the impact of biological and technological advances on humans and what actions are permissible, prohibited, or mandatory. Professional ethics related to healthcare professions has to do with understanding what is required for good professional action. Because healthcare professionals often use technology to provide good care, these areas overlap. A bioethical question might be "How do we decide who gets the one available heart of the four people who urgently need it?" Nursing ethics questions might be "What is my professional responsibility toward my patient whether or not he receives the heart? What is needed for his good care? How do I ensure that he gets what he needs for optimal well-being or to alleviate his suffering?" When Ethics or philosophical inquiry about good action is coupled with an area of human practice of some sort, for example, health care, business, or the law, it is called applied ethics. That is, theoretical understandings about what is good and/or the methods of philosophy (analysis and reasoning) are brought to bear upon a situation to both understand it and, if necessary, resolve it.

ETHICS: A FEW NECESSARY DISTINCTIONS

For the most part, in daily life when people discuss *ethics* they mean something very different from *ethics* as the word is being used here. In common language, *ethics* can merely mean how persons act in their daily lives and whether these actions accord with community values. In professional practice, *ethics* are sets of rules or standards, developed within the profession, that guide the actions of the professionals while working in their professional capacity. The American Nurses Association's (ANA) *Code of Ethics for Nurses with Interpretive Statements* (2001) is an example of this latter meaning of ethics. Nursing ethics scholars have recently provided more in-depth interpretations of the Code's interpretive statements (Fowler, 2010). These senses of *ethics* might be grasped more easily if a modifying term is added. For example, *personal ethics* is related to personal conduct, *nursing ethics* is related to the conduct of nurses as they engage in practice, *medical ethics* has to do with the conduct of physicians, and *bioethics* is concerned with the use of technological advances (and so might include a variety of health professionals, researchers, and technology professionals involved in using or propagating these).

Additionally, many people make a distinction between ethics and morals. They view *morals* as personal conduct that reflects personal values, whereas ethics is associated with critical reflection of the values (Weston, 2002). In fact, the root meaning of both terms is the same: "customs, mores, . . . conventions, institutions, laws" (Bahm, 1992, p. 8). For this text's purposes—considerations of professional judgment and action—the terms *ethical* and *moral* are used interchangeably to mean those actions most likely to further the goals of the profession.

Philosophy

The term *philosophy* can be used in a variety of ways. It can simply mean a personal view of a particular thing, as in "What is your philosophy about always telling the truth?," or, "What is your philosophy on balancing leisure and work?" Philosophy can also mean a group's view of the nature and purposes of its work; for example, there are a variety of philosophies of nursing practice. Philosophies of practice use the tools of philosophy to answer important questions about that practice. Florence Nightingale wrote hers as early as 1859 in *Notes on Nursing*. She believed that nurses attended to the patient's environment, making it conducive to natural healing. However, for the purposes of this discussion, *philosophy* means the overarching discipline, under which more specific philosophies belong.

Philosophy as a discipline encompasses the centuries-old endeavors of thinkers and scholars to find answers to the questions of existence. Philosophy, in this sense, has been concerned with a "search for wisdom about the universe and its workings," as well as the place and role of humans within the universe (Grace, 2004c, p. 280). The pre-Socratic (meaning before the time of Socrates) Greek philosophers such as Thales, Heraclitus, and Parmenides (around the 6th century B.C.) are considered the first philosophers (Russell, 1972). It is thought that before this time period people relied on mythological explanations for the mysterious and seemingly unpredictable workings of nature. The pre-Socratics, however, sought explanations using reason and observation.

For the purposes of this discussion, the discipline of philosophy uses reason and analysis to examine questions that are not answerable or not completely answerable by empirical science. As Nagel (1987) noted, "The main concern of philosophy is to question and understand very common ideas that all of us use every day" (p. 5) but often without giving much thought to their meanings. As an example, empirical science investigates the causes and effects of heart disease in the interests of both prevention and cures. Philosophical inquiry, however, would be concerned with questions such as "Is it possible to have a stable definition of health? Is health measurable?" If the answer to the question of "What is health?" is at all dependent on a subjective interpretation by a given individual, then it is not measurable by science.

Another way to look at this is to say philosophical inquiry highlights what cannot be true but does not necessarily give us truths. In fact, one major question of philosophy is "What is truth?" The main methods of philosophy are thinking and questioning. Reason is used to formulate and pose questions, seek out and examine possible answers, anticipate what objections could be made to the answers, or question whether counterexamples exist that would reveal a theory to be false. Philosophy also helps in understanding the limits of our knowledge.

The discipline of philosophy, then, can be seen to be the enterprise of inquiry itself. The major subareas of philosophical inquiry were presented earlier. The branch of philosophy most pertinent to the current discussion of healthcare professional responsibility is that of moral philosophy, also known as Ethics. From now on, when referring to that branch of philosophical inquiry that is concerned with human good, the terms *moral philosophy* or *Ethics* with a capital *"e" will be used* to distinguish it from the definition of ethics as rules or standards for action.

Moral Philosophy: The Study of Ethics

Ethics, as a term used to describe the area of philosophical inquiry concerned with what it means to say something is good, bad, or neutral in human activity, is also often referred to as moral philosophy. As explained earlier, this is a different view of ethics from that apparent in the term's use in everyday language. Philosophical inquiry is a theoretical endeavor; therefore, Ethics is also a theoretical endeavor. Ethics or moral philosophy is concerned with understanding human values. In fact, moral philosophy as a field of study often leads to the development of theories of value.

Value theories, often also called *moral theories*, try to answer such questions as "What do we mean when we say something is good, bad, praiseworthy, or blameworthy? What makes something, someone, or some action good or bad? Is something good because it is in line with divinely given rules using certain people as intermediaries (for example, Moses and the 10 commandments), or because it helps humans live a satisfying life? Are qualities of goodness and badness inherent in human nature? Are there some things that are absolutely right or wrong? Or are the understandings we have about right and wrong, good and bad, just conventions developed over the years to make it easier for humans to live in relative harmony with others?" Moral philosophers have different answers to these questions. The answers they give are meticulously thought through and provide important insights into the meaning and purposes of human life. It is, however, important to remember that these insights are always necessarily influenced by the lives and political times in which the philosophers engaged in their analyses, as well as by the philosophers' conscious or unconscious motivations for making sense of the world. Different theories can give conflicting directions related to a given situation depending on their premises and assumptions. Moral theories, then, are not capable of giving concrete direction in healthcare settings, because they are mostly theories about the conditions of living together within a society. Moreover, different moral theories give different answers to complex problems. Thus, what is considered "right" depends on which fundamental underlying premise is relied on to assert what is good for humans to strive for and why. In health care, however, the goal is to further the health and well-being of given persons or populations in the context of a particular goal. Moral theories serve to help explain the possible "considerations." They can provide clarity about a given situation, but they do not provide definitive answers. It might be desirable to have the comfort of relying on a particular theory for ethical decision making, but theories cannot serve this function. The following paragraphs are some examples of moral theories, along with critiques of their roles and limits in healthcare decision making.

Applied Ethics

As noted, the term *moral philosophy* is synonymous with Ethics viewed as a theoretical endeavor—the larger sense of ethics. When philosophical and theoretical concepts, suppositions, and skills are applied to practices or human action, the tendency is to refer to this as applied ethics rather than applied moral philosophy, although there is no particular reason for this—it is simply a convention. Applied ethics uses the theoretical knowledge and assumptions gained as a result of ethical theorizing, as well as the skills and tools of moral philosophy (analysis), to solve difficult problems of living. Applied ethics, as its name implies, is the application of moral philosophy to actual situations where it is important to determine good or appropriate actions and where a person or group can be held responsible for these actions. Thus, branches of applied ethics are many and varied and include such entities as ecoethics (good human actions related to the ecosystem), animal ethics, bioethics, and professional ethics.

The appropriate ethical conduct of a profession such as nursing is determined by a synthesis of philosophical inquiry about the ontology of the profession (what nursing is, why it exists, and what its goals are), what constitutes good practice for the discipline (moral philosophy), and what is the force of the responsibility of the profession, both as an organized body and via its individual members, to engage in actions that further its goals (applied or practice ethics). The result of this synthesis is *nursing ethics*. Nursing ethics is an applied ethics. It is the study of what constitutes good nursing practice, what obstacles to good nursing practice exist, and what the responsibilities of nurses are related to their professional conduct. Nursing ethics can be exploratory, descriptive, or normative (also called prescriptive). These distinctions and their importance are discussed in detail in later chapters.

Moral Reasoning in Health Care: Tools

"Ethics as a field of inquiry studies the foundation for distinguishing good from bad and right from wrong in human action" (Grace, 2004a, pp. 299–300). "The theoretical interest is concerned with knowing; the practical interest is concerned with doing" (Melden, 1967, p. 2). Thus, moral reasoning in health care uses theoretical understandings, reasoned assumptions, and proposals about what is the good for humans and applies these theoretical explanations to problematic or complex situations where it is not clear what actions should be taken. In addition to the tools of philosophy, personal characteristics and abilities are needed to apply theory to particular cases. The purpose of this section is to describe the scope and limits of various philosophical approaches in resolving ethical issues in healthcare settings. This section is designed to familiarize APNs with the language and techniques of ethics in the interest of facilitating communication and collaboration on behalf of their patients or patient groups.

An important point that is emphasized throughout this book is that nursing goals serve as the linchpin for decision making and are related to different aspects of promoting health and human functioning as determined by the specialty practice focus and/or the leadership, supervisory, educational, and policy roles of the DNP, nurse practitioner (NP), clinical nurse specialist (CNS), or other expanded nursing role. The tools of applied ethics, then, facilitate an understanding of what is required to promote professional goals. In this sense, the question, "What is the good?" has already been answered by nursing's scholars and theorists. Unlike the larger unanswered or unanswerable philosophical question "What is the ultimate good for human beings?" the nursing profession has an answer related to its practice and existence. Nurse scholars and practitioners have determined what constitutes the profession's good.

The four main types of philosophical tools that apply to morally ambiguous healthcare situations are moral theories, moral perspectives, moral principles, and analytic techniques. Additionally, skills of mediation are increasingly recognized as a way to keep moral spaces open (Blackall, Simms, & Green, 2009; Dubler & Liebman, 2011; Fiester, 2012; Walker, 1993). That is, mediation allows the voices of everyone involved to be heard in an unbiased fashion and in the interest of a mutually satisfactory resolution. An extensive discussion of ethical theory and principles is not possible (or desirable) here—whole books are devoted to any one of the theories or principles, and further books are dedicated to the critiques of these. However, a comprehensive summary of those aspects of previous work in moral theory that are important for our contemporary understanding of moral authority and responsibility follows.

Moral Theory

What is moral theory? The simple answer is that it is a systematic justified explanation of what good means in terms of how human beings *do* or *should* seek to live their lives. That is, it may be either a descriptive (this is what people do or seem to believe) or prescriptive theory (this is what people *should do if the precepts and assumptions of the theory are right*). The author of the theory has tried to formulate an answer to the unsolved question "What is the meaning of good as it relates to human lives and human living?" The theorist, using reasoning, observation, and questioning, formulates a hypothesis and systematically justifies it, all the while trying to anticipate and address possible objections that could be raised by critics of the theory or by those holding different views. Because one of the tasks of philosophy is to show what cannot logically be true (the logic branch of philosophy), every moral theory has many philosopher critics.

Theorizing about human lives and the nature of good has been a human pursuit since the times of the ancient Greek philosophers such as Socrates (circa 450 B.C.), Plato, and Aristotle. There has been an ongoing quest to find systematic explanations and/or unchangeable, irrefutable truths about what is valuable in human lives. One reason this has been seen as important is the human desire for stability, the need to dispel uncertainty about action, and also the need for clarity and direction about how people should live. As stated earlier, moral theory may sometimes be referred to as value theory because its subject matter has to do with what is taken to be valuable, or what should be valued. That is, if it is possible to know what is good for humans to pursue, what sorts of lives are good to live, and which human characteristics are good to develop, and humans have sound reasoning, then society can feel it has a relatively firm footing from which to move forward.

THERE IS NO THEORETICAL AGREEMENT ABOUT THE ULTIMATE GOOD

No theorist, however, has found a flawless answer to the question, "What is good?"; neither have any developed theories that can completely withstand critique. Contemporary thinkers argue that this quest to find the highest good for human beings, or in Latin the *summun bonum*, is misbegotten. In fact, Dewey (1980), a philosopher of the American Pragmatist School, noted the reason that philosophers have struggled so hard and long for answers is that "man who lives in a world of hazards is compelled to seek for security" (p. 3), but the nature of human life is such that it cannot be found. Thus, a paradox exists.

When relatively cohesive theories have been proposed, they often made sense because of the contexts and time periods in which the particular philosopher lived, but these same theories may not remain relevant in current times or may not be relevant in all situations. Additionally, moral theories for the most part come up with different answers to similar questions, as noted earlier.

> The ultimate "good" for persons (or that which persons should or do strive for as an end in itself) has been conceptualized variously as happiness (Bentham, 1789/1967; Mill, 1863/1967), duty (Kant 1785/1967; Ross, 1930), the cultivation of virtue (Aristotle, trans. 1967; MacIntyre, 1984), or something else. This variation is the result of fundamentally contrasting beliefs about the nature of human beings and their place and purpose in the world. (Grace, 2004a, p. 299)

Thus, it is not surprising that there will be many different answers to the hard questions of life. Significant time is not devoted here to discussing the different moral theories because nurses do not tend to rely on one or another of them in clinical or healthcare settings although, from my experiences in teaching ethics, it is evident that people often *want* to use a moral theory to frame a question or justify action. This desire arguably stems from the mistaken idea that theories such as utility or Kantian deontology are authoritative—there is security in "right" answers and "right" actions. However, people can only ever be *reasonably* sure that their actions will have good consequences.

Moral theories can be useful in clarifying an issue or highlighting underlying assumptions. They may provide the structure with which to examine an issue, but nurses—especially APNs—must always be clear about why they think a theoretical perspective is pertinent to use for the task at hand. That is, it is necessary to understand the limits of the theory and what its flaws are, rather than uncritically relying on theories to answer difficult issues in health care.

More frequently, people use ideas from an assortment of moral theories to help clarify their thinking. These ideas are referred to as *principles*. Principles that are particularly pertinent to use in health settings are discussed shortly. However, as noted earlier, the goals of decision making in advanced practice situations are usually concerned with the well-being of a patient, or patient group, directly in the APN's sphere of practice. This is true even when APNs are in supervisory, collaborative, or consultative relationships with other providers—decisions are ultimately being made with the interests of the patient in mind. Finally, the tools of moral reasoning also prompt APNs to ask questions about underlying conditions that give rise to the problems in front of them and help APNs to recognize the wide scope of professional responsibilities.

DESCRIPTIVE VERSUS NORMATIVE THEORIES

Moral theories such as David Hume's (1777/1967) are based on observations of what people seem to believe with regard to good actions and what reasons they give for their decisions or actions. Such theories do not prescribe what people ought to do. They are observational and explanatory rather than having any moral force. They make no claims about the existence of some universal underlying purpose that human beings should strive to fulfill but rather aim to describe human action. Lately, a number of research studies have looked at how nurses practice, what they think is good care, what characteristics are important, and/or how they address obstacles (Corley et al., 2005; Doane, Pauly, Brown, & McPherson, 2004; Hardingham, 2004; Pavlish, Brown-Saltzman, Hersh, Shirk, & Rounkle, 2011; Peter, Lunardi, & Macfarland, 2004; Varcoe et al., 2004). These result in *descriptive* conceptions of ethical practice. That is, they do not say what is right or wrong, but rather what people think is right and wrong and the reasons they give for their actions.

Normative theories, on the other hand, direct action. "They are either, reasoned and logically explored explanations of the moral purpose of human interactions, or they are divinely revealed truths about good action (religious ethics)" (Grace, 2005, p. 102). Essentially they argue that because this or that is the ultimate good for human beings, then humans should pursue that good; there is a responsibility to do so. For example, although the ANA's *Code of Ethics for Nurses with Interpretive Statements* (2001) is not a theory as such, it is a normative document. It tells nurses how they ought to practice and what their behavior or conduct should be. It has moral force.

NORMATIVE MORAL THEORIES: SOME EXAMPLES

Two types of normative moral theory familiar to most people are (1) consequentialist, that is, good consequences are the focus of action, and (2) duty based or deontological, where what matters more than actual consequences is that a person acts according to his or her duty. Perhaps the best known consequentialist theories are those of the utilitarians. Jeremy Bentham (1748–1832) and John Stuart Mill (1806–1873) both were instrumental in the development of utilitarianism. Both were social reformers reacting to the injustices of the time period in which they lived. The Industrial Revolution, which started around 1760 according to Ashton (1961/1997), caused oppression of the new working classes and mass poverty—it resulted in vast inequities in wealth. A few industrialists held all the power and wealth (Engels, 1845/1987).

Bentham was heavily influenced by Hume's descriptive moral theory, which proposed that most human values are socially constructed and stem both from intrinsic human characteristics such as the ability to sympathize with others and the pleasurable effects of benevolent acts as enacted, experienced, or observed (this is a greatly simplified explanation of Hume's work). Hume is credited with introducing the idea of a utility principle into the English language. It represents the idea that human responses are fortified in relation to perception of the usefulness of their actions to others and the pleasure gained from this (Hume, 1748/1963).

Bentham, a peer and friend of John Stuart Mill's father, James Mill, further developed the principle of utility, presenting it as one having moral force. That is, if it is true that humans desire happiness and shun pain and suffering, then that is the good toward which human beings *should* strive. Giving these ideas moral force allowed the social reformers to criticize inequities caused by the Industrial Revolution and to push for reform. Many reforms, "legal, political, social, and educational" (Flew, 1984, p. 41), did occur as a result of utilitarian ideas. As Melden (1967) notes, "Hume's principle of Utility was transformed [by Bentham] with unwavering consistency into 'the greatest happiness principle'" (p. 367).

Following Bentham, Mill (1861/1965) wrote that "pleasure and freedom from pain are the only things desirable as ends . . . all other desirable things (which are as numerous in the utilitarian as in any other scheme [*sic*]) are desirable either for the pleasure inherent in themselves, or as a means to the promotion of pleasure and the preventions of pain" (p. 281). Pleasure was characterized as qualitative in nature in Mill's view, so he distinguished between mere physical pleasures and higher level intellectual ones. Further, in his view the goals of action were to maximize overall happiness for a society and minimize overall pain or suffering. Each person's happiness is equally important; in this sense, the theory presents an impartial view. "Because of their focus on overall good, there are implications to these theories that many would find troubling" (Grace, 2004a, p. 300) and not in tune with common intuitions about good actions. For example, according to this approach, it would be permissible to cause harm to one innocent person if it would relieve 100 other sufferers from pain. However, when any one person becomes a means to achieving the good of another or others, all persons are in danger of becoming that person whose worth is being discounted. There are other critiques of utilitarianism, but the most salient for this text's purposes is that APNs are interested in the well-being of each patient, and this requires understanding who the patient is. Context and details, the "*who*" of nurses' patients, are important. Utilitarian considerations might require nurses to ignore individual details, deferring to an obligation to provide an overall good. Nevertheless, in social policy and justice settings, the ideas behind utilitarianism are important. People do not tend to think that social arrangements need benefit only a few when the majority is living in poverty. In healthcare settings, APNs obviously do think that the possible consequences of their actions are crucial considerations in planning actions—however, particular consequentialist theories do not provide a stable framework for APNs because of their flaws.

Deontologic or duty-based theories are also unsuitable as blanket frameworks for decision making in health care. Immanuel Kant's (1724–1804) moral philosophy is deontologic. It focuses on the idea that something other than consequences is the most important consideration in decision making. That something is duty. The main philosophical assumption underlying Kant's (1785/1967) theory is that human beings are rational animals. Humans have the ability to reason and therefore the capacity for self-governance. Indeed, "the hallmark of human beings is their innate reasoning ability" (Grace, 2004a, p. 300). Because humans have this capacity, Kant went further to say that people have a duty to do the action that their reason tells them is the most rational. How do we do this? We ask ourselves whether in all similar circumstances we would agree that people could act in the same way that we are proposing to act and whether we would be willing to support a rule to this effect. If the answer is yes, then it is permissible to act in this way. If the answer is no, then duty forbids the action. Duty forbids us because it would be irrational for us to act in a way that we would not wish others to act. Kant called this principle the Categorical Imperative because it is unwavering in its moral force. People must act from duty, regardless of consequences. For Kant, interestingly, it was this capacity of human beings to determine right from wrong actions that made them, in his eyes, worthy of respect as individuals; this capacity underlies the principle of autonomy, which will be discussed in more detail shortly.

Other versions of duty-based theories are derived from religious traditions. Kant's exquisitely argued and detailed theorizing was an attempt to avoid the criticisms leveled at religious theories by basing the idea of moral duties on the human capacity to reason. For Kant (1785/1967), then, there were absolute rules, such as truthfulness. He wrote that deviating from the truth even when it might not be convenient is irrational because if people cannot rely on the sincerity of others with whom they are conversing, then meaningful communication becomes impossible. Interestingly, Kant did not think that women and children had the same capacity for reasoning as men.

Criticisms of duty-based theories include: (1) The rules are too abstract to apply in practice; for example, how specific should we be in determining whether a situation is similar to another? What is truth telling and does it include withholding information that might be unpleasant to us and yet not necessary for us to know? (2) What if telling the truth might cause harm to another? Yet reason (Categorical Imperative) dictates that people should not harm each other. How do people decide between equally compelling duties?

Ethical Principles

It is clear that although moral theories exist as attempts to describe how human beings act or propose how human beings should act, and additionally provide justification for the soundness of the theory, they should not be treated as authoritative frameworks for action in healthcare settings. Nevertheless, they do provide some important insights about human values and characteristics: utilitarianism for its ability to critique social injustices, and deontology for its implications that there are general rules that all people can rationally agree on.

The APN's job is to determine both what are good professional actions in situations that require attention to nuance and particularities and what is needed to identify and address more entrenched problems related to inadequacies in the healthcare system. A key point is that certain principles derived from moral theories, together with analytic philosophical techniques, have proved helpful in healthcare settings for separating out aspects of complex situations, illuminating hidden assumptions and factors, and revealing gaps in information. Also, they are helpful in assisting clinicians as they reflect on why they feel uneasy about certain situations. It is important for collaboration and communication that the implications of certain principles are understood. Yet there is often confusion about the origins, definition, and implications of a given ethical principle. The next section explores some important principles in a little more depth, and in later chapters the principles are discussed relative to specialty practice problems.

WHAT ARE ETHICAL PRINCIPLES?

Ethical principles are rules, standards, or guidelines for action that are derived from theoretical propositions (different moral theories) about what is good for humans. Important principles emerge over time as their usefulness in imposing order on a situation, highlighting important considerations in solving complex issues, locating the proper object of decision making, or enhancing social harmony is realized. They reflect philosophical, cultural, religious, and societal beliefs about what is valuable. Thus, what are considered priority principles in one society may not be taken as important in another society. In Western cultures, particularly in relation to problems of healthcare delivery, several principles have retained importance over the last few decades. The most prominent examples of Western principles that are pertinent to healthcare settings have been explored and described in detail by Beauchamp and Childress (2009) and include autonomy, nonmaleficence, beneficence, and justice. These "four clusters of principles derive from considered judgments in the common morality and professional traditions in healthcare" (p. 25). APNs are charged with determining which, if any, apply in a given situation and whether clarity or insights about a dilemma or ethical issue can be gained by using these principles to explore the problem. Put another way, in healthcare practice professional judgment is still needed to determine whether a given principle applies and, if it does, how it will be honored. For example, most people understand that respect for another's autonomy is an important ethical principle, and that, all things being equal, this respect is likely to serve another's good. However, if the issue that the APN encounters is related to an incompetent colleague, then the pertinent principle to use as a guide is nonmaleficence (or how to prevent a patient from being harmed by an incompetent colleague).

In nursing practice, advocacy, caring, engagement with the patient, and knowing the patient within his or her context are also important principles derived from the profession's philosophies of practice, goals, and the roles of nurses. These principles are explored further in the next chapter.

USEFULNESS AND LIMITS OF ETHICAL PRINCIPLES

Ethical principles are useful in helping APNs identify salient issues, clarify important factors, uncover hidden assumptions, and affirm appropriate actions. However, the goals of nursing drive the principles used rather than the other way around. For example, the principle of beneficence (in general) exhorts APNs to provide a good, but the goals of nursing describe what that good is (e.g., promotion of health or relief of suffering), and nursing knowledge, skills, and experience provide the recipe for achieving the good. Motivation provides the impetus for action.

It is critical to understand that principles alone cannot solve healthcare problems because two or more principles pertinent to a situation can give conflicting direction. Additionally, principles tend to be too abstract and nonspecific to be practical. For example, no one is ever completely autonomous; everyone is influenced by conscious and unconsciously experienced pressures—so, what degree of autonomy is acceptable and how is this determined? Principles are not always sensitive to context. For example, what does *autonomous choice* mean when the patient is from a culture where family, not individual, decision making is the norm, or when a controlling relative is pressuring the patient? Finally, human decision making and the actions that flow from this process involve conscious and subconscious values and emotions as well as reasoning, so these are also considerations. In the next few paragraphs, the four major principles highlighted by Beauchamp and Childress (2009) are explored in more detail, as are other perspectives that serve as useful tools in clinical and practice ethics. Beauchamp and Childress's book is recommended for those who want to delve in some depth into a detailed analysis of the implications of these principles and their use in healthcare decision making. However, the unquestioning use of principles to analyze everyday as well as dilemmatic ethical issues in healthcare practice has been criticized by many ethicists as not giving a full enough picture of the issues at hand (Clouser & Gert, 1990; Engelhardt, 1996; Evans, 2000; Fiester, 2007; Gert, Culver, & Clouser, 2006; Macklin, 2003). Fiester (2007) argues that "the Principlist Paradigm is a tool that can only flag certain types of issues and considerations as morally salient in a case, and it leaves many others undetected" (p. 4). The next section will highlight both helpful and problematic aspects of these principles when used in nursing or healthcare practice settings. Other philosophical perspectives that can aid APNs in solving practice problems include feminist ethics, caring ethics, narrative ethics, and virtue ethics. These approaches can remind APNs to ask questions of the situations that permit the uncovering of hidden aspects. In later chapters, these concepts are illustrated in the specialty cases and case analyses.

THE PRINCIPLE OF AUTONOMY

If 20 people were randomly polled and asked about their understanding of the term *autonomy*, there would probably be several related but different answers. Autonomy is a term that is susceptible to a variety of interpretations. The word comes from Greek and literally means self-rule. It was originally used to describe the nature of governance in Hellenic cities (Beauchamp & Childress, 2009) rather than to describe individual capacities or rights. Subsequent understandings of autonomy are related to persons as individuals. Among the various meanings are self-determination, independence, freedom of the will, and a person's ability to regulate personal conduct using reason. It has become one of the more powerful moral principles in framing Western social and political systems and underlies ideas of universal human rights.

Because all of these different if overlapping meanings exist, it is important that clinicians clarify what definition of *autonomy* they are using when engaged in collaborative discussions or when presenting a patient's point of view. Transparency is necessary to avoid miscommunication. There are two main senses of the term *autonomy* as it is used in healthcare settings. In the first sense, autonomy means an attitude of respect for persons regardless of the incidental characteristics of any given human being. The principle charges people to respect all other persons as equally worthy of moral concern, simply because that person is a human being. This principle is justified by several different philosophical and theological arguments (it is beyond the purposes of this text to detail each argument). However, one branch of arguments asserts that the individual importance of human beings is derived from a divine, God-given or innate purpose. A second more secular string of arguments posits that all human beings share interests in being alive and flourishing, and thus all have a right to expect equal moral treatment. When individuals or groups of individuals are treated differently, it actually puts all persons at risk from a change in attitudes that then allows anyone to be treated as less than fully human, which in turn lessens the prohibition against being treated as a means to someone else's ends. For example, slavery treated a whole group as if it did not warrant the same respect as other groups of persons—slaves were a means to the economic and agricultural ends of the slave owners and possessed no individual rights. Autonomy as respect for persons, then, means that regardless of socioeconomic status and intellect, all people will receive equal consideration with others in social arrangements and interactions.

In the second sense, autonomy is the right to make personal decisions; historical arguments for this are based on the idea that human beings have the ability to reason and decide for themselves what actions are best, whether on behalf of themselves or in interactions with others. In current healthcare practice, the recognition that patients have rights to self-determine both acceptable treatment and with whom information may be shared is derived from the ethical principle of autonomy. However, autonomy is often interpreted by nurses and others as the right to make bad healthcare decisions. This is a distorted view of the concept and its use in healthcare settings. Honoring autonomy means the professional is responsible for evaluating what the person needs in the way of information and assisting the person to interpret all available knowledge in light of his or her own projects and desires.

Philosophical Theories of Autonomy

Immanuel Kant (1724–1804) is perhaps the best known proponent of autonomy as a moral principle. He wrote that because human beings have the capacity to reason, decide, and act, they should be free from the interference of others, at least as far as personal decision making is concerned. Moreover, "reason is the ruler of our will" (Kant, 1785/1967, p. 322). Our will is good in and of itself. This was evident to Kant because of "the common idea of duty and moral laws" that is evident in social life (p. 319). Kant gave the example that people know lying is wrong—they can reason this out for themselves—because lying works against social interests in being able to communicate and interact. Thus, it was self-evident to Kant that morality is an a priori condition, inherent in people. What he meant by this is that human beings are born with a capacity (and therefore are purposed) to determine what are moral actions and to carry these out. Kant believed that because man has the inherent capacity for moral decision making, he should never be used as a means to an end but always respected as having dignity and being equally worthy of moral consideration as any other man.

As previously mentioned, Kant did not view women and children as having the same capacity to reason as men.

For Kant there were two aspects to autonomy. Men, at least, are (1) capable of making their own decisions using reason, and (2) have the inherent structure to permit them to act morally (create moral rules) using the Categorical Imperative described earlier. Like Kant, "John Stuart Mill also argued that human beings—women included—have the capacity and the right to make their own decisions" (Grace, 2004b, p. 33). For Mill, diversity and creativity were to be welcomed. Freedom, he believed, is in the interests of society—it allows people to flourish and makes for better societies. Indeed, for Mill the only conditions under which it was permissible to interfere with the actions of persons was when their actions posed a serious threat of harm to another person, including restricting the other person's freedom. Mill did not believe that restricting an individual's actions for that person's own good was permissible. In healthcare settings, both theoretically and ideally, the proscription against overriding the autonomy of another cannot and does not go to this extreme. There are occasions when the ethical action is to stop a person who is at risk for serious harm from an action, at least until the APN can determine whether the person's act is informed, reasonable, and in line with his or her own values and preferences. Whether in actuality the APN always intervenes when there is ambiguity about a patient's decision-making capacity is a different issue that is discussed later in this book in relation to obstacles to good practice.

Contemporarily, there is agreement among moral philosophers that the reasoning process of human beings is never completely free from the influence of such things as culturally determined beliefs, emotions, lack of information, or other environmental conditions (Grace, 2004b). Autonomy is always a "more or less" condition: the more powerful and complex the influences we are subjected to, the less likely we are to be able to exercise our autonomy effectively. Decisions may seem to be autonomous when in actuality they are heavily influenced by overt or hidden influences. Recent research in cognitive, behavioral, and moral psychology highlights a more powerful role of subconscious mechanisms than previously recognized and accounted for in moral decision making (Doris, 2010; Eagleman, 2011). All people suffer from cognitive biases that prevent them from thinking as logically as they think they do (Kahneman, 2011). Therefore, people do not possess even the potential for the sort of detached reasoning that Kant theorized was inherent to human nature.

People are more or less capable of logical reasoning but never have absolute freedom to exercise reasoning that is divorced from unconscious, emotional, or powerful external influences.

Nevertheless, it is generally accepted that most people know themselves and their preferences better than other people can, and thus given certain conditions they have the right to exercise this freedom without interference. After all, they will live with the consequences of decisions made. Indeed, this moral right has been legislated as a legal right under the Patient Self-Determination Act of 1991 (PSDA) in the United States and is acknowledged as a moral right in many other countries (European Patients' Forum, 2009). Patients have the right to decide whether they will accept or refuse health care, including treatment and interventions. The PSDA as well as European patient rights guidelines and those of other countries are discussed in later chapters. It is important to note that many follow the prescriptions of the Universal Declaration of Human Rights adopted by member states of the United Nations in 1948. Two questions related to autonomy in either sense, respect for persons or the right to make one's own decisions, arise here. First, and in addition to the possibility of overt and hidden influences on decision making, some people are not capable of autonomous decision making because they either lack the developmental or cognitive skills necessary. This lack may be temporary or permanent. What is the responsibility of healthcare professionals in such cases? The short answer is that where possible, a healthcare providers responsibility is to try to discover what is known about the person and what his or her wishes would most likely be, so that actions are still predicated on the individual and the way that person has lived his or her life. However, in cases where health professionals are not able to determine what a person would have wanted, the *"reasonable person"* standard can be used. The healthcare provider tries, as a proxy, to decide what a reasonable person would want under similar circumstances. This issue of proxy decision makers is discussed in later chapters and also as related to specialty practice. Proxy decision makers cannot be said to be making autonomous decisions in the sense of autonomy discussed earlier, however. The decisions they make are on behalf of another, not themselves. Proxy or substitute decision makers are, nevertheless, supposed to support the autonomy of their wards by representing as accurately as possible what they would likely want.

The second question relates to the shifting nature of factors influencing the exercise of autonomy. This is often also referred to as *decision-making capacity.* For APNs, related questions are (1) How do we decide when and under what circumstances a person might be deemed capable of autonomous decision making? and (2) What is necessary to facilitate autonomous decision making? Criteria have been proposed that facilitate judgments about whether a person has sufficient decision-making capacity to make a decision that is likely to serve his or her interests. These criteria present their own challenges, but they do provide a framework for judging and thus for addressing impediments to decision making.

The President's Commission (1982) formulated from the pertinent literature, commission members' expertise, and discussions a minimum set of capacities needed for competent decision making. These are as follows:

- Possession of a set of values and goals
- The ability to communicate and to understand information
- The ability to reason and deliberate about one's choice (President's Commission, 1982, p. 57)

This means that for a voluntary choice to be made, professionals need to evaluate the cognitive maturity and abilities of the person. They must assess what information the person needs and how best to provide this—thus, a process of informing (rather than a singular presentation of information) is often needed. An evaluation of influences that might interfere with information processing is important. Interfering influences could include any of the following: unconscious or conscious psychological pressures; physiologic factors such as hypoxia, fever, pain; or contextual issues such as economics (personal and institutional), provider pressures, or wishing to please a provider. Finally, the patient should be able to describe how a given course of action is likely to map on to his or her own life trajectory.

Perhaps the most important thing to understand is that patients who obviously do not grasp the implications of proposed actions for their own goals and future life are not in a position to act autonomously. Thus, respecting autonomy in health care does not simply mean letting a patient make his or her own mistakes. Finally, in respecting autonomy there is a tendency not to interfere with people's decisions if providers are sure these are informed and/or if the risks are low. However, if the risks of a proposed course of action chosen by a patient are high, then providers must make a more concerted effort to ensure that these are autonomous decisions. Overriding a person's autonomy is a serious business but is sometimes necessary to serve the patient's interests. The rationale for overriding a patient's decision is that this is most likely to serve the patient's own interests and preserve autonomy (if the person dies—then no further autonomy is possible in this life anyway).

THE PRINCIPLE OF NONMALEFICENCE

Of the ethical principle nonmaleficence, Beauchamp and Childress (2009) note that "in medical ethics it has been closely associated with the maxim *primum non nocere:* 'Above all [or first] do no harm'" (p. 149). Some scholars have said that nonmaleficence means to do no *intentional* harm. In healthcare practice, and especially in APN practice settings, nonmaleficence is a nuanced principle with several implications. Some scholars treat nonmaleficence as a subcategory of beneficence (the obligation to do good or provide a good). However, exploring it separately facilitates better conceptual clarity. Moreover, healthcare professionals, by virtue of their interventional and therapeutic roles, are often in a position to cause harm in the course of attending to a patient's needs. First, what is meant by harm? Does psychological, spiritual, or economic distress count as harm, or does only physical distress count? Beauchamp and Childress (2009) construe harm as "thwarting, defeating, or setting back some party's interests . . . (A) *harmful action* by one party may not be wrong or unjustified (*on balance), although acts of harming in general are prima facie wrong*" (italics as in the original) (p. 152). *Prima facie* means on first sight. Thus, harms that are generally forbidden may occasionally be justified. In civilian life, this means a robber may be harmed by incarceration, but this harm is justified by the wrong actions of the robber and the robber's infringement on the rights of another. In healthcare settings, harms are not justifiable unless they set back the patient's interests temporarily to provide a longer term benefit. For example, inserting an intravenous catheter to provide fluids and antibiotics to someone in septic shock may be permissible even if the patient objects because not doing so risks irreversible damage, and APNs do not have time to evaluate the person's decision-making capacity.

For the purposes of this discussion, it is best to think of harm as either any avoidable distress caused to the patient in the course of providing care, or avoidable distress that is observed by the professional and/or experienced by the patient and brought to the attention of the professional but that is ignored or left unaddressed. Thus it is clear that harm can be caused both by actions and by inaction. APNs can do harm in several ways; most are *unintentional* but nevertheless often avoidable:

- APNs might fail to adequately understand a patient's needs and thus not protect him or her from preventable harms related to unmet needs.
- An APN's skills and competence might be inadequate to care for the patient's recognized needs, yet the APN fails to seek qualified assistance.
- The APN can neglect to anticipate foreseeable harmful effects from a proposed course of action.
- The APN can fail to intervene to protect a patient against the actions of an impaired, incompetent, or careless colleague.
- The APN can fail to assist the patient manage pressures from others that result in him or her accepting unwanted treatment.

In advanced practice roles, nurses can also cause harm by referring patients to inappropriate colleagues or not adequately training or supervising others who are caring for the patient under an APN's direction. Patients can also be harmed by ongoing interventions that are not likely to achieve desired effects (for example, chemotherapy that can only minimally prolong life and causes suffering in the process). Nonmaleficence, then, is closely aligned with ideas of accountability for the APN's own practice and for practice actions. Accountability means that care providers take responsibility for trying to anticipate foreseeable harms so that these can either be minimized or are balanced against the good that the actions are intended to achieve. Moreover, the effects on the nurse of causing or not preventing harms include moral distress, as noted earlier. Because moral distress can lead to a nurse distancing himself/herself from patients or even to leaving the profession, more diffuse harms to patients may result from the loss to the profession of experienced caring nurses. The APN can inadvertently cause harm through ignorance, incompetence, or failure to understand the patient's unique needs and desires. Harm can also be caused to patients when the APN cannot get them optimal treatment.

Additionally, nurses can cause harm indirectly. The principle of nonmaleficence provides what in legal terms would be called a duty of due care. "Due care is taking sufficient and appropriate care to avoid causing harm, as the circumstances demand of a reasonable and prudent person" (Beauchamp & Childress, 2009, p. 153). Another implication of this principle is that APNs are responsible for balancing the risks of interventions and treatments with the likely benefit. As illustrated with the chemotherapy example, within acute care settings harm can be caused by continuing life-sustaining treatments when the chances of recovery are minimal.

THE PRINCIPLE OF BENEFICENCE

For healthcare professionals the principle of beneficence might be viewed as a more active principle than nonmaleficence because it is the duty to provide a good or to benefit persons. In a sense the very reason for the existence of the healthcare professions is beneficence. These professions exist to provide a service that requires specialized training and skills. In public life, *beneficence* "connotes acts of mercy, kindness, and charity" toward others (Beauchamp & Childress, 2009, p. 166). It concerns the duty one person has to provide benefit to another. Certain moral theories, such as utilitarianism, have as their singular underlying premise the idea that people have a duty to maximize the good in society. Beneficence is unlike nonmaleficence in that it is not morally required of societal members except in special circumstances such as parents or guardians toward their wards. "Whether beneficence is viewed as a moral requirement of societal members very much depends upon [the] philosophical beliefs," culture, and values of the individual or prevalent societal values (Grace, 2004a, p. 317). Although beneficent actions may not be morally required, they do serve a purpose in maintaining the cohesiveness of society. In Western countries at least, and to greater or lesser extent in other countries, people tend to think that if they can easily help someone who is struggling then they should. This is the basis for charitable actions.

In healthcare settings, though, beneficence is viewed as the duty to maximize benefits and minimize harm to patients. It is morally required of the clinician acting as clinician, whether they are physicians, nurses, physical therapists, respiratory therapists, and so on. The goals of healthcare professionals are beneficent—they are inherently for the patient's good, and more broadly, to further societal health. As argued earlier, healthcare professions exist because they provide a critical good for persons. Therefore, beneficence underlies all actions of the professional while engaging in role-related activities.

Paternalism

Paternalism is often taken to be a derogatory attitude that connotes one person's attempts to control another or condescension toward another. However, in its original or legal sense, the principle of paternalism is both an ethical and legal principle that protects the interests of one who cannot be self-protective. The principle is derived from the term "parens patriae," or the state's interests in protecting the vulnerable in society from neglect or abuse. There are extensive philosophical and political debates about whether and when legislative or governmental paternalism is permissible (for the collected arguments see Coons & Weber [2013], *Paternalism: Theory and Practice*). However, in healthcare settings paternalistic actions are ethically permissible or even obligatory—depending on the circumstances—if they serve an incapacitated person's best interests. A person is incapacitated when he or she is unable to make a substantially informed decision as described under the principle of autonomy. Paternalistic actions, then, are beneficent actions. They promote the good for a person who is unable, whether because of cognitive or developmental status, to advocate for his or her own best interests. These best interests can be served by using the person's own history, values, and beliefs where possible. However, in the case of a person who has never had capacity or whose history is unknown or unknowable, the standard used is that of a "reasonable person." Beauchamp and Childress (2009) define paternalism as "the intentional overriding of one person's known preferences or actions by another person, where the person who overrides justifies the action by the goal of benefiting or avoiding harm to the person whose preferences or actions are overridden" (p. 208). Thus, the patient's own interests are the main focus of paternalistic actions. In viewing paternalism this way, it becomes clear that knowledge of the patient in context and as an individual with a life history, beliefs, and values, where this is possible, is a crucial goal of paternalism. Beauchamp and Childress (2009) propose five criteria for justifying paternalistic actions:

1. A patient is at risk of a significant preventable harm.
2. The paternalistic action will probably prevent the harm.
3. The projected benefits to the patient of the paternalistic action outweigh its risks to the patient.
4. There is no reasonable alternative to the limitation of autonomy.
5. The least autonomy-restrictive alternative that will secure the benefits and reduce the risks is adopted. (p. 216)

To summarize, paternalism is sometimes understood differently in healthcare settings than warranted by a fuller understanding of the principle. It has assumed negative connotations in many instances. Some people, nurses and others, have used it to label the condescending, arrogant, or even self-interested behavior of healthcare providers toward patients who they think are making bad decisions. Patients may be persuaded to accept certain treatments, important information may be withheld from them, or a competent patient may have his or her decision overridden. Understanding the real nature of paternalistic actions as both beneficent (patient's best interests) and supportive in the long run of autonomy (restoring the patient to a state where autonomy can be exercised) keeps the focus on the needs of the patient and away from the lure of expediency or other conflicts of interest.

CONFLICTS BETWEEN BENEFICENCE AND AUTONOMY

Sometimes ensuring beneficence seems to be in conflict with the principle of autonomy. For example, a patient with impending sepsis refuses to have a cannula inserted so that treatment with fluids and antibiotics can begin. At first sight, it seems as if there is a dilemma: honor her autonomy or override it and give the fluids because this is what will save her life. The conflict, however, may be false. If the patient does not meet all of the criteria for voluntary informed consent, then she is not capable of exercising her autonomy. She is not adequately aware of the risks and benefits of refusal. Thus, the beneficent action is to treat but to minimize the harms that may stem from overriding her decision. She may, for instance, feel disrespected or that her trust was undermined. Additionally, beneficence supports the idea that as soon as the patient regains decision-making capacity, she resumes her right to make her own decisions, as long as these are adequately informed and align with her own life values and goals. Beneficence does not, as some have assumed, mean that providers know what is best for the patient, but rather that decisions are made based on the individual patient and his or her values, beliefs, and what is known about the patient's life and preferences. In overriding a person's autonomy, health professionals are still charged with formulating actions that accord with an understanding of the patient as an individual with unique characteristics.

THE PRINCIPLE OF JUSTICE

Several different conceptions of justice exist. In Western societies, *retributive justice* has to do with punishment for problematic actions; *restorative or compensatory justice* has to do with restoring to people what they lost in being harmed by another or others. These two forms can be considered noncomparative stances or perspectives. They both are concerned with "seeing to it that people receive that to which they are entitled, that their rights are recognized and protected" (Munson, 2008, p. 774). *Comparative justice*, on the other hand, has to do with how the benefits and burdens of living in a social context—where people are dependent on one another for certain goods and services—should be distributed across a society. For health care and healthcare delivery purposes, distributive justice can also be conflated with *social justice*. It is an important ethical principle in times or circumstances of limited resources.

Philosophical theories of justice try to show what are or would be sound justifications for the rules of distribution. In this sense, comparative justice is social justice. Theories try to delineate which formal social systems will result in the fairest conception of deciding who should get what in terms of social goods such as education, food, shelter, and health care. Buchanan (2000) reports that social justice has been an important concept for centuries and continues to be "central to human understandings of socially significant values" (p. 155).

> There are two broad socially oriented ideas regarding justice. One perspective views justice as being based on deserving it—those who are more worthy of merit or who contribute more are viewed as deserving of better social benefits. The other perspective views justice as equalizing benefits across society regardless of merit. This latter view is "justice as fairness." (Grace, 2005, p. 120)

In the literature related to health care, the predominant accounts are of justice as fairness. The principle of equality underlies accounts of justice as fairness. Justice is impartial in the sense that each person is considered initially as equally worthy of concern. Underlying the various theories is a basic principle that "similar cases ought to be treated in similar ways" (Munson, 2008, p. 774). The conception of distributive justice that is probably most often cited contemporarily is that of John Rawls. His work, *A Theory of Justice* (1971), is a systematic look at the sort of social structures that would need to exist for justice as fairness to prevail. Rawls takes as a starting point Kant's ideas about people as rational and able to divine which actions are morally permissible, obligatory, or forbidden. Rawls's method is a hypothetical device. That is, he wants to show what the underpinnings of a just social system would be and what just institutions would look like. Because man is his own lawmaker, as we have seen from the idea of the Categorical Imperative (the right action is the one that I could agree everyone else *should* take in similar circumstances—that is, it is ethically sound), the design of the system will be dependent on a "group of persons" in the "original position" (Rawls, 1971, p. 12) who do not know their standing in society, or what physical characteristics or material goods they would possess, nor what their "natural assets, and abilities" (p. 12) would be. The hypothesis is that such a group would come up with the rules and standards necessary for the initiation and arrangement of institutions that would ensure everybody is served fairly. That is, if one did not know whether one would be rich or poor, one would be more likely to build in remedies for those who are the least well off even if that did somewhat disadvantage those who are well endowed with worldly goods.

Rawls identifies two rules of justice that he believes would emerge from a group's deliberations taking place behind this "veil of ignorance" about their individual states and traits (Rawls, 1971, p. 136). "First: each person is to have an equal right to the most extensive liberty compatible with a similar liberty for others. Second: social and economic inequalities are to be arranged such that they are both (a) reasonably expected to be to everyone's advantage, and (b) attached to positions and offices open to all" (Rawls, 1971, p. 60).

As might be expected, Rawls's theory is subject to a variety of criticisms, including that the nature of human beings is such that this would not eliminate jockeying for power and advantage and thus upset any ethical system initiated. However, the salient aspects of the theory for the purposes of this discussion are that justice in this sense means being alert to inequities and being willing to address them. Any inequities within a society's arrangements should be slanted toward benefiting the least well off. In contemporary U.S. health care, most would agree that justice as fairness might be accepted in spirit but not in reality. Nevertheless, for APNs the ideas behind justice as fairness cohere with the premises of the ANA's (2003) *Social Policy Statement* and its *Code of Ethics for Nurses with Interpretive Statements* (ANA, 2001). Therefore, it is among APNs' professional responsibilities to promote justice in health care because without this, the most vulnerable will remain most at risk for not receiving good care.

Justice is an important concept related to research, managed care, and health disparities. The important thing to keep in mind about justice as fairness is that it is an impartial look at inequities. It might be a requirement of justice as fairness that the special needs of a disadvantaged group are considered, but each member of the group is impartially and equally accorded that consideration. The nature of justice in health care, then, is that in some circumstances it might give rise to tensions for the APN. For example, a nurse's clinical judgment leads her to believe that her patient needs an expensive drug that is not on formulary, perhaps because of prior sensitivities to other drugs or because current drugs are detrimental in some other way. She feels that she must advocate for her patient to get this drug and that other patients might also benefit but not to the same degree. In advocating for this treatment, resources may be diverted away from others in her care.

Others have argued that although justice as fairness is meant to ensure equal consideration for like cases, in practice people who are perceived as the most meritorious sometimes receive priority over those with a higher need. For example, celebrities seem to get moved up the waiting list for organs more rapidly that others who may be in more immediate need or have fewer resources (Simmerling, 2007).

The justice as fairness perspective in healthcare settings also tends to be directed toward the allocation of scarce resources in terms of technologically or biologically based innovations and interventions and as arising within the healthcare institution or as a result of the types of insurance or funding available. The disease model of health care predominates in the United States in a way that it does not (or not so much) in other countries with universal healthcare coverage. This sometimes directs attention away from looking for inequalities as arising from the "fabric of society" (Grace & Willis, 2012). Therefore more than just redistribution of resources is necessary to rectify injustices and to promote health and healing. In a recent article in *Nursing Outlook* my colleague Danny Willis and I (2012) critiqued the problem that social justice viewed as fairness does not necessarily facilitate looking for the source of intractable injustices in the fabric of societal institutions and arrangements. Moreover, injustices can seriously affect health or the ability of persons to heal. We used an alternate conception of social justice to look at the problem of child abuse and its long-range effects on health. Powers and Faden's (2006) model takes the job of social justice as being concerned with ensuring a basic minimum level of six essential dimensions of well-being needed for living a "minimally decent" life (Grace & Willis, 2012). This conception matches the responsibility of the nursing profession for individual and societal health as outlined in the nursing code of ethics for various countries, including the ANA (2001) and the International Council of Nurses (ICN, 2012). Chapter 4 on human rights and responsibilities expands on the discussion of justice presented here. For the purposes of this text, it is necessary to have a foundational understanding of justice in order to optimize health, both for individuals and the larger society.

THE PRINCIPLES OF VERACITY AND FIDELITY

These two principles, while not achieving the same status in healthcare ethical decision making as Beauchamp and Childress's framework of the four ethical ideals discussed earlier, are nevertheless important in professional ethics. They represent professional characteristics or intents that support the realization of autonomy, beneficence, nonmaleficence, and even justice. Veracity is about the duty to be truthful. The term has its origins in the French *véracité* and medieval Latin *veritas* and means "the quality or character of speaking the truth . . . truthfulness, honesty, trustworthiness" (Brown, 1993, Vol. 2). A related principle is that of fidelity. Fidelity means "loyalty, faithfulness, unswerving allegiance" to another (Brown, 1993, Vol. 1).

Veracity

Although it might seem that veracity is a simple concept—of course APNs should be truthful in their dealings with patients, families, and others—this is not always so easy to accomplish, especially in light of trying to honor the principles of beneficence and nonmaleficence. What does it mean to be truthful? Truthfulness is generally thought to be supportive of autonomy, but is it always? Beauchamp and Childress (2009) note, "[v]eracity in the health care setting refers to comprehensive, accurate, and objective transmission of information, as well as to the way the professional fosters the patient's or subject's understanding" (p. 289). But stark veracity can be harmful to some patients in certain circumstances. Additionally, APNs do not always know what interventions work under what circumstances. How then can APNs decide when, if ever, the standard of veracity should be bent for the good of the patient? Sissela Bok (1999), in her seminal work, *Lying: Moral Choice in Public and Private Lives*, pointed out "the lack of a theory of moral choice which can help in quandaries of truth-telling and lying" (p. xxxi). How do APNs determine what and how much information accomplishes professional goals of providing for patient good? Bok (1989) delineates three arguments that are generally given to support less than full disclosure to patients: "truthfulness is impossible; that patients do not want bad news; and that that truthful information (can cause) harms (to patients)" (p. 129). Each of these stances is susceptible to argument. During the course of the book, the issue of using ethically supportive clinical judgment in decision making is illustrated via cases. The extent and intent of veracity, nuances of veracity, and exploring the permissibility, nature, and role of deception are explored in more detail also in later chapters. In giving honest information the delivery and extent of information are necessarily tailored to the knowledge of the patient, who he or she is, and what he or she wants to know, as far as this is possible. All of the following can be used in determining how to use truthfulness to benefit the patient and uphold his or her autonomy: clinical judgment, collaboration, evidence, knowledge of the patient including cultural needs, and a clinical decision-making framework. Self-reflection related to biases and prejudices as well as reflection on practice are important elements of decision making related to the continuum of veracity. In general, veracity supports trust in the professional, other professionals, and the institution.

Fidelity

The duty of allegiance to the patient is closely aligned with the idea that healthcare professional relationships are fiduciary or trust relationships, as discussed earlier. Provision 2 of the ANA's *Code of Ethics for Nurses with Interpretive Statements* (2001) states "The nurse's primary commitment is to the patient, whether and individual, family, group, or community." Element 1 of the ICN's (2006) *Code of Ethics for Nurses* asserts, "[T]he nurse's primary professional responsibility is to people requiring nursing care." There are many opportunities for nurses and other healthcare professionals to be sidetracked from this priority. Nurses working within institutions and practices may experience pressures to follow the wishes of their employers, supervising physicians, or administrators. There are many other conflicts of interest that arise within healthcare settings that must be negotiated. Additionally, for providers who work within the prison system or the armed forces, there may be overt priorities that work in opposition to a focus on the good of the patients.

Other Approaches

Several other helpful approaches can assist in ethical decision making. These are discussed briefly in the following section. They are not theories; rather they are added dimensions that permit looking more deeply into the underlying conditions that give rise to practice problems. They help clarify the dimensions of an issue or dilemma.

FEMINIST ETHICS AND THE ETHICS OF CARE

Over the past few decades, feminist philosophers have criticized analytic philosophical theory and its methods as they are applied in healthcare settings (Donchin & Purdy, 1999; Tong, 1997; Warren, 2001). They suggest that in addition to moral theory and reasoning, ethical decision making in health care requires the "unearthing of buried assumptions about the influence of power in relationships and situations" (Grace, 2004a, p. 302). *Feminist ethics*, then, is not a singular approach but an assortment of perspectives. "A feminist approach is defined by taking as its starting point the experience of women, by acknowledging that this experience is characterized by oppression and domination" (Peter & Liaschenko, 2003, p. 33). Feminist ethics approaches do not limit themselves only to the concerns of women but address oppression and domination wherever they occur. Other issues of concern are "race, class, class, disability, sexual orientation, and so forth" (Peter & Liaschenko, 2003, p. 37).

This is different from the focus of many of the theories explored thus far. The traditional moral theories tend to view persons as isolated individuals with the right to have their autonomous actions protected or to pursue happiness. Davis, Aroskar, Liaschenko, and Drought (1997) note that Gilligan's research on moral development revealed women's moral concerns to be focused more on "care and responsibility in relationships rather than on the application of abstract principles such as respect for individual autonomy and justice" (p. 58). This is an important insight for nurses because their work is most frequently with individuals and the goals of the profession include caring for the individual as a unique being in all of his or her complexity. Good nursing care involves engagement with the patient and a willingness to focus on the whole person in context. This means that nurses understand the place and importance of significant others in the patient's life.

Feminist perspectives are also helpful in looking at the contexts within which nurses work. Feminist ethics supports the idea that "moral decision-making must include an investigation of both hidden and overt power relationships implicit in ethical problems" (Grace, 2005, p. 105). Questions to pose from a feminist perspective, when involved in ethically challenging situations, include: What are the power structures—social, institutional, or interpersonal? Is there an imbalance? Who has an interest in keeping a power imbalance? How is this affecting the patient or the decision making?

How can we change the focus of power or empower the person who is the primary focus of the issue?

NARRATIVE ETHICS

Narrative ethics represents another contemporary approach to addressing ethical issues. Narratives are stories of people's lives or situations told with rich detail and often from different perspectives. They are most frequently used either in a teaching/learning environment or as an after-the-fact exploration of a difficult case. In narrative ethics, stories are used to explore hidden facets of morally worrisome cases. They may portray the experiences of different persons involved in the story, giving fuller dimensions than usually available in a clinical case presentation. Narrative explorations permit the fleshing out of nuances in a given situation as well as stimulating further questions to be asked. Stories also permit people to vicariously engage in the experience of another from their own subjective stance. This can enhance empathy and compassion, which in turn facilitates understanding of how the person or situation got to a certain point in time. Stories are attentive to context and evolve over the time period of the narrative rather than being a static time slice. Narrative ethics is also a way of learning from situations that have already occurred. Criticisms of narrative ethics include the problem that it is difficult to apply ethical norms or determine what the good action would be.

Summary

This chapter systematically introduced the idea that professional nursing practice is intimately related to philosophy, moral philosophy, and applied ethics. Theories and principles of ethics were discussed in light of their uses, scope, and limits for good decision making in healthcare settings. These ideas will be elaborated on, put into context, and become more familiar as they are used to explore or analyze cases in this text. The following discussion questions are designed to help you understand your own professional values. There are no right or wrong answers, only thoughtful and interesting ones.

Discussion Questions

1. Preventive ethics is the anticipation of potential problems, followed by actions taken to stop their further development. For critically

or chronically ill patients, inadequate consideration of end-of-life options can give rise to patients receiving care and treatments they do not want or not receiving the care and treatments that they do want.

Mrs. Durant is a 75-year-old patient who has experienced a return of breast cancer that was successfully treated 20 years earlier. She now has bone metastases. She is eligible for a chemotherapy protocol that may extend her life for up to a year, but it is not expected to be curative. As an oncology nurse specialist, you are charged with discussing options with Mrs. Durant.

In what ways do the principles and concepts explored in this chapter permit gaining clarity about the situation and thus facilitate preventive ethics? The goal of preventive ethics is to facilitate good patient care and prevent the development of dilemmas or ethical crises.

2. Virtue ethics is another approach. In virtue ethics, the idea is that a person can cultivate a good character. The argument is that "a person of good character will engage in good actions." Thus, the actions of a good nurse would necessarily be good.

Do you think a good character can be cultivated?
Does the nurses' code of ethics from your country or the ICN code support this idea?
What is a good person?
What is a good nurse?
Would a good nurse necessarily be a good person?
What characteristics would a good nurse possess?

Present counterexamples (examples that would point to flaws in virtue ethics theory) and discuss these with your peers.

3. How has this chapter changed your understanding of nursing or healthcare ethics?

4. Knowledge of theories and principles is necessary for dialogue and collaboration with other professionals in the interest of good care for the patient. Do you agree with this statement or not? Defend your answer.

References

American Nurses Association. (2001). *Code of ethics for nurses with interpretive statements*. Washington, DC: Author.

American Nurses Association. (2003). *Social policy statement*. Washington, DC: Author.

Aristotle. (1967). The Nichomachean Ethics, Books I, II, III (chapters 1–5), VI & X. In A. I. Melden (Ed.), W. D. Ross (Trans.), *Ethical theories: A book of readings* (2nd ed., pp. 88–142). Englewood Cliffs, NJ: Prentice Hall. (Date of original work uncertain.)

Ashton, T. S. (1997). *The Industrial Revolution, 1760–1830*. New York, NY: Oxford University Press. (Original work published in 1961.)

Bahm, A. J. (1992). *Why be moral?* (2nd ed.). Albuquerque, NM: World Books.

Ballou, K. A. (2000). A historical-philosophical analysis of the professional nurse obligation to participate in sociopolitical activities. *Policy, Politics, & Nursing Practice, 1*(3), 172–184.

Beauchamp, T. L., & Childress, J. F. (2009). *Principles of biomedical ethics* (6th ed.). New York, NY: Oxford University Press.

Bentham, J. (1967). An introduction to the principles of morals and legislation. In A. I. Melden (Ed.), *Ethical theories: A book of readings* (pp. 367–390). Englewood Cliffs, NJ: Prentice Hall. (Original work published in 1789.)

Blackall, G. F., Simms, S., & Green, M. J. (2009). *Breaking the cycle: How to turn conflict into collaboration*. Philadelphia, PA: American College of Physicians.

Bok, S. (1989). Lies to the sick and dying. In P. Y. Windt et al. (Eds.), *Ethical issues in the professions* (pp. 127–133). Englewood Cliffs, NJ: Prentice Hall.

Bok, S. (1999). *Lying: Moral choice in public and private life* (2nd ed.). New York, NY: Random House.

Brown, L. (Ed.). (1993). *The new shorter Oxford English Dictionary*. New York, NY: Oxford Clarendon Press.

Buchanan, D. R. (2000). *An ethic for health promotion*. New York, NY: Oxford University Press.

Chambliss, D. F. (1996). *Beyond caring: Hospitals, nurses, and the social organization of ethics*. Chicago, IL: University of Chicago Press.

Clouser, K. D., & Gert, B. (1990). A critique of principlism. *Journal of Medical Philosophy, 15*, 219–236.

Coons, C., & Weber, M. (2013). *Paternalism: Theory and practice*. New York, NY: Cambridge University Press.

Corley, M. C. (2002). Nurses' moral distress: A proposed theory and research agenda. *Nursing Ethics, 9*(6), 636–650.

Corley, M. C., Minick, P., Elswick, R. K., & Jacobs, M. (2005). Nurse moral distress and ethical work environment. *Nursing Ethics, 12*(4), 381–390.

Davis, A. J., Aroskar, M. A., Liaschenko, J., & Drought, T. S. (1997). *Ethical dilemmas and nursing practice* (4th ed.). Upper Saddle River, NJ: Appleton & Lange.

Dewey, J. (1980). *The quest for certainty: A study of the relation of action knowledge and action*. New York, NY: Perigee Books. (Original work published in 1929.)

Doane, G., Pauly, B., Brown, H., & McPherson, G. (2004). Exploring the heart of ethical nursing practice: Implications for ethics education. *Nursing Ethics, 11*(3), 240–253.

Donchin, A., & Purdy, L. (Eds.). (1999). *Embodying bioethics: Recent feminist advances*. Lanham, MD: Roman & Littlefield.

Doris, J. M., & the Moral Psychology Research Group. (2010). *The moral psychology handbook.* New York, NY: Oxford University Press.

Dubler, N., & Liebmann, C. B. (2001). *Bioethics mediation: A guide to shaping shared solutions.* Nashville, TN: Vanderbilt University Press.

Eagleman, D. (2011). *Incognito: The secret lives of the brain.* New York, NY: Random House.

Engelhardt, H. T. (1996). *The foundations of bioethics.* New York, NY: Oxford University Press.

Engels, F. (1987). *The condition of the working class in England.* (Edited with an introduction by V. Kiernan.) Middlesex, UK: Penguin Books. (Original work published in Germany in 1845.)

European Patients' Forum. (2009). Patients' rights in the European Union. Retrieved from http://www.eu-patient.eu/Documents/Projects/Valueplus/Patients_Rights.pdf

Evans, J. H. (2000). A sociological account of the growth of principlism. *Hastings Center Report, 30*(5), 31–38.

Fiester, A. (2007). The principlist paradigm and the problem of the false negative: Why the clinical ethics we teach fails patients. *Academic Medicine, 82*(7), 684–689.

Fiester, A. (2012). Mediation and advocacy. *The American Journal of Bioethics, 12*(8), 10–11.

Flew, A. (1984). *A dictionary of philosophy* (2nd ed.). New York, NY: St. Martin's Press.

Fowler, M. D. M. (2010). *Guide to the code of ethics for nurses: Interpretation and application.* Silver Spring, MD: ANA.

Gallagher, A. (2011). Moral distress and moral courage in everyday nursing practice. *Online Journal of Issues in Nursing, 16*(2). doi: 10.3912/OJIN.Vol16No02PPT03

Gert, B., Culver, C. M., & Clouser, K. D. (2006). *Bioethics: A systematic approach.* New York, NY: Oxford University Press.

Gide, A. (1959). *So be it, or The chips are down (Ainsi soit-il; ou, Les jeux sont faits).* New York, NY: Knopf.

Grace, P. J. (1998). *A philosophical analysis of the concept 'advocacy': Implications for professional–patient relationships.* Unpublished doctoral dissertation. University of Tennessee, Knoxville. Retrieved from http://proquest.umi.com. Publication number AAT9923287, Proquest Document ID No. 734421751.

Grace, P. J. (2001). Professional advocacy: Widening the scope of accountability. *Nursing Philosophy, 2*(2), 151–162.

Grace, P. J. (2004a). Ethics in the clinical encounter. In S. K. Chase (Ed.), *Clinical judgment and communication in nurse practitioner practice* (pp. 295–332). Philadelphia, PA: F. A. Davis.

Grace, P. J. (2004b). Patient safety and the limits of confidentiality. *American Journal of Nursing, 104*(11), 33, 35–37.

Grace, P. J. (2004c). Philosophical considerations in nurse practitioner practice. In S. K. Chase (Ed.), *Clinical judgment and communication in nurse practitioner practice* (pp. 279–294). Philadelphia, PA: F. A. Davis.

Grace, P. J. (2005). Ethical issues relevant to health promotion. In C. Edelman & C. L. Mandle (Eds.), *Health promotion throughout the lifespan* (6th ed., pp. 100–125). St. Louis, MO: Elsevier/Mosby.

Grace, P. J., Fry, S. T., & Schultz, G. (2003). Ethics and human rights issues experienced by psychiatric-mental health and substance abuse registered nurses. *Journal of the American Psychiatric Nurses Association, 9*(1), 17–23.

Grace, P. J., & Willis, D. G. (2012). Nursing responsibilities and social justice: An analysis in support of disciplinary goals. *Nursing Outlook, 60*(4), 198–207.

Hardingham, L. (2004). Integrity and moral residue: Nurses as participants in a moral community. *Nursing Philosophy, 5*, 127–134.

Hume, D. (1963). *An enquiry concerning human understanding and other essays.* New York, NY: Washington Square Press. (Original work published in 1748 by A. Millar, London.)

Hume, D. (1967). An enquiry concerning the principles of morals. In A. I. Melden (Ed.), *Ethical theories: A book of readings* (pp. 273–316). Englewood Cliffs, NJ: Prentice Hall. (Original work published in 1777.)

International Council of Nurses. (2012). *Code of ethics for nurses.* Geneva, Switzerland: Author.

Jameton, A. (1984). *Nursing practice: The ethical issues.* Upper Saddle River, NJ: Prentice Hall.

Kahneman, D. (2011). *Thinking fast and slow.* New York, NY: Farrar, Straus & Giroux.

Kant, I. (1967). Foundations of the metaphysics of morals. In A. I. Melden (Ed.), *Ethical theories: A book of readings* (pp. 317–366). Englewood Cliffs, NJ: Prentice Hall. (Original work published in 1785.)

MacIntyre, A. C. (1984). *After virtue: A study in moral theory* (2nd ed.). Notre Dame, IN: University of Notre Dame Press.

Macklin, R. (2003). Applying the four principles. *Journal of Medical Ethics, 29*(5), 275–280.

Melden, A. I. (1967). On the nature and problems of ethics. In A. I. Melden (Ed.), *Ethical theories: A book of readings.* Englewood Cliffs, NJ: Prentice Hall.

Mill, J. S. (1965). *Mill's ethical writings.* (Edited with an introduction by J. B. Schneewind.) New York, NY: Macmillan. (Original work published in 1861.)

Mill, J. S. (1967). Utilitarianism. In A. I. Melden (Ed.), *Ethical theories: A book of readings* (pp. 391–434). Englewood Cliffs, NJ: Prentice Hall. (Original work published in 1863.)

Mohr, W. K., & Mahon, M. M. (1996). Dirty hands: The underside of marketplace health care. *Advances in Nursing Science, 119*(1), 28–37.

Munson, R. (2008). *Intervention and reflection: Basic issues in medical ethics* (8th ed.). Belmont, CA: Wadsworth.

Nagel, T. (1987). *What does it all mean?* New York, NY: Oxford University Press.

Newton, L. H. (1988). Lawgiving for professional life: Reflections on the place of the professional code. In A. Flores (Ed.), *Professional ideals* (pp. 47–56). Belmont, CA: Wadsworth.

Nightingale, F. (1859). *Notes on nursing: What it is and what it is not.* London, England: Harrison. (Reprint Philadelphia, PA: Lippincott)

Pavlish, C., Brown-Saltzman, C., Hersh, M., Shirk, M., & Rounkle, A. (2011). Nursing priorities, actions, and regrets for ethical situations in clinical practice. *Journal of Nursing Scholarship, 43*(4), 385–395.

Pellegrino, E. D. (2001). Trust and distrust in professional ethics. In W. Teays & L. Purdy (Eds.), *Bioethics, justice, and health care* (pp. 24–30). Belmont, CA: Wadsworth. (Reprinted from *Ethics, trust, and the professions: Philosophical and cultural aspects,* by E. D. Pellegrino, R. M. Veatch, & J. P. Langan, Eds., 1991, Washington, DC: Georgetown University Press.)

Peter, E., & Liaschenko, J. (2003). Feminist ethics. In V. Tschudin (Ed.), *Approaches to ethics: Nursing beyond boundaries* (pp. 33–44). New York, NY: Butterworth-Heinemann.

Peter, E., Lunardi, V. L., & Macfarland, A. (2004). Nursing resistance as ethical action: Literature review. *Journal of Advanced Nursing, 46*(4), 403–413.

Powers, M., & Faden, R. (2006). *Social justice: The moral foundations of public health and health policy.* New York, NY: Oxford University Press.

President's Commission for the Study of Ethical Problems in Medicine and Biomedical and Behavioral Research. (1982). *Making health care decisions.* Washington, DC: U.S. Government Printing Office. 33. PB83236703.

Rawls, J. (1971). *A theory of justice.* Cambridge, MA: Harvard University Press.

Ross, D. (1930). *The right and the good.* Oxford, England: Oxford University Press.

Russell, B. (1972). *A history of Western philosophy.* New York, NY: Simon & Schuster.

Simmerling, M. (2007). Beyond scarcity: Poverty as a contraindication for organ transplantation. *Virtual Mentor, 9*(6), 441–444.

Spenceley, S. M., Reutter, L., & Allen, M. N. (2006). The road less traveled: Advocacy at the policy level. *Policy, Politics, and Nursing Practice, 7*(3), 180–194.

Tong, R. (1997). *Feminist approaches to bioethics: Theoretical reflections and practical applications.* Boulder, CO: Westview Press.

Varcoe, C., Doane, G., Pauly, B., Rodney, P., Storch, J. L., Mahoney, K., . . . Starzomski, R. (2004). Ethical practice in nursing: Working the in-betweens. *Nursing Philosophy, 45*(3), 316–325.

Walker, M. U. (1993). Keeping moral spaces open: New images of ethics consulting. *The Hastings Center Report, 23*(2), 33–40.

Warren, V. L. (2001). From autonomy to empowerment: Health care ethics from a feminist perspective. In W. Teays & L. Purdy (Eds.), *Bioethics, justice, and health care* (pp. 49–53). Belmont, CA: Wadsworth.

Weston, A. (2002). *A practical companion to ethics* (2nd ed.). New York, NY: Oxford University Press.

Zaner, R. M. (1991). The phenomenon of trust and the physician–patient relationship. In E. D. Pellegrino, R. M. Veatch, & J. P. Langan (Eds.), *Ethics, trust and the professions: Philosophical and cultural aspects* (pp. 45–67). Washington, DC: Georgetown University Press.

CHAPTER 2

Nursing Ethics

Pamela J. Grace

The professional must respond . . . if practices in his field are inadequate at any stage of the rendering of the service: if the client the ultimate consumer is unhappy; if he is happy, but unknowing, badly served by shabby products or service; or if he is happy and well served by the best available product but the state of the art is not adequate to his real needs.
— L. H. Newton, "Lawgiving for Professional Life:
Reflections on the Place of the Professional Code," 1988

Let whoever is in charge keep this simple question in her head (not, how can I always do this right thing myself, but) how can I provide for this right thing to be always done?
— Florence Nightingale, *Notes on Nursing:*
What It Is and What It Is Not, 1946

Introduction

The purposes of this chapter are several. The primary intent is to reinforce advanced practice nurses' (APNs') understanding of the different senses of nursing ethics, its conceptual origins, its relationship to practice, and the importance of this understanding for good patient care. It locates the foundation of APN responsibilities securely within the goals of the profession and the responsibilities of human service professions to individuals and society. An understanding of how and why professions developed and what purposes they served and now serve provides a basis for grasping the importance of contemporary professions to individual security and the relatively smooth running of societies. While the authors' contexts of practice are mostly within the U.S. healthcare system, implications for nurses practicing in advanced roles internationally have been researched and are highlighted when evidence was available. Some characteristics and concepts that have gained importance in professional nursing and in nursing ethics are discussed. Finally, a decision-making heuristic (helpful device) is applied to a deceptively simple case to demonstrate how all of the following are essential elements in meeting nursing goals of good patient care. These essential elements include nursing knowledge, a basic understanding of the language of ethics, certain personal characteristics (discussed later), personal and professional experiences, and the philosophical tools of exploration, analysis, and clarification. The goals of nursing have been articulated in terms of responsibilities "to promote health, to prevent illness, to restore health and to alleviate suffering" (International Council of Nurses [ICN], 2012, p. 2). Additionally, Willis, Grace, and Roy (2008) recently synthesized from nursing literature an implicit central unifying focus for the discipline that gives nursing its unique perspective. This focus, "facilitating humanization, meaning, choice, quality of life and healing in living and dying" (p. E28), provides a basis for clinical/ethical judgments and action and is aligned with the principle of beneficence.

Table 2-1 describes some habits that are vital for critical appraisals both of practice situations and reading material. Many readers will have already acquired such habits as a result of life and practice experiences; if so, these tips will serve as a refresher, and hopefully as reinforcement. The first task, though, is to be clear about what is meant by the term *nursing ethics*. This is necessary because, although the term is used widely in the nursing literature, it is not always clear from the topic or content discussed exactly what is meant.

Two Senses of Nursing Ethics

For many people working in health care, the term *ethics* has come to be associated with bioethical dilemmas or with other extremely difficult situations. A dilemma is a special sort of problem that requires a choice to be made between two or more equally undesirable options. The origin of the term is in the Greek *di,* meaning two, and *lemma,* meaning premises or assumptions (Brown, 1993). One reason for the association between bioethics and dilemmas is that the sorts of problems typically brought to public attention are those raised by technological or biological innovations. Nurses may well be involved in decision-making situations involving dilemmas; however, these situations are far from the most common issues that they face in daily practice.

■ Table 2-1   Habits of Critique

Questioning Authority	**Assumptions:** Authorities are human beings. Authoritative texts are the interpretations of human beings. The orders of superiors, managers, and leaders can be mistaken or misinformed. Important details of a situation can been missed, time may be an issue, or conflicts of interest may supplant goals.
	Case: The chief nursing officer (CNO) is under pressure to cut costs and urges her clinical nurse specialists (CNSs) to limit the time spent mentoring new staff in favor of completing more administrative work. The CNSs understand that in the long run spending the time to mentor staff will result in better patient outcomes and be more likely to meet professional goals.
	Actions: CNSs should ask themselves what assumptions the CNO is making in proposing the plan and whether these are supportable given available data, not supportable for other reasons, or require more data. CNSs must gather needed data and present the data to the CNO. They should consider eliciting peer support, weighing the risks and benefits of this.
Self-reflection	It follows that the APN's authority and expertise are also subject to critique. Thus a second important (and sometimes painful) habit is that of genuine self-reflection. Genuineness refers to willingness to recognize and admit that a person's position may not be the only valid one, that others may have equally valid positions, even if they radically differ. It is possible to learn from listening carefully to these alternate perspectives. Asking what is underlying these perspectives provides further insights.
	Many people believe themselves to be self-reflective although actually they are more interested in molding the facts and details to fit their original belief (rationalization).
	Self-reflection allows a person to both assume that biases and prejudices exist and try to discover what these might be in relation to a particular situation in the interests of controlling for them.

(continues)

■ Table 2-1   Habits of Critique (*continued*)

Logical Critique	Throughout this text reasoned argument is used to support positions taken. A reasoned argument is not a dispute; it is the presentation of concept, or an assertion that results from a chain of reasoning about a specific entity. It entails questioning underlying assumptions, discarding irrelevant information, and ensuring that the tentative conclusion can be supported by facts, logical reasoning, and/or sound assumptions. Sound assumptions are those that have stood up to critique and for which no counterexample can be given. There is an area of philosophy that actually studies the logic of arguments. When the premises of a logically sound argument are true, a conclusion derived from the premises will be true. A simple example of a sound argument is this: Premise: Human beings need nutrition for survival. Premise: Mr. Jones is unable to eat and refuses to take in nutrition by any other route. (*Assuming this is true . . .*) Conclusion: Mr. Jones will not survive. Sometimes, however, in the course of presenting an argument, a person discovers that an important aspect has been overlooked or that an assertion is made that is not true of all situations. In this example, if some persons were known to have survived without nutrition, it would not be possible to conclude that Mr. Jones would not survive.
Reading Critically	As you read, ask yourself, "Does this ring true?" If it does not, then try to isolate what is troubling. Are there counterexamples that would disprove the statement being made? Is the author missing some important facts? Discuss your thoughts with your peers. Refuse to take anything at face value. There are no moral experts in health care. No group of professionals has superior ethics knowledge; someone might have superior technical or content knowledge, but this is no preparation for ethical reasoning.
Living with Nuance	There will always be some uncertainty in ethical decision making because of the complex nature of human beings. Absolute security in having the right answer is not possible. Dewey's (1929/1980) insight is, "The distinctive characteristic of practical activity, one which is so inherent that it cannot be eliminated, is the uncertainty which attends it" (p. 6).

■ Table 2-1   Habits of Critique (*continued*)

Keeping Professional Goals in Mind	However, nursing ethics assumes that the application of nursing judgment and action can positively influence patient well-being and reduce the likelihood of harm.
	A basic foundation for ethical professional action is the knowledge developed by the practitioner's discipline and/or knowledge from other sources that is then filtered through the discipline's lens and modified to meet the discipline's goals. Additionally, the possession or development of certain characteristics is important to good practice. In nursing, these include the willingness to be self-reflective, reflect on practice, and engage with patients as individuals whose needs differ in important ways from those of others. The process of furthering nursing's goals often also requires willingness to tackle difficult systemic problems arising from unjust societal healthcare arrangements. Thus, the political skills of negotiation and collaboration are also crucial to hone.

Professional responsibility and nursing ethics may be understood as equivalent concepts. This statement requires some further explanation. The term *nursing ethics,* like the term *ethics* can represent either a field of inquiry about nursing's responsibilities or nurses' actual practice-related actions (that is, those actions nurses undertake in the role of nurse and the extent to which these both flow from nursing knowledge and are anchored in nursing goals). Nursing ethics as a field of inquiry and nursing ethics as rules of professional conduct are, of course, closely related and inform each other. Here is a common example—if an intensive care nurse is asked to provide care for three critically ill patients during the same shift, each of whom realistically requires the attention of one nurse, he or she cannot fulfill nursing goals for all or, probably, for any of the patients. No matter how experienced a nurse, the situation is impossible. The best the nurse can do is to try and head off disaster. He or she cannot give what is considered good or optimal care to each patient. How is Nursing Ethics as a field of inquiry helpful in this situation? It investigates what a nurse's options are for the immediate circumstances and what changes might need to be made in the environment so that such problems do not recur. Nursing Ethics as inquiry, then, seeks to understand the following: What is an individual nurse's responsibility in such situations, and how should such problems be addressed so that the conditions that gave rise to it are changed or removed? Additionally, the profession's collective responsibility to address underlying or accompanying environmental concerns is the subject of critique and investigation by Nursing Ethics, when viewed as a field of study. Fry (2002) succinctly summarized the main concerns of Nursing Ethics as being about "describing the characteristics of the 'good' nurse, and identifying nurses' ethical practices" (p. 1). Implicit in this definition is the further political task of critiquing environments of practice and describing the necessary educational strategies to prepare ethical nurses. However, for the nurse involved in the example situation given, nursing ethics is her professional responsibility to recognize the ethical nature of the problem while trying to minimize possible harms and maximize patient good using available resources and within the limits of the immediate situation. It may also mean working after the fact (probably in concert with others) to address the conditions that led to this patient care problem.

In Nursing Ethics as a field of inquiry, the situation described explores why the nurse is being asked to do the seemingly impossible, what this means to the nurse, what this means to individual patients and society, and what the legitimate avenues of response are. These are questions for nursing's philosophers, scholars, and other interested parties to address (with input from practice). In contrast, nursing ethics, viewed as professional responsibility to further nursing's goals of practice in individual situations, pertains to the nurse being and acting within the context of actual practice or perhaps in the interests of actual practice (for example, political action to change inadequate practice settings as discussed in Chapter 4). This may also be termed *professional advocacy* (Grace, 1998, 2001). Professional advocacy is the nurse's responsibility both to address immediate situations of inadequate practice and to be active in addressing the environmental conditions that give rise to practice problems. (Professional advocacy is addressed in more detail later in this chapter.)

This chapter uses the convention of capitalizing the term Nursing Ethics when referring to the field of inquiry and will leave in lowercase the term nursing ethics when discussing the ethical conduct of nurses. Nursing Ethics, then, is a field of study involved in theorizing about, or researching, what nursing practice is, what good it provides, and how nurses should or do act. It has exploratory, descriptive, and prescriptive interests. The exploratory task of Nursing Ethics includes philosophical and theoretical investigations about professional goals and ways to further these. The descriptive task involves the use of research or observation to understand how nurses act in practice, what nurses think are good ways of acting, and how they recognize and address problems. Finally, the prescriptive or normative aspect provides guidelines for nurses about what actions are expected of the nurse. For example, the American Nurses Association's (ANA, 2001) *Code of Ethics for Nurses with Interpretive Statements* (**Table 2-2**) or the ICN's (2012) *Code of Ethics for Nurses* (**Table 2-3**) both provide guidelines for ethical conduct that are derived from disciplinary goals. More recently, the European Council

■ **Table 2-2**   American Nurses Association *Code of Ethics for Nurses*

---

1. The nurse, in all professional relationships, practices with compassion and respect for the inherent dignity, worth, and uniqueness of every individual, unrestricted by considerations of social or economic status, personal attributes, or the nature of health problems.

2. The nurse's primary commitment is to the patient, whether an individual, family, group, or community.

3. The nurse promotes, advocates for, and strives to protect the health, safety, and rights of the patient.

4. The nurse is responsible and accountable for individual nursing practice and determines the appropriate delegation of tasks consistent with the nurse's obligation to provide optimum patient care.

5. The nurse owes the same duties to self as to others, including the responsibility to preserve integrity and safety, to maintain competence, and to continue personal and professional growth.

6. The nurse participates in establishing, maintaining, and improving health care environments and conditions of employment conducive to the provision of quality health care and consistent with the values of the profession through individual and collective action.

7. The nurse participates in the advancement of the profession through contributions to practice, education, administration, and knowledge development.

8. The nurse collaborates with other health professionals and the public in promoting community, national, and international efforts to meet health needs.

9. The profession of nursing, as represented by associations and their members, is responsible for articulating nursing values, for maintaining the integrity of the profession and its practice, and for shaping social policy.

Source: Reprinted with permission from American Nurses Association, *Code of Ethics for Nurses with Interpretative Statements*, © 2001 Nursesbooks.org, Silver Spring, MD.

■ Table 2-3 The International Council of Nurses' *Code of Ethics for Nurses*

Section of the Code	Text
Preamble	Nurses have four fundamental responsibilities: to promote health, to prevent illness, to restore health and to alleviate suffering. The need for nursing is universal. Inherent in nursing is a respect for human rights, including cultural rights, the right to life and choice, to dignity and to be treated with respect. Nursing care is respectful of and unrestricted by considerations of age, colour, creed, culture, disability or illness, gender, sexual orientation, nationality, politics, race or social status. Nurses render health services to the individual, the family and the community and coordinate their services with those of related groups.
Element 1 Nurses and People	■ The nurse's primary professional responsibility is to people requiring nursing care. ■ In providing care, the nurse promotes an environment in which the human rights, values, customs and spiritual beliefs of the individual, family and community are respected. ■ The nurse ensures that the individual receives accurate, sufficient and timely information in a culturally appropriate manner on which to base consent for care and related treatment. ■ The nurse holds in confidence personal information and uses judgement in sharing this information. ■ The nurse shares with society the responsibility for initiating and supporting action to meet the health and social needs of the public, in particular those of vulnerable populations. ■ The nurse advocates for equity and social justice in resource allocation, access to health care and other social and economic services. ■ The nurse demonstrates professional values such as respectfulness, responsiveness, compassion, trustworthiness and integrity.
Element 2 Nurses and Practice	■ The nurse carries personal responsibility and accountability for nursing practice, and for maintaining competence by continual learning. ■ The nurse maintains a standard of personal health such that the ability to provide care is not compromised.

■ Table 2-3   The International Council of Nurses' *Code of Ethics for Nurses* (*continued*)

Section of the Code	Text
	■ The nurse uses judgement regarding individual competence when accepting and delegating responsibility. ■ The nurse at all times maintains standards of personal conduct which reflect well on the profession and enhance its image and public confidence. ■ The nurse, in providing care, ensures that use of technology and scientific advances are compatible with the safety, dignity and rights of people. ■ The nurse strives to foster and maintain a practice culture promoting ethical behaviour and open dialogue.
Element 3 Nurses and the Profession	■ The nurse assumes the major role in determining and implementing acceptable standards of clinical nursing practice, management, research and education. ■ The nurse is active in developing a core of research-based professional knowledge that supports evidence-based practice. ■ The nurse is active in developing and sustaining a core of professional values. ■ The nurse, acting through the professional organisation, participates in creating a positive practice environment and maintaining safe, equitable social and economic working conditions in nursing. ■ The nurse practices to sustain and protect the natural environment and is aware of its consequences on health. ■ The nurse contributes to an ethical organisational environment and challenges unethical practices and settings.
Element 4 Nurses and Co-workers	■ The nurse sustains a collaborative and respectful relationship with co-workers in nursing and other fields. ■ The nurse takes appropriate action to safeguard individuals, families and communities when their health is endangered by a co-worker or any other person. ■ The nurse takes appropriate action to support and guide co-workers to advance ethical conduct.

Source: Courtesy of the International Council of Nurses—Four Elements of the ICN *Code of Ethics for Nurses* © 2012. Geneva, Switzerland: Author.

of regulatory bodies and competent authorities for nursing (FEPI) formed in 2004 and has proposed a *European Code of Ethics and Conduct* (FEPI, 2012) aimed to provide consistency in standards across the increasingly fluid nursing work boundaries of the European Union. The development of a code of ethics is one of the hallmarks of a contemporary service profession and is an especially important characteristic of what are often called crucial professions (Windt, 1989), or those that address an important societal need such as health care. These codes of ethics and their implications for APNs internationally are discussed again later.

Nursing as a Profession

Characteristics of Professions

For the purposes of this text on ethical issues associated with advanced practice roles, nursing is characterized as a profession. The responsibilities of a profession's members are more extensive than those of a technical occupation or vocation. Although nursing has not reached the level of profession in many developing countries (for reasons given shortly), in those countries where the nursing role includes responsibility and accountability for professional judgment and action and/or has expanded as a result of advanced education and skills, it can be considered a profession. What does it mean to say that nursing is a profession? Why is this an important point? These questions can be answered through a brief review of what professions are and what purposes they are supposed to serve. In everyday circumstances almost any vocational group may refer to itself as a profession. For example, dry cleaning businesses advertise themselves to be professional, and in the business section of any phone book there are many instances of plumbers, carpenters, and others all advertising their professional status. Historically, however, the term *profession* meant something very specific, and contemporarily this meaning remains important for individuals and society. This is especially true of those disciplines that provide crucial human services; services that individuals do not have the knowledge, skills, or capacity to provide for themselves but that are necessary for both existing and flourishing.

The earliest organized occupational groups were the craftsmen's guilds. They are noted to have formed in medieval times and perhaps earlier (Carr-Saunders & Wilson, 1933). They consisted of groups of technically accomplished artisans who banded together to hone and protect their skills and knowledge in order to make a living. Out of these beginnings some groups began to affiliate themselves with religious orders, which besides engaging in ministerial duties often also had educational and intellectual aims. Much university education in medieval times and later was ecclesiastical in origin.

The original professions were ministry, medicine, and the law. These three disciplines often required members to take a vow to be accountable for actions, to profess their sincerity, abilities, and/or motivations. These Church-affiliated groups supposedly had altruistic motivations behind their educational endeavors and a service focus. They were less inclined toward substantial monetary awards and more inclined toward developing virtues than many other occupational groups (Carr-Saunders & Wilson, 1933). Thus, a distinction evolved that separated the artisan or tradesman from the professional. Gradually professions such as medicine and law withdrew from their theological origins, yet they maintained their service goals and mission.

Contemporary professions emerged from this background. Perhaps the most well-known attempt to describe the essential characteristics and purposes of professions emerged from Flexner's (1915) extensive study of medical education in the United States and Germany, which resulted in major reforms in medical education in the United States and elsewhere. Flexner, an educator, proposed that professions have an extensive and specialized knowledge base, take responsibility for developing and using their knowledge, have a practice or action orientation that is used for the good of the population served, and autonomously set standards for and monitor the actions of their members.

Following Flexner, further attempts have been made to identify essential characteristics of professions. Kepler (1981) notes that "professions are organized . . . [and] a high level of education is necessary to provide knowledge not readily available or capable of being understood by all. Professions normally interact with clients for whom they provide services rather than goods" (pp. 17–18). The profession is also self-reflective so that it can adapt to changing needs. It is, however, the possession of not readily available knowledge that persuades societies to grant a certain level of prestige and autonomy to professions (Grace, 1998). Perhaps the aspect of contemporary professions that is both the most important to those served and to the membership is the explicit formulation of codes of conduct or ethics.

In reviewing historical accounts of the traditional professions— ministry, law, medicine, and later the professoriate—less noble accounts of their purposes emerge. Some have argued that professions are self-serving and deliberately protective of their knowledge in order to benefit their memberships. My doctoral dissertation (Grace, 1998) investigates such claims in more detail than there is room for here. However, a synthesis of the literature reveals that, though historically some disciplines were protective of their power and prestige, modern helping professions do not see their goals as being primarily self-serving. Nor do they view themselves as engaged in promoting the interests of their membership. Rather it is evident from their published codes of ethics that they view themselves as existing for the primary purpose of serving the public good via their areas of knowledge, skills, and expertise.

CODES OF ETHICS

The codes of ethics of contemporary healthcare professions in essence represent the discipline's promises to society (Grace, 2004b). These codes were developed over time and are periodically revised by the profession's leadership, with membership input, in response to how well they continue to address professional goals and the evolution of societal needs. Although they tend to be abstract rather than specific (the exception to this is lawyers' codes of professional conduct, which are more specific and directive), they provide general direction and guidance to their membership related to professional conduct and the scope of practice. Some, such as the ANA's *Code of Ethics for Nurses with Interpretive Statements* (2001), are accompanied by interpretive statements that provide more detailed explanations of each provision or tenet.

Importantly, professions and their members can be held accountable by the public through such agencies as professional licensure boards for the promises made (Grace, 2004b, p. 284). Curtin (2001) notes that historically "codes of ethics came into being—as did almost all early laws—to protect the vulnerable from the powerful; the unwary from the unscrupulous" (p. 1). However, the public is typically not cognizant of the existence, never mind the content, of professional codes of ethics. Nevertheless, were these to be broadly publicized, they could serve as a potent tool for political action. (This idea is discussed in more detail later.)

Helping Professions and the Public Good

Codes of ethics, formulated as they are from within a profession, also serve as a profession's check on what it expects of its members related to the primary focus of actions. For example, the preamble to the American Medical Association's *Principles of Medical Ethics* (2001) asserts that "a physician must recognize responsibility to patients first and foremost, as well as to society." The ANA's (2001) and ICN's (2012) codes of ethics for nurses likewise assert that nurses' primary interest is the service of individual and societal well-being. The relatively new *Code of Ethics and Conduct for European Nurses* was thought necessary for "the establishment of ethical and deontological principles [that could be] shared throughout Europe [and] would give better protection to European citizens and enhance professional development" (Sasso, Steviano, Jurado, & Rocco, 2008, p. 821). The National Association of Social Workers (1999) in its preamble promises, "A historic and defining feature of social work is the profession's focus on individual well-being in a social context and the well-being of society."

In an earlier work, I noted that "the philosophical roots of the helping professions are imbedded in the idea that humans are not solely self-interested individuals but also have the capacity for altruism" (Grace, 2004b, p. 283). *Altruism* is the ability to understand that others have aims, projects, and life ambitions just as we do and to feel sympathy for someone who is suffering as a result of being unable to fulfill his or her own needs. Humans understand that others sometimes require assistance in achieving their aims and are willing to assist, even if doing so does not necessarily result in a direct gain or primary benefit (Nagel, 1970). That is, the philosophical aims of the helping professions are directed not primarily at furthering the needs of the professional to make a living (as they might be in retail or business settings) but toward the well-being of the individuals served (of course, it is also important that nurses are able to achieve a reasonable standard of living). This is one meaning of altruism. It has been extensively documented as well as supported in the research literature that what draws many people to a profession such as nursing is the desire to contribute to the well-being of others.

Societal Importance of Professions

As has already been pointed out, nursing, medicine, and other professions such as law and education provide services that are crucial in some way to the functioning of individuals and the societies in which they live. Looking at the relationship of what Windt (1989) terms a crucial profession to the population served might shed some light on the persistent importance to society of having professions, given the existence of ongoing debates about what exactly these are and what groups qualify for the designation.

The explanation for the importance of professions hinges on the idea of human vulnerability. Crucial professions serve a specific human need that left unserved would make people, as Sellman (2005) terms it, "more-than-ordinarily vulnerable" to the environment in which they live. Moreover, this vulnerability is widespread. Lack of education (teaching profession) disadvantages people in all sorts of ways. An inability to hold people accountable for infringing on the property or other rights of people (law) would cause security and safety problems for civilians, and everyone is susceptible to ill health or less than optimal functioning. Healthcare professions, such as nursing and medicine, supply services that promote human functioning and flourishing, albeit they have different perspectives on this.

Society should be able to trust professions to provide the services that they profess to be capable of delivering (see the discussion in Chapter 1 related to trust and fiduciary relationships). The existence and privileges of certain professions are sanctioned by society in exchange for their specialized services. In return for these services, society awards professions and professionals a certain standing. It places a high value on the information and skills that professionals contribute and supports the education of professionals (often) by subsidizing their training costs. Professionals are trusted to provide what they promise in exchange for financial or other types of compensation. In return, professionals are held to standards of practice that support the betterment of society as a whole (Grace, 2004b, p. 284).

Some philosophers, sociologists, and political commentators have expressed concern about the dangers to society should crucial professions lose their professional status. This phenomenon has been termed *deprofessionalization* (Bruhn, 2001; Dougherty, 1990; Sullivan, 1999). In deprofessionalization, the professions lose the ability and right to control their own practice—two of the most essential aspects of professions. These are essential aspects for many reasons, but most especially because professionals understand what is needed to meet individual and societal goals. Professional goals are focused on a good that is not primarily economic or business oriented, and the results of inadequate services are generally more immediately perceived and more concerning to the professional than to others with commercial rather than service interests.

The current global financial crisis, healthcare delivery reform in the United States, and cost-containment initiatives in other countries that have varying methods of healthcare financing have led or may lead to the focus of healthcare delivery being diverted away from patients and society and toward cost containment and/or profit making. In addition, the contemporary disease focus fails to adequately account for the roots of ill health in societal conditions. Many scholars and critics in the United States have pointed to problems for society when business models are used to structure healthcare delivery (Fineberg, 2012; Reid, 2009; Relman, 2007). Although many other countries do not rely on business models to structure their healthcare systems and do not have profit as a driving force, nevertheless there is a trend toward cost containment and away from patient-centered or societal concerns in recent initiatives. These issues as well as the question of whether health and thus healthcare are human rights are taken up again in Chapter 4. Market and/or cost-containment forces tend to work against professional autonomy. What this means is that persons other than healthcare professionals make decisions about who needs what in terms of protecting and promoting health. However, for a professional to be held accountable for his or her clinical judgments and the actions that follow from them, there must be a choice of action. If someone else is dictating what will or can be done, and what cannot, then it is not reasonable to hold the professional responsible for performing impossible actions. That is not to say that the profession has no further ethical responsibilities, but it does shift the focus of responsibility toward the systemic, economic, or political issues that are constraining clinical judgment.

In philosophical circles this is termed the problem of "ought implies can," meaning that, if it is dictated that someone ought to provide the appropriate care for a patient, then the care needed must be available. It is unreasonable to hold someone responsible for carrying out an impossible task. However, a professional who does not attempt to locate and remedy the source of a problem after the fact might be held responsible. What it boils down to is that although sometimes health professionals do not have a choice of action in a problematic situation, they must still try to work with others after the fact to ensure that better options are available in the future. For example, in the case of the critical care nurse who is asked to care for three patients, the nurse must do what he or she can until reinforcements arrive; however, the nurse also has a responsibility to try to change the underlying conditions that led to this current situation. The idea is that professionals, perhaps especially healthcare professionals, understand the end results and implications of poor care for their population, perhaps better than any other group.

The Status of Nursing as a Profession

CONCERNS

Why should nurses be concerned with the quality and intent of all clinical judgments and the actions that follow from them? Is it not true that some actions are purely routine? Why should everything about nursing practice be subject to ethical appraisal (nursing ethics)? The answer lies partly in the idea that nursing is one of those professions that caters to the sorts of human needs that left unmet make subjects more than ordinarily vulnerable to their environments and partly in the idea that all actions are in some way directed toward the care of a human individual with unique needs. Thus, even tasks that at first glance seem simple, such as giving an intravenous (IV) medicine or taking a blood pressure, will have a different meaning for that patient than for any other. APNs are responsible for responding to patients as unique individuals with unique needs. And when circumstances do not allow for this, for whatever reason, nurses are responsible for recognizing the ethical nature of the obstruction to what they know to be good care. In addition, problems that have often been assumed to be out of the purview of nurses, such as institutional obstructions to patient care, inadequate staffing, poor inter- and/or intradisciplinary communication about a patient, all have ethical aspects for the same reason: they obstruct efforts to provide good care.

Therefore, in addition to responsibilities related to direct care, there is logical support for the idea that nurses have broader societal responsibilities as outlined in the ICN's (2012) and ANA's (2001) codes of ethics and in the ANA's (2010) *Social Policy Statement*. Furthermore, individuals on entering a profession and achieving professional status are implicitly promising to fulfill the goals of the profession. The profession's code of ethics applies to the practice of each professional. It supersedes all other institutional policies and cannot be negated by other professions, by administrators, or by the demands of the workplace (ANA, 1994). In advanced practice settings, where APNs so often find themselves working side by side and on a par with colleagues from other disciplines, they may find it hard to resist the "pull" of the other profession's particular aims, or of economic interests, and lose sight of the importance to individual and societal health of prioritizing nursing goals (Bryant-Lukosius, DiCensio, Browne, & Pinelli, 2004; Hagedorn & Quinn, 2004). Additionally, nurses working in research and correctional facilities may experience pressures to prioritize the goals of research or of the prison system over nursing goals.

Therefore, it is critically important that APNs understand that advanced practice, although it may bring with it augmented responsibilities, is nevertheless specific to nursing practice, and they must be able to articulate what this means. One way to think about this is that further education enables nurses to meet professional goals of good patient care more comprehensively because they are then able to provide for a wider array of patient needs. This lessens the fragmentation that can occur with multiple providers attending to different problems or systems and makes it easier to elicit the real needs of patients both for care and information.

Finally, some have noted the problem of dual loyalties arising for professionals working in certain circumstances such as military service (Gross, 2010; Williams, 2009). The question revolves around primary duties. Is the military nurse a nurse first—subject to the nursing code of ethics—or a member of the armed forces first and subject to military rules as a priority? The practical answer is probably that military service (unlike correctional service) provides an exception to the rules of professional (medical, nursing, or allied healthcare) conduct. A military nurse is bound first by military ethics rules and nursing ethics rules second. Moreover, the military nurse is not free to change her job and is subject to different legal sanctions than civilian nurses. The problem of military nursing and divided loyalties has not been sufficiently explored in the philosophical or ethics literature. Nevertheless, the ethical decision-making tools provided throughout this text provide strategies for military nurses to practice well in spite of their sometimes conflicting loyalties.

Changes in Contemporary Healthcare Settings

Changes in contemporary healthcare settings both in the United States and elsewhere, resulting from a shift of emphasis to the economic bottom line and expediency and away from the patient and/or societal good, lend urgency to the need for all professional nurses to understand that the basis for their work is firmly attached to the goals of their profession. Unless this is taken seriously, the goals of other professions or institutions will dominate nursing work at all levels—this is a problem for the reasons given in more detail shortly but mostly because nursing serves a distinct purpose and has a distinct perspective that is crucial to the well-being of individuals and for societal health. Should nursing merge with another healthcare profession or its goals become subsumed under the goals of another profession, the gains that have been made over the last century in professional autonomy, and thus the ability to directly influence nursing care, will be lost.

Not only do contemporary healthcare delivery systems both in the United States and elsewhere present a danger that nursing will lose its hard-won autonomy, but the autonomy of other professions is also at risk. Thus it is more vital than ever that the healthcare professions in general, including nursing, retain their societal status as professions—they are, arguably, the last line of defense against the political and/or business interests of contemporary health care and other major shifts that have been projected in healthcare delivery internationally (Anscombe, 2008; Bruhn, 2001; Dougherty, 1992; Mechanic, 1998).

Interdisciplinary work and action are becoming more common because collaboration is often needed to address or research complex health issues. The danger is that a blurring of professional boundaries will occur. Nursing is perhaps more vulnerable to this than other professions, yet nursing's perspective is important because of its unique emphasis on the person as contextual and continuously evolving.

Ambiguity About Nursing as a Profession

The question of whether nursing is a full-fledged or mature profession is still somewhat open for debate. Achieving generally accepted professional status within a society is important because it is accompanied by a certain amount of control or autonomy of practice. In some countries nursing is accorded professional status and with that status the ability to regulate itself. In some countries other more established professions have ignored or are unaware of nursing's particular knowledge about, and contributions to, the health of persons and the larger society. The troubled history of nursing as a female profession, the progress of which "has echoed the status of women in society" (Grace, 2004b, p. 285) as an oppressed group, is well documented (Andrist, Nicholas, & Wolf, 2006; Group & Roberts, 2001). Nursing as a predominantly female discipline has been subject to "gender discrimination" (Andrist et al., 2006, p. 1), lessening its ability either to realize its political potential or be taken seriously by others as a political force. Wuest (2006) highlights the paradox that a key factor of professions historically is that they excluded women. When women did enter professions such as nursing, their motivations did not tend to include the acquisition of power. This has led to relatively easy domination by other groups working within the same environments, such as physicians and administrators. This statement is not intended to denigrate the significant contributions of some eminent members of the profession who managed Herculean tasks of nursing and healthcare reform, but rather to highlight the idea that nurses as the largest workforce within most healthcare systems could have significant power to improve the lot of individuals and society related to health.

Multiple Entry Levels

A further problem for the development of the nursing profession, in the United States at least, is lack of internal cohesiveness caused in part by the multiple levels of entry and multiple grades of practice. A registered nurse in the United States, for example, may have completed a 2-year associate's degree program, a 3-year diploma program, a baccalaureate degree, or have entered nursing as a second-career nurse with degrees in another field. This lack of a unified entry level is suspected to have contributed to the delayed progress of nursing as a driving force for change in health care. Additionally, specialization has tended to cause the formation of special interest groups, the focus of which is addressing concerns that arise within those practice areas or settings. Nursing's scholars and leaders continue their struggle for disciplinary unification. By using insights from nursing's history, the feminist movement, sources of nursing knowledge development, and a changing professional body with its increasingly more highly educated membership, it is hoped nursing will be more equipped to meet its goals related to the health of individuals and society. Arguably, an important unifying force for the good of individuals and society is recognition of the profession's social responsibilities to further its shared goals.

NURSING POSSESSES THE ESSENTIAL CHARACTERISTICS OF A PROFESSION

Although no agreement has been reached about the precise nature of professions, there is nevertheless a general consensus that professions serve an important purpose in democratic societies and that they have certain characteristics in common. The discipline of nursing possesses these characteristics and thus fits the description of a profession. Professions have responsibilities to society that should not be circumvented by economic or business interests. Professions direct and monitor their own activities independent of those who might wish to subvert professional goals. The loss of professional status would not bode well for the population nursing serves, for reasons highlighted later. And yet there is great concern among nursing scholars that nursing, instead of realizing its potential for societal good, is in danger of becoming weakened by lack of attention to, or concern for, the philosophical and theoretical work that draws upon and contributes to nursing practice (Fawcett, Newman, & McAllister, 2004).

The Relationship of Nursing's Goals and Nursing Ethics

In the preceding discussion, not much distinction was made between medicine and nursing in regard to goals because the greater point of focus was the importance of certain professions to individuals and society. This section concentrates more on laying out the distinct nature of nursing goals and nursing perspectives as they have developed over the last century or so.

There is an inevitable relationship between nursing's goals and nursing ethics that has not always been as well recognized as it is currently. Nursing's philosophers and scholars over the past 150 years or so have been diligently involved in trying to determine and describe what the purpose of nursing is, who is served, what knowledge is needed for addressing these goals, and the responsibilities of nursing's membership in keeping these goals as the focus of their endeavors. This quest to define nursing and its unifying purpose is well documented in nursing literature (Donaldson & Crowley, 1978; Milton, 2005; Newman, Sime, & Corcoran-Perry, 1991; Packard & Polifroni, 1992; Willis et al., 2008) and represents the self-reflective nature of the discipline. Interestingly, medicine as a discipline has not been so self-reflective—much of what has been written about the nature and goals of medicine has come from philosophers and historians who for the most part are not physicians.

Fowler (1997) draws attention to the fact that ethics has "been at the foundation of nursing practice since the inception of modern nursing in the United States in the late 1870s" (p. 17). Fry (1995) has documented the development of nursing ethics. She describes its evolution as "paralleling the development of nursing as a profession" in that early nursing ethics resembled rules of etiquette and duties that included such things as "neatness, punctuality, courtesy, and quiet attendance to the physician" (p. 1822).

It is clear that nursing ethics in the early days was less about nurses' autonomous actions than it was about good personal conduct in carrying out physician orders. Part of the reason for this was that a hierarchy existed. Nurse educators in the United States and elsewhere were drawn from an elite group of privileged women from the higher classes. They were influenced by Florence Nightingale's ideas about nursing as a virtuous activity. Coburn (1987) notes that it was difficult to attract the numbers of refined women to institutional nursing that were needed. Working-class women were attracted because they had limited work options. Thus, nurse educators attempted to instill in the women from the lower classes the characteristics thought necessary for the care of the sick.

On a personal note and in support of the historical account, my own mother, who was from a working-class family in Manchester, England, told her family that she wanted to become a nurse. She was 18 years old at the time. Her parents refused to sanction this because of the long working hours (72 hours per week) and the arduous nature of the work. So, for 4 years she worked as a secretary in a factory, at which point she applied for nurse training; she was accepted in 1942, and graduated in 1945. Later she became a midwife (perhaps the earliest version of advanced practice nursing). Anecdotal accounts of her training period echoed historical accounts.

The reason that ladylike characteristics were promoted, nevertheless, was directly related to the interests of the patient. It was thought that quiet diligence and competence in the tasks of caregiving would provide the most beneficial environment for a patient's recovery. This view of nursing conduct was heavily influenced by Nightingale's (1859/1946) theory of good nursing. As evidenced in her writings, she believed that the right environment was crucial to the healing process and nursing's job was to manage the environment to facilitate healing.

Since Nightingale's era, the nature and substance of nursing ethics literature has, not surprisingly, closely followed developments in the profession and in nursing education. As nursing has evolved and become increasingly differentiated from medicine in terms both of goals and of practice autonomy, the subject matter of Nursing Ethics has evolved and nurses' understanding about what constitutes good practice actions (nursing ethics) has developed.

Evolution of Nursing and Consolidation of Nursing Goals

IMPORTANT QUESTIONS

What is nursing's particular knowledge base and how does this differ from that of other professions? The question of whether nursing has a unique knowledge base continues to be argued in contemporary nursing literature. Many scholars believe the question has been answered; however, many more practicing nurses remain unsure of the theoretical bases for their practice. This is a problem at all levels of nursing but most especially at the level of advanced practice. Cody (2006) notes, "The practice of nursing at an advanced level requires a deep understanding of theory and the ability to apply theory effectively in providing healthcare services to people. Indeed, if such understanding and ability is not found within a given nurse, in any specialty whatsoever, his or her practice *cannot* be considered to be advanced at all" (p. ix).

The acceptance and proliferation of advanced nursing roles in the United States, parts of Europe and Scandinavia, and certain Eastern countries such as Korea, Japan, Taiwan, and Thailand (Chiang-Hanisko, Ross, Boonyanurak, Ozawa, & Chiang, 2008) makes an understanding of the particular and unique nature of nursing concerns ever more critical if individual and societal needs for holistic nursing care are to be met. The role of advanced practice nursing is crucial in "fostering better health around the world" (Chiang-Hanisko et al., 2008, para. 1). In the United States there was a concerted effort by the American Association of Colleges of Nursing (AACN) to move toward acceptance of a doctor of nursing practice (DNP) degree as the primary advanced practice qualification by 2015 (Cronenwett et al., 2011). This proposal has been tempered by several factors, including the economic downturn and its effects on education. Nevertheless, there is a proliferation of DNP programs in the United States (over 120 as of this writing), the contents of which are guided by the AACN's list of essential inclusions for the program (AACN, 2006). A lengthy discussion of the pros and cons of nursing practice doctorates is beyond the purposes of this text. The salient point is that all nurses, regardless of level of education, remain focused on the goals and purposes of nursing as a profession and use their advanced education to these purposes and not the purposes of other professions except where there are mutual goals. Nurses need to recognize that the profession's unique nature may become diluted or lost and guard against this (Dracup, Cronenwett, Meleis, & Benner, 2005; Silva & Ludwick, 2006). Concerns exist about the possibility that instead of advanced nursing practice, DNPs will be used to make up for shortages of physicians in both specialist and generalist medical settings. There are also worries that the control of these clinicians will fall under the department of medicine rather than belong to nursing's services. Although the central unifying focus of the discipline has been identified and highlights nursing's unique perspective on patient and society needs, it will, nevertheless, take a concerted effort for nurses to keep nursing perspectives and goals at the core of their work, regardless of the level and type of their preparation. It remains to be seen how doctorally prepared nurse clinicians augment the nursing profession and support professional goals—there is a growing but immature body of literature that can provide insights.

> Contemporary developments in nursing and the movement of nursing toward professional maturity have occurred partly because nursing's scholars, theorists, and even researchers have been willing to ask the hard questions about nursing. They have been willing to ask, "What is it we are doing when we are doing nursing? How is what we do different than what other professionals do? What is our unique purpose?" (Grace, 2004b, p. 288)

Present-day APNs, regardless of their level of preparation, will have an important role in keeping and promulgating a nursing perspective. Most readers engaged in higher nursing education are exposed to nursing's conceptual bases for practice and will have had courses or modules that trace and critique the theoretical works of nursing's scholars. This chapter does not explore these works in detail for that reason. However, a brief overview will help those who have not yet been exposed; it can also serve as a refresher for those who have and will facilitate an understanding of the inevitable link between theory development and the evolution of nursing ethics.

NURSING THEORY AND DISCIPLINARY KNOWLEDGE DEVELOPMENT

Florence Nightingale is generally considered the first person to have asked and answered the question "What is nursing?" In her *Notes on Nursing: What It Is and What It Is Not* (1859/1946), she clearly articulates her philosophy of nursing. Her philosophy embraced the idea that nurses, in appropriately manipulating the patient's environment, "put the patient in the best condition for nature to act upon him" (p. 75). She used previous knowledge, research, and current conditions to conceptualize good nursing actions. Thus, her particular focus proves very different from those followed by the medical and surgical establishments of the era. The focuses of the medical professions actually did very little to change conditions in spite of gains in empirical knowledge about disease and illness that were available. Nightingale's influence both on public health and on the education of nurses was significant and led to the development of schools of nursing in Europe and eventually the United States.

Nursing, for several decades after Nightingale, was vocational rather than professional. Cody (2006) writes that it was not until Hildegarde Peplau published *Interpersonal Relations in Nursing* as a theory of nursing in 1952 that a shift in the development of nursing into a more professional endeavor commenced in earnest. This development coincided with the post–World II implementation of tax-supported college education for veterans funded by the G.I. Bill of Rights of 1944. More opportunities arose for nurses to receive baccalaureate-level or higher nursing education.

In the 1950s and 1960s, "additions to the literature on philosophy and theory in nursing began to appear" (Cody, 2006, p. 2). The important idea that nursing was concerned with "the *whole person* and *health in all its dimensions*" (Cody, 2006, p. 2) emerged. In 1991, Virginia Henderson's definition of nursing was published by the ICN. She notes that the definition represents the crystallization of her ideas about nursing over a period of time.

> The unique function of the nurse is to assist the individual sick or well, in the performance of those activities contributing to health or its recovery (or to peaceful death) that he would perform unaided if he had the necessary strength, will or knowledge. And to do this in such a way as to help him gain independence as quickly as possible. (Henderson, 1991, p. 21)

In 1970, Rogers's account of human beings as consisting of more than the sum of their parts and inseparable from their environments was published. She termed this view of persons "unitary man." Cody (2006) points out that over the next 20 years or so "at least 20 significant frameworks intended to guide practice were published" (p. 3). Thus, he asserts, "The distinctiveness of nursing's disciplinary knowledge base is a reality that cannot be ignored" (p. 3). Nursing's knowledge base constitutes a science in this sense—that is, it is a developed body of knowledge about a phenomenon. The development of nursing's knowledge base has been directly informed by practice. Nursing's scholars and philosophers, almost all of whom have at some point been immersed in practice, have in turn used the questions and problems of practice to theorize about what it is that nurses do and how they might do it to meet professional goals more effectively.

"The (foundational) goal of the nursing profession is generally agreed to be that of promoting a 'good' which is health. Health may be variously defined depending on philosophical and theoretical perspectives guiding practice" (Grace, 2001, p. 155) and on the particular contexts of practice. Nevertheless, nursing has espoused a perspective of human beings that grounds the discipline's activity in the assumption that humans are contextual beings whose needs cannot be conceptualized in isolation from the larger contexts of their lives, histories, relationships, projects, and values. Additionally, many of nursing's philosophers have noted the importance of the nurse–patient relationship and engagement with patients to facilitate meaning-making in difficult and fluid circumstances. The relationship and engagement are important even in cases of those who have profound cognitive challenges that prevent the individual's direct input.

Some have criticized nursing's perspective, noting that certain allied professions could also lay claim to this perspective. Indeed, in the past 20 years or so, some physicians have moved to adopt what they call the "new medicine" or an "integrative medicine" approach to patient care (Blumer & Meyer, 2006). This is good for patients. Even so, the new medicine fails to draw on the copious previous work done in nursing, and "new medicine" practitioners cannot necessarily be found in all the disparate settings where nurses practice in advanced roles, and they do not stand in the same relationships to patients. Additionally, it is doubtful that many physicians see integrative medicine as a realistic approach, given the limits of current healthcare environments and their emphasis on cure, along with a narrow view of what constitutes a good outcome. Still, it is an encouraging movement and one where nurses are well equipped to provide leadership.

REVISITING NURSING ETHICS AS PROFESSIONAL RESPONSIBILITY

In light of the preceding discussion, it is clear that an examination of nursing ethics is appropriately addressed "via the explications of nursing's theorists and scholars" (Grace, 2006, p. 68). In turn, nursing's theorists and scholars can realistically be called nursing philosophers because their theories or thoughts emerge from their philosophical attempts (informed by practice experiences) to find reasonable answers to the following questions: What is nursing? Why is nursing necessary? How can it best be done? What is needed to do it (including knowledge, characteristics, and skills required of practitioners as well as the environments in which it can be done)? Hence the two main goals of theorizing in nursing are (1) "To describe and explain (all levels of) nursing" (Grace, 2006, p. 68), and (2) to provide a structure or framework that facilitates practice, guides research endeavors aimed at expanding nursing's knowledge base, and underpins practitioner development and education.

The use of philosophies, models, and theories as guides for nursing practice and the reverse influence of practice experiences on theory development are factors critical to the development of nursing's knowledge base and thus to the maturation and evolution of the discipline. However, it is the discipline's explicit aim of contributing both to the health of individuals and the overall health of society that makes nursing itself a moral endeavor.

Flaming (2004) has argued that because theories of nursing say what nursing is (ontology), they represent ethical imperatives. Take, for example, the goal of nursing to promote an individual's health. Because nursing views of health all include the understanding that human beings are complex entities, inseparable from the environment in which they live and connected to countless important others in their lives, promoting health means taking into account the person in context. Failure to do so represents a failure of nursing ethics or, alternatively stated, a failure of professional responsibility. Willis and colleagues (2008) synthesized a central unifying focus of the discipline that is implicit in almost all theoretical and philosophical nursing works and that gives nurses a way to articulate their work. This focus, as noted earlier, is facilitating humanization, meaning, choice, quality of life, and healing in living and dying. The central theme evident in the historical nursing literature is that nurses facilitate humanization for patients and patient groups. "Nursing facilitates humanization by engaging experiential human beings [persons who experience life and its events] in practice and modeling humane relating for other human beings. Humanization . . . is manifested when the nurse works with [any] human being [and views them as] relational, experiential, valuable, respectworthy, meaning-oriented, flawed, imperfect, vulnerable, fragile, complex, and capable of health and healing even if not capable of being cured" (p. E34).

Critical Questions

Given that there are quite a few nursing philosophers and theorists and as many philosophical, conceptual, or theoretical approaches to nursing knowledge development in the interests of nursing care, how does the APN know which perspective to follow to ensure professionally responsible care? The answer is that the perspective and knowledge brought to bear on a practice issue will, to a certain extent, depend on the nature of the problem, the patient or group involved, the nature of the practice setting, and the personal and professional characteristics and experiences of the clinician. The point is not so much that following a particular theory or perspective will result in ethical action, although having a structure to a nurse's practice definitely helps with consistency of data gathering and approach to care and so forth, but rather that much work has been accomplished in identifying nursing's goals, and that there is agreement among nursing scholars on certain key points.

There is implicit or explicit agreement that nursing's metaparadigm concepts, or the overarching concepts of the discipline, include person, environment, health, and nursing (Fawcett & Malinski, 1999). What this means, roughly, is that there is unity about the fact that "nursing has to do with assisting humans, who are viewed as complex individuals who interact with their environment and have health needs that nursing can address" (Grace, 2004b, p. 288).

THE GOALS OF NURSING

The authors of the current ANA *Code of Ethics for Nurses with Interpretive Statements* (2001)— informed by practicing nurses and contemporary societal developments—synthesized historical and current literature. In the preface to the code, the goals of nursing are stated as follows: "The prevention of illness, the alleviation of suffering, and the protection, promotion, and restoration of health." Similarly, the ICN affirms the goals of nursing in terms of the responsibilities of nurses and nursing "to promote health, to prevent illness, to restore health and to alleviate suffering" (ICN, 2012). These agreed-on goals of nursing should be kept in mind as the discussion moves to the skills and characteristics needed to practice ethically.

However, there are other factors that are important to ethical practice that apply regardless of what philosophical or theoretical approach to care is used. These factors include understanding the role of bias in data gathering or relationships, the boundaries of knowledge and skills possessed, moral development, and motivation to engage with patients and to act (refer to Table 2-1).

Nursing Ethics: State of the Science

THREE PHASES

To recap, the status of Nursing Ethics as a field of inquiry can be categorized into three phases, as described by Sara Fry (2002). The first phase covers the early days of nursing's formal development via training or apprenticeships in line with Florence Nightingale's vision. Fry (2002) notes that "during the early days of the 20th century, nursing ethics was understood as the articulation of the customs, habits and moral rules that nurses follow in the care of the sick" (p. 1). The transition to the second phase began after World War II. During this time, more nurses were able to gain access to university education, started to become more independent (from physicians) in their practice, and thus assumed more accountability for actions that resulted from their clinical judgments. "This new expectation of accountability created changes in how nurses' ethical duties and behaviours were understood"

(Fry, 2002, p. 1). Much earlier, nursing leaders had begun to recognize the need for a formalized code of ethics that would serve as a unifying guide for action. However, it took 53 years between recognition that a code was needed and the actual adoption of the 1950 *Code for Nurses* (Fowler, 1997). Following the ANA, in 1953 the ICN, a federation of nursing groups from several countries (now more than 128), also developed and published a document entitled *The Code of Ethics for Nurses* that reflected the "shared values of nurses" across borders (Curtin, 2001).

Finally, the current or third Nursing Ethics phase is concerned with exploration and analyzing contemporary nursing practice for its ability to meet nursing goals. The concerns of contemporary Nursing Ethics reflect the maturing of the discipline. Nursing Ethics explores the meaning of being a good nurse and good nursing practice in increasingly complex settings. This contemporary phase has seen an increase in research activities. See **Table 2-4** for a synopsis of nursing ethics research phases.

IMPORTANT CONCEPTS

Fry (2002) identifies four concepts that are important to contemporary practice and that apply also to advanced practice. These concepts are "co-operation, accountability, caring, and advocacy" (p. 2). These four related concepts are discussed in more detail in the following chapters. They are especially important in advanced practice because of the expanded nature of such practice and the leadership roles assumed by APNs. Briefly, cooperation and collaboration are responsibilities to work with others within and outside the profession to get what is needed for patient care on the individual as well as the societal levels. The problem for APNs in collaborative relationships is how to maintain their disciplinary perspective while taking into account other perspectives. That is, how do nurses ensure that the collaboration is egalitarian in view of nursing's history of subservience? Accountability was discussed earlier and refers to responsibility for one's professional actions. This discussion uses a modified conception of advocacy termed *professional advocacy* (Grace, 2001) to denote actions required to ensure good care at the level of the individual and at increasingly broader levels as necessary to demolish obstacles to good practice. This is a panoramic conception of advocacy that goes beyond mere protection of human rights. Many argue that the political activities required by conceiving the scope of professional responsibilities this way are not possible for most nurses, who do not possess the knowledge, skills, energy, or necessary supports.

■ Table 2-4   Phases of Nursing Ethics Empirical Research

Phase	Research Details
Earliest Nursing Ethics Research	In 1935 Rose Vaughan studied the diaries of student and graduate nurses related to ethical problems encountered for her dissertation (Fry & Grace, 2007).
1980s: Ethics Research Expands	Content related to nurses' ethical reasoning, judgments, and behaviors.
1990s: Nursing Ethics Research Focus	As in earlier phase, plus concepts such as advocacy, participation in end-of-life decision making, patient values, influence of education on moral reasoning, and nurses' experiences of ethical issues
1994 Nursing ethics research – dedicated publication venue	Inception of the *International Journal of Nursing Ethics* (Tschudin, 2006). Early issues featured research on advocacy, quality care, nurses' decision making, and ethical issues experienced by nurses. There was an increase in qualitative studies: reflective practice and experiences of moral unease and moral distress.
Contemporary Nursing Ethics Research	Qualitative and quantitative studies: Obstacles to care, the meaning of experiences, moral distress, nurse–patient relationships, characteristics of good nurses, patient decision making, collaboration, nurses engagement in preventive ethics, ethical decision making especially around end-of-life care, and political activity. Some studies on advanced practice: conflicts of interest, collaboration, specialty practice.

Finally, caring requires a little more discussion because contemporarily it has received a lot of attention both within and outside of the discipline. Indeed, nursing has been heavily criticized by feminists and other ethicists for framing caring as an ideal of practice. Defining caring in the nursing context provides an important foundation for the ensuing section.

Care and Nursing Practice: Ethical Implications
Care is a concept that highlights the relational aspects of human interactions. As an ethic of nursing practice, it has its origins in insights from

feminist ethics and related research (Gilligan, 1982). These insights expose the idea that women consider context and relationships to be important in reasoning about ethically difficult situations. They do not rely purely on principle-based reasoning.

For example, a nursing home patient, Mr. Jones, wants to be allowed to walk to the bathroom unattended even though he is unsteady on his feet and has been evaluated as a falls risk. The adult nurse practitioner (ANP) reasoning about his autonomy and how best to facilitate this request would do a risk–benefit assessment and make a decision that balances protecting Mr. Jones's autonomy and the likelihood of a fall—this is the same assessment that would be made of any other patient whose autonomy was threatened. However, from a care perspective, the ANP is interested in knowing about Mr. Jones within this particular context, what it means to him to walk unaided, and how his wishes could be accommodated in a way that makes sense to him. The ANP would engage with Mr. Jones in the decision-making process. "The ethic of care means a responsibility to attend to the individual as individual in all of his or her complexities" (Grace, 2005, p. 105). Indeed the goals of nursing practice require that the clinician has, or cultivates, a predisposition to engage with the patient to understand that person's particular needs. Benner, Tanner, and Chesla (1996) note that care facilitates "the alleviation of vulnerability; the promotion of growth and health; the facilitation of comfort, dignity or a good and peaceful death" (p. 233).

Care as a facet of nursing requires engagement on the part of the nurse with the patient in a relationship that permits the meaning and context of the person's need to be exposed. This is not a purely emotional sense of care; it is not, for example, the same meaning as "I care about my friend." Rather, knowledge, skills, and motivation are all needed for an engaged knowing of the person. In their research, Benner and colleagues (1996) note that it appears as "the dominant ethic found in [nurses'] stories of everyday practice" (p. 233).

Of course, there are criticisms of the ethic of care. Nelson (1992), a bioethicist, notes the problem of moral predictability. That is, she wonders how to determine right actions from within the nurse–patient care relationship. Another criticism is that a care ethic does not permit a critique of morally suspect environments. Further, feminists have cautioned that adoption of an ethic of care as the dominant nursing ethic could further jeopardize nursing's power to effect change on behalf of patient care; nurses, they argue, could be manipulated by powerful patients. One other important criticism has to do with the fact that nurses have responsibility for more than one patient, so excessive care for one might disadvantage another.

These are all valid criticisms and represent worrisome issues if the ethic of care is taken to be the only important consideration in clinical decision making. However, an ethic of care is an important concept where knowledge of the patient as an individual is needed for the goals of the profession to be furthered. Ethical decision making, like sound clinical judgment, requires nurses to take into account both the larger context and the context of the individual. It includes determining which tools are appropriate to employ in identifying the ethical content of everyday practice.

Ethical Decision Making and Action for Good Care

Clinical and Moral Reasoning

So far, this chapter has traced the development of nursing into a profession and made the argument that membership in the profession leads to responsibility and accountability for practice actions and that all practice actions are subject to critique related to how well they are likely or able to fulfill the profession's goals as these have been developed over time. At this point, then, it is appropriate to gain clarity about practical applications. As articulated so far, the argument can be made that in many ways clinical and moral (ethical) reasoning are inseparable concepts. "Good or 'ethical' nursing practice results from the use of theoretical, conceptual, and practical knowledge in formulating clinical judgments, and evaluating ensuing actions for their ability to meet patient needs" (Grace, 2004a, p. 296). The "conceptual or theoretical knowledge may be derived from other disciplines as well as nursing" (Grace, 2004a, p. 296); however, this knowledge should still be filtered through a nursing lens (perhaps by asking "How will this facilitate the patient's good in the context of nursing practice?" or "How should I work to influence needed practice or societal changes?").

Clinically good actions, it can be argued, are synonymous with ethically good actions. It is even possible to go one step further and assert that when clinically good actions (those most likely to further the patient's good) are obstructed in some way, good clinical judgment would conceptualize what nonclinical actions are needed to circumvent or tear down the obstruction—these actions highlight what professional responsibility requires of nurses. Strategies for addressing obstacles are suggested and proposed throughout the following chapters. As synthesized from extant nursing, philosophical, and research literature, good or ethical practice requires all of the following:

- An ongoing focus on the goals of the discipline and the ethical nature of these goals
- Disciplinary knowledge and skills related to the practice setting and role assumed
- Adherence to the scope and limits of nursing or nursing specialty practice as well as a nurse's own knowledge and experience (entails knowing personal limits and being willing to seek assistance from knowledgeable or skilled others)
- Ability to communicate a nursing perspective using the language of ethics to convey a patient's or group's needs
- Understanding of personal and professional values (self-reflection and reflection on practice)
- Willingness and capacity to engage with patients where possible regardless of level of cognitive functioning (there may be some patients with whom a nurse cannot engage because of unresolved or unresolvable prior personal or life experiences; in this case, good practice permits turning care of the person over to another)
- Ability to make sound decisions
- Motivation to act
- Perseverance in carrying out ethical actions despite or in spite of obstacles

The next section explores in more detail the cognitive and affective processes that underlie ethically appropriate actions. Ethically appropriate means those actions that are required by nursing's goals and the role responsibilities of nurses.

Processes of Moral Action

James Rest (1941–1999) gleaned his views on the cognitive and affective processes that must underlie moral behavior from the contemporary theory and literature of disparate disciplines. He noted that there are at least four, but perhaps more, interrelated activities of a person's mind and ways of thinking that lead to that person acting to achieve a "good." This conceptualization of the "good" action is internal—it is not a predetermined good. That is, his theory does not presuppose that there is an ultimate good that only the most moral people are able to achieve or that there is some sort of factual principle that if followed would always lead to a good. There is no agreement about whether there is an "ultimate good" for humans to pursue, and many doubt that one exists. However, there is general agreement that human beings have interests in living a meaningful life without undue interference or obstruction from others (Weston, 2011).

Rest's theory of moral action is based in the idea that persons can be engaged in a process of considered intention to do good. His insights derived from accumulated research cohere, for the most part, with the list of attributes given earlier as synthesized from nursing and allied literature. Rest (1982, 1983), an educational psychologist, noted that research or inquiry about cognitive and affective processes underlying moral action is in its infancy. Approaches tend to be scattered or fragmented, often focused on only one of the following: moral thought, moral emotion, or moral behavior, but not the interfaces between these. Additionally, the different disciplines tend to be concerned only with their perspective, causing further fragmentation. Yet a coherent understanding of the processes of moral behavior is needed to know what can and cannot be fostered and what strategies are most likely to work. To be clear, Rest's quest was not about discovering absolute or universal truths; it was about the psychology of human action, that is, about what cognitive and affective factors are in play when a person acts morally, given some predetermined moral goal of action. More recently, Doris and colleagues (2010), in *The Moral Psychology Handbook*, describe the state of the science related to interdisciplinary research on human action. Unprecedented knowledge about how the human mind works is now available because of collaborative studies undertaken by disparate disciplines. Knowing more about human capacities and predispositions allows people to guard against certain errors of judgment that are common but not well understood. The assumption of all professional education is that it is, for the most part, possible to foster the sorts of characteristics needed for moral practice and moral decision making. That is, education can prepare professionals to achieve professional goals. Therefore, continuing to investigate how these processes are integrated or integral to each other is necessary for us to know more about how to foster moral behavior. Rest's assumption, derived from a thorough review of work done so far in a variety of sciences and disciplines, is that the processes are interrelated, and all are necessary for a moral action or moral behavior to result. A failure in just one area or one process may result in a failure to behave morally. Many disciplines have undertaken ongoing research related to moral behavior, including nursing (see Table 2-4 for examples of contemporary nursing ethics research). Although integrative approaches that look at the relationships of all processes are included, and work in moral and behavioral psychology as well as in the cognitive and physiological sciences has advanced our understanding, the state of the science remains immature.

Rest's tentative framework is also helpful in artificially delineating important aspects of moral action while understanding the necessary interdependence of these aspects. Appreciating that there are limits and hindrances to moral decision making and moral action alerts professionals to those factors that can interfere with their decision making and allows them to guard against these. Rest suggests four questions that have been partly addressed by contemporary philosophical and empirical research and that correspond to the probable internal processes behind moral decision making and action: "(1) How does the person interpret the situation and how does he or she view any possible action as affecting people's welfare? (2) How does the person figure out what the morally ideal course of action would be? (3) How does he or she decide what to do? and (4) Does the person implement what he or she intends to do?" (Rest, 1982, p. 29).

There are both affective (emotion) and cognitive (thought) components to these processes that may not be separable for the purposes of studying how people actually act. An implication is that good action results from all of these processes working together and that emotion and reason are both crucial elements. This is helpful in defining the characteristics of good clinicians. In **Table 2-5**, Rest's explanations of the nature of each process or aspect are modified by applying them to direct patient care situations to provide a clearer idea of what is meant. This illustrates how a nursing ethics course or book, together with group reflections on practice, might facilitate the development of or highlight already possessed attributes that are supportive of an APN's confidence in moral decision making and action. Table 2-5 also synthesizes the research and theoretical literature to present some factors that have been discovered to obstruct each process. The list of obstructing factors is not meant to be exhaustive.

Self-Reflection, Values Clarification, and Reflection on Practice

Gaining confidence in one's moral decision making is admittedly a slow process. My colleagues, Drs. Ellen Robinson (Project Director) and Martha Jurchak, Clinical Ethics Directors at Massachusetts General Hospital (MGH)

■ Table 2-5   Four Aspects of Moral Action and Interfering Factors

Rest's Processes (1982)	Practical Implications	Interfering Factors
1. **Interpretation of the situation**	APNs' understanding of the inherently ethical nature of any practice situation; APNs are responsible for their actions, and their professional actions are to facilitate the profession's goals directly or indirectly Assessment of this particular situation and what is needed to achieve optimal care for the person or persons in need	Personal troubles Energy level Time available Knowledge level No understanding of the inherently moral nature of practice Lack of connection with the patient/inability to engage Perception/sensitivity affected by age and life experiences Lack of self-reflection
2. **Discerning the morally ideal action—what ought to be done**	Using appropriate tools, methods, resources, and collaborations for decision making Identifying the beneficiary, the goal, appropriate actions	Level of moral development Level of independence Level and types of education Personal values conflict with patient/significant other/other professionals' values Lack of reflection on practice
3. **Deciding what to do**	Deciding among competing courses of action What ought to be done may not always be possible or consensus not reachable	Situational ambiguity Theoretical ambiguity Uncertainty about outcome Lack of institutional or peer support

(*continues*)

■ Table 2-5   Four Aspects of Moral Action and Interfering Factors (*continued*)

Rest's Processes (1982)	Practical Implications	Interfering Factors
4. Implementation and perseverance	Envisioning the steps and anticipating problems Addressing and overcoming problems and barriers Taking sociopolitical actions to get what is needed Keeping sight of the goal Reminding others of the goal	Too many obstacles Fear of personal consequences, peer/colleague disapproval Fatigue Frustration Lack of resources and supports

and Brigham and Women's hospital (BWH), respectively, and the Reverend Angelika Zollfrank, Director of Pastoral Education at MGH, have been working under a U.S. Department of Health and Human Services, Health Resources and Services Administration (HRSA) grant to build nurses' confidence and capacity in clinical ethics at the bedside. This is a 1-year program consisting of 8 hours per month of didactic, experiential (role play and simulation), and practice components—it is offered to select bedside nurses and APNs (*N* = 18–25 per year). The program is currently working with its third cohort. Data analysis of its efficacy in improving confidence and capability in addressing practice issues and speaking up on behalf of patients and families is ongoing. However, overwhelmingly nurses report verbally and in their course evaluations increased confidence in speaking up on behalf of good patient care and engaging in a variety of ethics-related projects such as organizing unit-based ethics rounds and participating in ethics committees and interdisciplinary ethics forums. Nurses unanimously note the importance of being able to discuss issues with others and the insights this permits, as well as gaining clarity about important aspects of the ethical crises and situations they face. Nursing research studies and scholarly literature reveal that many nurses at all levels of practice remain unsure of the validity or importance of their point of view in ethically difficult situations (Ceci, 2004; Dierckx de Casterlé, Izumi, Godfrey, & Denhaerynck, 2008; Dodd, Jansson, Brown-Saltzman, & Wunch, 2004; Duffy & Currier, 1999; Hardingham, 2004; Helft, Chamness, Terry, & Uhrich, 2011; Kelly, 1998; Pavlish, Brown-Saltzman, Hersh, Shirk, & Rounkle, 2011; Varcoe et al., 2004; Whitney et al., 2006). One explanation is the idea that ethics belongs in the realm of the obscure or difficult. There is a common belief that ethics in healthcare settings is about difficult dilemmas that require esoteric knowledge brought to bear by high-minded individuals. What I realized as a result of my studies in philosophy and medical ethics is that most ethical issues arise in daily healthcare practice and are the result of lack of focus on either the goals or the recipient of care. Thus, nurses, as the clinicians who tend to spend the most time with patients, are often the ones who have the most comprehensive version of the patient's story. Moreover, nurses probably have the best opportunity to diffuse situations that have the potential to develop into crises, in some cases simply by gathering important parties together to talk about goals in view of patient desires and preferences. APNs can serve as important resources both within institutional settings and in primary care settings.

CASE STUDY: MS. KNIGHT

Although this chapter clearly states that all practice actions, from the simple to the complex, are subject to ethical appraisal, that is, they can be judged good or bad according to whether they are focused on furthering nursing's goals, this slightly more complex case demonstrates how to approach moral decision making using the tools and skills described throughout the chapter, as well as in the accompanying tables. **Table 2-6** lists some key factors in any healthcare decision-making process. However, there are many different frameworks available in the literature, and you may well find one of these is more in concert with your style of analysis. The important thing to remember is that there will never be enough information to unquestionably confirm that a decision is flawless, but it is possible to gain reasonable clarity on most situations by asking the questions posed in Table 2-6.

Ms. Knight

Ms. Jean Knight is an 80-year-old patient who was successfully treated for breast cancer 5 years ago. Her cancer has returned, however, and she now

■ Table 2-6 Ethical Decision Making in Difficult Situations: Important Considerations

In the course of *daily practice,* what is needed for ethical action is the thoughtful exercise of knowledge, experience, and skill, together with a constant focus on the good of the patient or group in need of services and an understanding of the nurse's own biases.

In more *complex* situations, where what is good is not so clearly seen, a more in-depth analysis may be needed. This is not necessarily a linear process, nor will all of the following considerations always be pertinent. There are other decision-making models available, but all have similar considerations.

Steps	Questions
Identify the major problem(s)—relate these to professional goals.	■ What are the facts: clinical, social, environmental?
Pay attention to the "trigger"— you feel uneasy about a situation—try to discover why, what is bothering you. This is a good starting point for exploration.	■ What implicit assumptions are being made? ■ What ethical principles or perspectives are pertinent? Examples: autonomous decision making is in question, conflict of values among providers and patient/significant others, economic versus patient good ■ Are there power imbalances? What are these? Who has an interest in maintaining them?
Identify information gaps.	■ Do you need more information? ■ From whom or where might you get this information?
Determine who is involved.	■ Who is the main focus? Is there more than one important party? Who has (or thinks they have) an interest in the outcome (relatives, staff, other)? Who will be affected by the outcome?
Decide what the prevalent values are.	■ Values held by patient, staff, institution ■ Are there value conflicts?—interpersonal, interprofessional, personal versus professional, patient versus professional.

■ Table 2-6   Ethical Decision Making in Difficult Situations: Important
Considerations (*continued*)

Steps	Questions
Determine if an interpreter is necessary (for cultural or language issues). Who would be the most appropriate interpreter (knowledgeable and neutral)? Often this is not the family member!	■ Are there cultural perspectives? Who can help with these?
Identify possible courses of action and probable consequences.	■ Which course of action is likely to be the most beneficial and the least harmful to those involved, including you? ■ Can safeguards be put in place in case of unforeseen consequences?
Implement the selected course of action. Conduct an ongoing evaluation.	■ Does the actual outcome correlate with the anticipated outcome? What was unexpected? Was this foreseeable given more data? ■ Do similar problems keep reoccurring? If so, why (requires a look at underlying environmental or societal issues perhaps)? Does this point to the need for policy changes or development at the site, institution, or societal level? What further actions might be needed? ■ Are there continuing staff provider education needs related to the issue?
Engage in self-reflection, reflection on practice (individually, in an interdisciplinary group debriefing session, or in a specialty group forum).	■ Could you have done things differently? What would you have liked to understand better? ■ Would a consultation with colleagues or an ethics resource person have altered your conception of the issue or the course of action taken? ■ What valuable insights did you gain that should be shared with others and may be applicable to the approach used for future problems?

has bone and liver metastases. She was admitted 2 days ago from a local nursing home, to Clarion, a medical floor, for pain management and pneumonia. She is being treated with IV antibiotics and fentanyl patches for her pain. She occasionally experiences breakthrough pain, for which she is prescribed oral hydromorphone. Her IV site has become obstructed and she is refusing to have a new IV inserted.

Gina Jenks is Ms. Knight's primary nurse. She has been working as a staff nurse for only 8 months and sometimes is not very confident in her skills. However, this is her second day with Ms. Knight, and she thought that she had developed a good rapport with her patient. She tries to reason with Ms. Knight about the importance of receiving the IV antibiotics, but Ms. Knight remained opposed to having the IV inserted.

Ms. Sandy Norton is the clinical nurse specialist (CNS) for this busy unit. Recently, Sandy Norton has been trying to encourage some of the newer nurses like Gina to take a more active role in presenting their patient's point of view to physicians, allied providers, and family members as needed. Gina seeks Sandy out to ask her advice. She tells her that Ms. Knight's exact words were, "I don't want any more medicines and I don't want any more fluids. I am ready to die. Just let me die, won't you?" Gina appears shaken.

Discussion

The decision-making considerations from Table 2-6 are italicized in the following discussion because, as with explorations of many difficult issues, they do not proceed in a linear fashion; rather, considerations or questions suggest themselves as the story unfolds. Not all considerations are pertinent in all cases; however, a cursory review of them permits relative confidence that no important aspect of analysis is overlooked.

The *main problem* seems relatively straightforward: Ms. Knight is refusing care that her providers deem to be in her best interests. Providing IV antibiotics is the standard treatment for her immediate medical problem of pneumonia and can also be used to give pain medicines if needed. The *underlying assumptions* being made are that (1) Ms. Knight will physically benefit from the IV antibiotics (beneficence), (2) without the antibiotics she will worsen and die (nonmaleficence), and (3) death is a bad outcome for Ms. Knight.

Although premise 1 is true, premises 2 and 3 are more questionable. Premise 2 depends on there being no alternative treatments for the pneumonia, and premise 3 requires more information about *Ms. Knight, her preferences, and values*. Additionally, Ms. Knight wants her autonomy respected. She appears to understand that she might die and, if her understanding is adequately informed as discussed in Chapter 1, she has both the moral and the legal right to decide for herself what treatments she will or will not accept.

However, nurses' responsibilities do not end even if a determination of decision-making capacity is made. *Professional goals* require that nurses find out more about how the patient feels and what alternatives are available that might be acceptable to her, thus not abandoning her to her autonomy. From the narrative it is not clear whether any overt *power imbalances* exist; however, implicit in most provider–patient relationships is an imbalance related to knowledge. The fact is that the provider serves as a gatekeeper for further care and interventions, and sometimes to setting. Power influences are likely present in the case of Ms. Knight, who is dependent on the nurses and institution to meet all of her other daily living needs. She has no relatives in the local area, and she has lost touch with many of her friends since entering the nursing home 2 years prior because of mild mobility issues. This power differential does need to be taken into consideration in communicating with her. The nurses must keep in mind that she might be susceptible to caregivers' influence if she thinks they will neglect her other needs, the most salient of which may be pain control.

Sandy (CNS) talks to *Gina (novice nurse)* about her feelings in the situation because Gina is visibly shaken by the event. Sandy's responsibilities as a CNS include staff support and education, both of which ultimately affect patient care. Gina says she is worried that Ms. Knight will deteriorate just when the nurses feel she is doing better. She hopes that there is something more that can be done—she does not want to "have to watch her die needlessly." Gina and Sandy must try to ascertain what Ms. Knight's understanding of the situation is, that is, what information gaps exist and how these could be filled in.

Gina and Sandy are charged with discovering whether Ms. Knight does actually have decision-making capacity. If decision-making capacity is impaired, her ability to understand the implications of the choices she makes will be limited. Autonomous action depends on her ability to take in information, digest it, and convey that what she understands and wishes is in line with her previous life choices and desires for the future. Sandy decides that the best way to proceed is to role model for Gina how such an assessment can be made, acknowledging the need for discussion later. First, she talks to Gina about her feelings, reassuring her they are normal, that she knows more than she thinks she does, and that increased experience in handling such situations will help her develop confidence in decision making.

Before approaching Ms. Knight, Sandy emphasizes the importance of first making sure that there are no obvious physiologic or psychological impediments to information processing. Gina reports that although Ms. Knight did have some confusion the previous day when her oxygen saturation levels were borderline and her temperature was 101.4°F, today she has been lucid and oriented. Additionally, her pain is being well controlled with the fentanyl patch, with only one additional dose of hydromorphone needed during the night. However, she did tell Gina that the management of her nursing home had changed and the residents were not getting the same quality of attention as they were previously. This made her very unhappy, and she was worried about the quality of her care on her return. Sandy asked Gina to consider how this information might be relevant to the current situation and something to investigate further.

Sandy and Gina approach Ms. Knight and find her crying. Sandy says, "Ms. Knight, Gina tells me that you don't want to have your IV reinserted. I am so sorry that you are experiencing these problems. I am here to help figure out what can be done to ensure that you are comfortable and your needs are taken care of. Tell me more about what you are thinking."

Ms. Knight accurately recounts what went on and in response to further questions admits that she does not *necessarily want to die but is not happy with her life lately*, is afraid that if she goes back to the nursing home she will not get her pain needs met, and thinks that if this is the way it has to be then she is prepared to die. She turns to Gina and says, "I am sorry I yelled—you have been so good to me—you didn't deserve it, but I am at the end of my rope. I really do not want any more IVs sticks—they always have trouble with my IVs."

Sandy talks to Ms. Knight about some of the *alternatives,* both to having the IV reinserted and to ongoing care in the nursing home. She also asks about her mood, suspecting that she may be depressed. They discuss the possibility of oral antibiotics and the need for Ms. Knight to drink plenty of fluids. Sandy also talks about other options that can be explored such as having hospice or palliative care services visit her at her nursing home. They can provide staff education related to pain management and the existential needs of a person facing death as well as extra patient care services. She suggests having a social worker come and talk to Ms. Knight so that arrangements can be made in advance of her discharge.

During the conversation, Ms. Knight stops crying and is agreeable both to the idea of oral antibiotics and a visit from the social worker. She admits to feeling "down what with the cancer coming back and everything, but isn't that to be expected?" Gina says, "Ms. Knight, I remember you talking to me about the pastor from your church and how she had visited you in the nursing home and been very helpful. Would you like me to contact her and ask her to visit?" Ms. Knight says, "Yes I would, I hadn't thought that she could come here to see me."

Back in Sandy's office, Sandy and Gina revisit the interaction. Sandy reassures Gina that her actions were appropriate, and that it was important that she recognized the limits of her experience and knowledge and sought appropriate advice, but that it was also apparent that she had her own resources to draw on—she indeed knew Ms. Knight better than anyone else. In Sandy's experience, events could have gone very differently if, for example, there had been an urgent need to restart the IV (for example, a dehydration issue) before anyone had talked to Ms. Knight about her preferences for care and interventions in the event of an emergency. Because the situation was not an emergency, Ms. Knight's wishes could be heard and conveyed to the physician. Gina said she would be comfortable phoning Ms. Knight's attending physician and explaining the situation, what had been discussed, and what Ms. Knight wanted. However, she thought that it would be helpful for the floor nurses to have a meeting to discuss the situation. Additionally, in her college classes they had discussed the problems of advance directives and how to talk to patients about their preferences should an emergency arise and thought this would be good time to reinforce the importance of these.

Summary

This chapter explores the status of nursing as a profession with its accompanying responsibilities. The relationship of clinical and moral reasoning was highlighted and supported. Finally, the exercise of clinical and moral decision making in advanced practice was exemplified by a case study and case analysis. An important facet of moral decision making in difficult situations is processing the event after the fact. This is a time when reflection and self-reflection can be crucial to the development of confidence in decision making and when the insights of others can broaden a nurse's perspective.

Yet, perhaps understandably, this is often the most neglected part of ethical practice. Time constraints, fiscal constraints, and the relative isolation of many advanced practice settings all conspire against collegial meetings of these kinds. Important tips for the conduct of such meetings include neutral settings, confidentiality, and sensitivity to the feelings of those presenting so that they are not made to feel that they "did it wrong." Rather, the emphasis should be on the idea that such sessions help further professional goals by facilitation of new tools, strategies, and approaches.

Discussion Questions

1. Does your country have its own code of ethics or does it rely on that of the ICN (over 130 member states)? What guidance is provided in your code of ethics or conduct related to restrictive contexts and environments? What are the responsibilities of the professional or professions?

2. Think of a simple case or situation you were involved in that left you feeling troubled. Explore this with colleagues using Table 2-6 or another decision-making heuristic (helpful framework). What new insights do you have? Would you have done things differently in light of what you learned in this chapter?

3. Preventive ethics is the process of anticipating and addressing potential problems before they arise. Many of the issues in health care that progress to the dilemma stage (choice between two or more equally bad alternatives) start off as minor communication problems. Think of one or more occasions from your practice when recognizing or addressing something early on would have defused an incipient difficult situation. For example, in my past experience with a patient critically ill with toxic shock syndrome, I believe that early honest conversations with her family would have prevented the loss of trust with its subsequent suspicion and anger.

References

American Association of Colleges of Nursing. (2006). *The essentials of doctoral education for advanced nursing practice*. Washington, DC: Author. Retrieved from http://www.aacn .nche.edu/publications/position/DNPEssentials.pdf

American Medical Association. (2001). *Principles of medical ethics.* Retrieved from http://www .ama-assn.org/ama/pub/category/2512.html

American Nurses Association. (1994). *Ethics and human rights position statements: The nonnegotiable nature of the ANA Code for Nurses with interpretive statements.* Washington, DC: Author. Retrieved from http://www.nursingworld.org/positionstatements

American Nurses Association. (2001). *Code of ethics for nurses with interpretive statements.* Washington, DC: Author.

American Nurses Association. (2010). *Social policy statement.* Washington, DC: Author.

Andrist, L. C., Nicholas, P. K., & Wolf, K. A. (2006). *A history of nursing ideas.* Sudbury, MA: Jones and Bartlett.

Anscombe, J. (2008). Healthcare out of balance: How global forces will reshape the health of nations. Report of A. T. Kearney Inc. Retrieved from http://www.atkearney.com /documents/10192/dced09b1-745b-4934-be20-3dec90d8195e

Benner, P., Tanner, C. A., & Chesla, C. A. (1996). *Expertise in nursing practice: Caring, clinical judgment and ethics.* New York, NY: Springer.

Blumer, R. H., & Meyer, M. (2006). *The new medicine.* Ashland, OH: Atlas Books.

Brown, L. (1993). (Ed.). *The new shorter Oxford English Dictionary.* New York, NY: Oxford Clarendon Press.

Bruhn, J. G. (2001). Being good and doing good: The culture of professionalism in the health professions. *Health Care Manager, 19*(4), 47–58.

Bryant-Lukosius, D., DiCensio, A., Browne, G., & Pinelli, J. (2004). Advanced practice nursing roles: Development, implementation and evaluation. *Nursing and Healthcare Management and Policy, 48*(5), 519–529.

Carr-Saunders, A. M., & Wilson, P. A. (1933). *The professions.* Oxford, England: Clarendon.

Ceci, C. (2004). Nursing, knowledge and power: A case analysis. *Social Science and Medicine, 59*, 1879–1889.

Chiang-Hanisko, L., Ross., R., Boonyanurak., P., Ozawa, M., & Chiang., L. (2008). Pathways to progress in nursing: Understanding career patterns in Japan, Taiwan, and Thailand. *The Online Journal of Issues in Nursing, 13*(3), Manuscript 4. doi: 10.3912/OJIN. Vol13No03Man04

Coburn, J. (1987). "I See and Am Silent." A Short History of Nursing in Ontario, 1850–1930. In D. Coburn, C. D'Arcy, G. Torrance, & P. New (Eds.), *Health and Canadian society* (2nd ed.). Markham, Ontario: Fitzhenry and Whiteside.

Cody, W. K. (2006). *Philosophical and theoretical perspectives for advanced practice nursing.* (4th ed.). Sudbury, MA: Jones and Bartlett.

Cronenwett, L., Dracup, K., Grey, M., McCauley, L., Meleis, A., & Salmon, M. (2011). The Doctor of Nursing Practice: A national workforce perspective. *Nursing Outlook, 59*, 9–17.

Curtin, L. (2001). Guest editorial: The ICN Code of Ethics for Nurses: Shared values in a troubled world. *ICN International Nursing Review, 48*(1), 1–2.

Dewey, J. (1980). *The quest for certainty: A study of the relation of action knowledge and action.* New York, NY: Perigree Books. (Original work published in 1929.)

Dierckx de Casterlé, B., Izumi, S., Godfrey, N. S., & Denhaerynck, K. (2008). Nurses' responses to ethical dilemmas in nursing practice: Meta-analysis. *Journal of Advanced Nursing, 63*(6), 540–549.

Dodd, S. J., Jansson, B. S., Brown-Saltzman, M. S., & Wunch, K. (2004). Expanding nurses' participation in ethics: An empirical examination of ethical activism and ethical assertiveness. *Nursing Ethics, 11*(1), 15–27.

Donaldson, S. K., & Crowley, D. M. (1978). The discipline of nursing. *Nursing Outlook, 26*(2), 113–120.

Doris, J. M., & The Moral Psychology Research Group. (2010). *The moral psychology handbook.* New York, NY: Oxford University Press.

Dougherty, C. J. (1990). The costs of commercial medicine. *Theoretical Medicine, 11,* 275–286.

Dougherty, C. J. (1992). The excesses of individualism. For meaningful healthcare reform, the United States needs a renewed sense of community. *Health Progress Journal, 73*(1), 22–28.

Dracup, K., Cronenwett, L., Meleis, A. I., & Benner, P. E. (2005). Reflections on the doctorate of nursing practice. *Nursing Outlook, 53,* 177–182.

Duffy, M. E., & Currier, S. (1999). *Ethics and human rights in nursing practice: A survey of New England nurses. Unpublished report of the survey.* Principal investigators: Sara Fry, Henry Luce Professor of Nursing Ethics, Boston College, Chestnut Hill; & Joan Riley, Director, Department of Nursing Emmanuel College, Boston, MA.

Fawcett, J., & Malinski, V. M. (1999). On the requirements for a metaparadigm: An invitation to dialogue. In J. W. Kenney (Ed.), *Philosophical and theoretical perspectives for advanced nursing practice* (2nd ed., pp. 111–116). Sudbury, MA: Jones and Bartlett.

Fawcett, J., Newman, D. M. L., & McAllister, M. (2004). Advanced practice nursing and conceptual models of nursing. *Nursing Science Quarterly, 17*(2), 135–138.

FEPI. (2012). *Code of Ethics and Conduct for European Nurses.* Brussels, Belgium: Author. Retrieved from http://www.fepi.org/userfiles/file/FEPI_Code_of_Ethics_and_Conducts_170908 .pdf

Fineberg, H. V. (2012). A successful and sustainable healthcare system: How to get there from here? *New England Journal of Medicine, 366*(11), 1020–1027.

Flaming, D. (2004). Nursing theories as nursing ontologies. *Nursing Philosophy, 5*(3), 224–229.

Flexner, A. (1915). Is social work a profession? *Proceedings of the National Conference of Charities and Correction, 581,* 584–588, 590. Retrieved from http://darkwing.uoregon .edu/~adoption/archive/FlexnerISWAP.htm

Fowler, M. (1997). Nursing's ethics. In A. J. Davis, M. A. Aroskar, J. Liaschenko, & T. S. Drought (Eds.), *Ethical dilemmas and nursing practice* (4th ed.). Stamford, CT: Appleton & Lange.

Fry, S. T. (1995). Nursing ethics. In W. T. Reich (Ed.), *Encyclopedia of bioethics* (Rev. ed., Vol. 2, pp. 1822–1827). New York, NY: Simon & Schuster Macmillan.

Fry, S. T. (2002). Guest editorial: Defining nurses' ethical practices in the 21st century. *International Nursing Review, 49,* 1–3.

Fry, S. T., & Grace, P. J. (2007). Ethical dimensions of nursing and health care. In J. L. Creasia & B. Parker (Eds.), *Conceptual foundations: The bridge to professional practice* (4th ed.). Philadelphia, PA: Mosby, Elsevier.

Gilligan, C. (1982). *In a different voice: Psychological theory and women's development.* Cambridge, MA: Harvard University Press.

Grace, P. J. (1998). *A philosophical analysis of the concept "advocacy": Implications for professional–patient relationships.* Unpublished doctoral dissertation, University of Tennessee: Knoxville, TN. Retrieved from http://proquest.umi.com. Publication Number AAT9923287, Proquest Document ID No. 734421751.

Grace, P. J. (2001). Professional advocacy: Widening the scope of accountability. *Nursing Philosophy, 2*(2), 151–162.

Grace, P. J. (2004a). Ethics in the clinical encounter. In S. K. Chase (Ed.), *Clinical judgment and communication in nurse practitioner practice* (pp. 295–332). Philadelphia, PA: F. A. Davis.

Grace, P. J. (2004b). Philosophical considerations in nurse practitioner practice. In S. K. Chase (Ed.), *Clinical judgment and communication in nurse practitioner practice* (pp. 279–294). Philadelphia, PA: F. A. Davis.

Grace, P. J. (2005). Ethical issues relevant to health promotion. In C. Edelman & C. L. Mandle (Eds.), *Health promotion throughout the lifespan* (6th ed., pp. 100–125). St. Louis, MO: Elsevier/Mosby.

Grace, P. J. (2006). Philosophies, models, and theories: Moral obligations. In M. R. Alligood & A. Marriner-Tomey (Eds.), *Nursing theory: Utilization and application* (3rd ed., pp. 67–85). St. Louis, MO: Elsevier/Mosby.

Gross, M. L. (2010). Teaching military medical ethics: Another look at dual loyalty and triage. Cambridge *Quarterly of Healthcare Ethics, 19*, 458–464.

Group, T. M., & Roberts, J. I. (2001). *Nursing, physician control and the medical monopoly.* Bloomington, IN: Indiana University Press.

Hagedorn, S., & Quinn, A. A. (2004). Theory-based nurse practitioner practice: Caring in action. *Topics in Advanced Practice Nursing, 4*(4).

Hardingham, L. (2004). Integrity and moral residue: Nurses as participants in a moral community. *Nursing Philosophy, 5,* 127–134.

Helft, P. R., Chamness, A., Terry, C., & Uhrich, M. (2011). Oncology nurses' attitudes toward prognosis-related communication: A pilot mailed survey of oncology nursing society members. *Oncology Nursing Forum, 38*(4), 468–474.

Henderson, V. A. (1991). *The nature of nursing.* New York, NY: National League for Nursing.

International Council of Nurses. (2012). *Code of ethics for nurses.* Geneva, Switzerland: Author. Retrieved from http://www.icn.ch/icncode.pdf

Kelly, B. (1998). Preserving moral integrity: A follow-up study with new graduate nurses. *Journal of Advanced Nursing, 25*(8), 1134–1145.

Kepler, M. O. (1981). *Medical stewardship: Fulfilling the Hippocratic legacy.* Westport, CT: Greenwood Press.

Mechanic, D. (1998). The functions and limitations of trust in the provision of medical care. *Journal of Health Politics, Policy and Law, 23,* 661–686.

Milton, C. (2005). Scholarship in nursing: Ethics of a practice doctorate. *Nursing Science Quarterly, 18*(2), 113–116.

Nagel, T. (1970). *The possibility of altruism.* Oxford, England: Clarendon.

National Association of Social Workers. (1999). Code of ethics. Retrieved from http://www .socialworkers.org/pubs/code/code.asp

Nelson, H. L. (1992). Against caring. *Journal of Clinical Ethics, 3,* 8–15.

Newman, M. A., Sime, A. M., & Corcoran-Perry, S. A. (1991). The focus of the discipline of nursing. *Advances in Nursing Science, 14*(1), 1–6.

Newton, L. H. (1988). Lawgiving for professional life: Reflections on the place of the professional code. In A. Flores (Ed.), *Professional ideals* (pp. 47–56). Belmont, CA: Wadsworth.

Nightingale, F. (1946). *Notes on nursing: What it is and what it is not.* Philadelphia, PA: Lippincott. (Original work published in 1859.)

Packard, S. A., & Polifroni, E. C. (1992). The nature of scientific truth. *Nursing Science Quarterly, 5*(4), 158–163.

Paley, J. (2012). Book review: The moral psychology handbook. (Edited by John Doris and the Moral Psychology Research Group. Oxford University Press.) *Nursing Philosophy, 13,* 18–22.

Pavlish, C., Brown-Saltzman, K., Hersh, M., Shirk, M., & Rounkle, A. (2011). Nursing priorities, actions, and regrets for ethical situations in clinical practice. *Journal of Nursing Scholarship, 43*(4), 385–395.

Pelau, H. E. (1952). *Interpersonal relations in nursing.* New York, NY: G. P. Putnam's Sons.

Reid, T. R. (2009). *The healing of America: A global quest for better, cheaper, and fairer health care.* New York, NY: Penguin.

Relman, A. S. (2007). Medical professionalism in a commercialized health care market. *Cleveland Clinic Journal of Medicine, 75* (Suppl. 6), S33–S36.

Rest, J. (1983). The major components of morality. In P. Mussen (Ed.), *Manual of child psychology* (Vol. Cognitive Development). New York, NY: Wiley.

Rest, J. R. (1982). A psychologist looks at the teaching of ethics. *Hastings Center Report, 12*(1), 29–36.

Rogers, M. E. (1970). *An introduction to the theoretical basis of nursing.* Philadelphia, PA: F. A. Davis.

Sasso, L., Steviano, A., Jurado, M. G., & Rocco, G. (2008). Code of Ethics and Conduct for European Nurses. *Nursing Ethics, 15*(6), 821–836.

Sellman, D. (2005). Towards an understanding of nursing as a response to vulnerability. *Nursing Philosophy, 6*(1), 2–10.

Silva, M. C., & Ludwick, R. (2006, March 20). Is the Doctor of Nursing Practice ethical? *Online Journal of Issues in Nursing.* Retrieved from http://www.nursingworld.org /MainMenuCategories/ANAMarketplace/ANAPeriodicals/OJIN/Columns/Ethics /DNPEthical.aspx

Sullivan, W. M. (1999). What is left of professionalism after managed care? *Hastings Center Report, 29*(2), 7–13.

Tschudin, V. (2006). How nursing ethics as a subject changes: An analysis of the first 11 years of publication of the *Journal of Nursing Ethics. Nursing Ethics, 13*(1), 66–82.

Varcoe, C., Doane, G., Pauly, B., Rodney, P., Storch, J. L., Mahoney, K., . . . Starzomski, R. (2004). Ethical practice in nursing: Working the in-betweens. *Nursing Philosophy, 45*(3), 316–325.

Weston, A. (2011). *A practical companion to ethics* (4th ed.). New York, NY: Oxford.

Whitney, S. N., Ethier, A. M., Fruge, E., Berg, S., McCullough, L. B., & Hockenbury, M. (2006). Decision making in pediatric oncology: Who should take the lead? The decisional priority in pediatric oncology model. *Journal of Clinical Oncology, 24*(1), 160–165.

Williams, J. R. (2009). Dual loyalties: How to resolve ethical conflict. *South African Journal of Bioethics and Law, 2*(1), 8–11.

Willis, D. B., Grace, P. J., & Roy, C. (2008). A central unifying focus for the discipline: Facilitating humanization, meaning, choice, quality of life and healing in living and dying. *Advances in Nursing Science, 31*(1), E28–E40.

Windt, P. Y. (1989). Introductory essay. In P. Y. Windt, P. C. Appleby, M. P. Battin, L. P. Francis, & B. M. Landesman (Eds.), *Ethical issues in the professions* (pp. 1–24). Englewood Cliffs, NJ: Prentice Hall.

Wuest, J. (2006). Professionalism and the evolution of nursing as a discipline: A feminist perspective. In W. K. Cody (Ed.), *Philosophical and theoretical perspectives for advanced nursing practice* (4th ed., pp. 85–98). Sudbury, MA: Jones and Bartlett.

COMMON ETHICAL ISSUES ACROSS PRACTICE SPECIALTIES

CHAPTER 3

Advanced Practice Nursing: The Nurse–Patient Relationship and General Ethical Concerns

Pamela J. Grace

Our privileges can be no greater than our obligations. The protection of our rights can endure no longer than the performance of our responsibilities.
—John F. Kennedy, "The Educated Citizen,"
Vanderbilt University 90th Convocation Address, May 18, 1963

Introduction

This edition of the text intends to be inclusive of issues related to advanced practice nursing regardless of country of practice. An estimated 24 countries have nurses practicing in advanced roles (Nieminen, Mannevaara, & Fagerström, 2011). Where possible, the expertise of colleagues from countries outside the United States has been solicited to help understand and account both for similarities and differences in ethical issues faced by persons who are in a variety of roles and designations. For North America, the acronym APN is used for advanced practice nurses to avoid confusion because the acronym for advanced nursing practice (ANP)—the term used by the International Council of Nurses (ICN)—denotes specialty certification as an adult nurse practitioner in the United States, which is just one of many possible advanced practice designations globally.

The first two chapters of this text laid the groundwork for APNs' understanding of their ethical responsibilities. Here it is important to consider the essence of the advanced practice role. Are there commonalities across countries and settings? Contemporarily, there is wide interest in describing the scope and boundaries of such roles, and deriving a coherent internationally acceptable definition is seen as a necessary step in professional development to meet the needs of diverse patients and communities and across country boundaries. Hanson and Hamric (2003) have synthesized a definition of advanced practice nursing from several important resource documents and their own experiences of the development of advanced practice: "Advanced nursing practice is the application of an expanded range of practical, theoretical, and research-based therapeutics to phenomena experienced by patients within a specialized clinical area of the larger discipline of nursing" (p. 205). The ICN's publication on advanced practice nursing (Schober & Affara, 2006) cites the 2002 ICN definition of the advanced practice nurse as:

> a registered nurse who has acquired the expert knowledge base, complex decision-making skills and clinical competencies for expanded practice, the characteristics of which are shaped by the context and/or country in which s/he is credentialed to practice. [Further the ICN recommends] a masters degree ... for entry level (practice). (Schober & Affara, 2006, p. 210)

Advanced nursing roles have existed for several decades in many countries, for example midwifery and health visitors in the United Kingdom and other countries and nurse anesthetists in the United States. However, the first officially designated advanced practice role in the United States was that of nurse practitioner (NP) in the mid-1960s (Schober & Affara, 2006). Ketefian, Redman, Hanucharurnkul, Masterson, and Neves (2001) identified several critical factors that have been conducive to the development of these roles internationally. These are: "environment; the health needs of society; the health workforce supply and demand; governmental policy and support; intra- and interprofessional collaboration; the development of nursing education; and documentation of effectiveness of the advanced role" (p. 152).

The APN role is nevertheless a nursing role that is distinguishable from other nursing roles only by the breadth and depth of responsibility to patients implied by the term *advanced practice*. This means, for example, that APNs often oversee a patient's total care in a given practice setting (e.g., primary care, anesthesia, midwifery, gerontology, etc.), and in alternate settings they also have expanded responsibilities. For example, in acute care they may be responsible for handling emergencies and ordering and carrying out invasive interventions. For this reason and in this sense, their moral responsibilities can sometimes seem more complex and onerous "than, those of nurses who share [patient] oversight with other health-care professionals" (Grace, 2004b, pp. 321–322). Effective exploration of ethical issues faced in advanced practice, then, should reflect the implications of these broad role obligations. That is, although the ethical substance of situations may not differ from that faced by nurses in nonexpanded roles, advanced practice nursing ethics account for the more extensive duties incurred in these roles.

The following inquiry focuses on a variety of ethical problems and concerns that are common across many advanced practice settings. Such concerns are also discussed in general nursing ethics textbooks and will not be unfamiliar to the seasoned clinician. Here, however, the implications of these issues are discussed specifically in terms of the APN's augmented responsibilities. Illustrative examples are drawn from a variety of advanced practice sources and from my experiences as an APN, as well as from cases shared by nurses in the master's level ethics course I teach. A more focused application of particular ethical issues and strategies for their resolution may be found in the later specialty chapters. Because it is not feasible to cover all issues that an APN is likely to encounter, it is suggested that any troubling issues that the student or graduated APN faces that are not directly addressed in this text be brought up for in-class exploration with faculty and peers or explored with colleagues using the insights and strategies provided here or in other resources. Other helpful resources include clinical ethicists, philosophers who have ethics expertise, ethics websites, and networking groups.

An appropriate start to the next section is a comprehensive discussion of the demands of the nurse–patient relationship. Characteristics discovered to be essential for consistently good patient care and decision making are explored, with suggestions for the development of these. These qualities are sometimes called virtues and include the use of both intellect (thinking) and affect (emotions and motivation) in decision making and ensuing action. Certain philosophers, such as Aristotle and more contemporarily Alasdair MacIntyre (2007), have argued that virtues can be developed through habitual practice. A person who develops a virtuous personality through habitual practice is predisposed to consistently engage in "good" actions. It is debatable whether all persons can become virtuous in this way or even that people who might be considered "good" persons always act in "good" ways. It is useful to focus on developing existing qualities that facilitate professional–patient relationships and equally useful to be mindful that circumstances can sometimes get in the way of this focus. Examples of important qualities are discussed in more depth later in the chapter; they include such characteristics as empathy, veracity, transparency of purpose, cultural sensitivity, motivation to act, courage to act, and perseverance in carrying an act through.

A further important issue for all clinical and research settings is that of adequately informing patients (or their surrogate decision makers) about their options for care, treatments, and procedures. Thus, the parameters and demands of informed consent are explicated in this chapter with the exception of informed consent in human subjects' protection, which is discussed in detail in Chapter 6. Problems associated with the adequacy of informed consent to the provision of care and therapeutics include the issue of patients who lack decision-making capacity for a variety of reasons, persons who are difficult to engage with, and people who are making decisions that seem to be at odds with their own values. A further topic investigated is that of privacy and confidentiality related to patients' health information. In this highly technological age, it is becoming increasingly difficult to adequately protect patient information from entities that do not necessarily have a patient's best interests in mind when seeking it. Additionally, inadvertent breaches of confidentiality can occur via the use of social media. Unethical use of social media can also lead to loss of trust in the involved profession (an example of this is provided later). The protection of information is multifaceted. One important aspect is transparency. The person at risk should be told for what purposes the data are required and to what uses they will be put, and in so far as these are known, the risks and benefits of sharing the data. This is in addition to being careful about who can have access to a person's data.

Additionally, APNs often have concerns about how to maintain their personal integrity. Sometimes this is related to patient or peer requests to engage in something that is at odds with a nurse's values, or it may be related to conflicts within the healthcare system, such as managed care or institutional pressures to limit care. Some of the sources of these concerns, along with strategies to address them, are presented. Finally, because some practice problems end up as complex and extremely difficult to sort out, the issue of preventive ethics is woven throughout this section. Many so-called dilemmas actually can be prevented or diffused by good communication or an early understanding of the likelihood that unaddressed problems might cause critical difficulties for the patient in question and/or the patient's significant others.

Virtue Ethics: The Characteristics of Good APNs

Many people are attracted to the nursing profession because they see it as a practice that contributes to individuals, as well as the greater societal good. This is true not just at the undergraduate level but also for those who choose nursing as a second career and take an accelerated route to ANP. Thus, the personal values of nurses are often congruent with the values of the nursing profession—for example, nascent nurses are drawn to the idea of contributing to the well-being of others. The desire to contribute to the welfare of others is often considered a virtue (as opposed to the desire to hurt someone, which would be considered a vice). As Feldman (1978) writes, in acknowledging that something is good, we are noting its qualities "relative to some class of comparison . . . some feature of that thing in virtue of which [we] hold it to be good. This feature is its virtue, or good-making characteristic" (p. 234). This section explores the issue of virtue ethics as it relates to good APNs, where "*good*" is taken to be synonymous with ethical. Virtue ethics in healthcare practice is essentially the idea that a person can cultivate certain characteristics (virtues) that will predispose him or her to good actions related to the profession's predetermined goals.

Contemporary proponents of virtue ethics almost all trace their influences back to Aristotle, although ideas about virtue can also be discovered in ancient texts on Eastern philosophy. Aristotle's idea is that a good or virtuous person is someone who possesses practical wisdom or prudence. The Greek term for this is *phronesis*. Practical wisdom permits a man (in ancient times women were considered subordinate to men) both to understand what is a good way to live and that living a good life necessarily means developing mutually beneficial relationships with others. To act well, a man must learn to habitually moderate emotional impulses by using reasoning. This is what is required to achieve the desired purpose of living a good life. Eventually, a person will habituate himself to always engaging in good action—he will become a good or virtuous person. The desirable or virtuous purpose of all human beings, according to Aristotle, is to live in accordance with their human nature. The essential characteristic of human nature—that which distinguishes human nature from the nature of all other beings—is rationality. The ability of human beings to use logical reasoning gives human beings purpose, and that purpose is the pursuit of a satisfying life. The Greek term for this is *eudaimonia,* often also referred to as happiness, although it loses something in the translation and does not mean happiness in any superficial sense of the term (Hutchinson, 1995).

Practical reason acts as a constraint on emotional and instinctual drives that can result in harmful actions on the one hand, and on the other hand in a lack of needed action or inadequate action. Reason mediates a balance between extremes of action. For example, according to Aristotle, courage is a virtue. Unrestrained courage can cause unnecessarily risky behavior, which is therefore irrational. Alternatively, timidity in the face of doing something important is problematic and also requires reason to moderate action. Practicing the development of virtue eventually leads to the formation of a virtuous character. Additionally, a satisfying life is necessarily lived within society and in relationships with others and facilitates harmony in these relationships. It is noteworthy that for Aristotle being virtuous has a self-focus, but nonetheless a harmonious society is also requisite for a satisfying life. Thus, the actions of a virtuous man have the serendipitous result of contributing to the good of others.

How does this explanation of virtue pertain to the current project of understanding what characteristics are necessary for good practice? The answer is that contemporary moral philosophers, such as Elizabeth Anscombe (1958/1981), Bernard Williams (1985), and Alasdair MacIntyre (2007), have been interested in resurrecting the idea of virtue as a way to understand peoples' relationships to each other and to inform provider-patient relationships. This move represents, in part at least, a way around the problem that deontological and consequentialist ethical theories do not account for the contextual and relationship-dependent nature of human life in situations where moral decision making is needed. Neither do these theories always capture contingencies of healthcare providers' multifaceted and relationally oriented roles.

MacIntyre's work, although not resulting in a theory that can be applied directly to action, does provide some unifying ideas about virtues (Sellman, 2000, p. 27). The constituents of virtue, or those characteristics that make a person virtuous in MacIntyre's view, are context dependent. Thus, virtues may be "seen as supporting and maintaining particular ends" (Sellman, 2000, p. 27). Because virtues are seen as those characteristics necessary to support a particular end, goal, or practice, some common objections to the idea that a virtue ethic is helpful in healthcare practice are overcome (Armstrong, 2006; Begley, 2005; Sellman, 2000). Criticisms of virtue ethics include the observation that what is virtuous in one situation or in a given culture may not be considered virtuous in another. Therefore, there is no stable footing for the idea of a virtuous person and neither is there a list of virtues a person must possess to be virtuous.

An additional and potentially serious criticism is that there is no external criterion (within virtue theory) for judging whether the actions of a virtuous person are actually good. There is no "gold standard" for good actions. Additionally, the actions of someone who is thought to be virtuous will not necessarily always be good; that is, they may not meet a predetermined goal. Many factors can interfere with a good person's ability to do good actions, as listed in **Table 3-1**.

However, if certain virtues are viewed as pertaining to a particular professional practice and necessary for meeting the goals of that practice, then it

■ Table 3-1   Factors That Interfere with Ethical Nursing Action

Locus	Factors
Agent related	Level of moral development
	Capacity to recognize ethical content. Chambliss (1996) discusses the phenomenon "routinization of disaster."
	Openness to reflection
	Personal or emotional issues
	Energy levels
	Creativity
	Locus of control (powerfulness/powerlessness)
	Unable to connect with patient
	Fear of disapproval (peer or other)
	Disapproval of patient's choice
	Time of day—complexity of preceding workload or decisions
	Level of knowledge related to the issue
	Subconscious cognitive processes—effects of unexamined "universal" cognitive biases—overreliance on intuitions (Doris, 2010; Kahnemann, 2011)
Environmental	Pressures from peers—supervisors
	Competing demands (peers/patients/relatives/institution)
	Social sanction
	Economic and institutional conditions
	Time or resource constraints
	Conflicts of interest
	Job insecurity
	Catastrophic conditions

is possible to evaluate a given action based on how well it addresses those goals. Because nursing is a practice profession with relatively well articulated goals, it is possible to agree that persons who possess certain characteristics are more likely than those who do not, to routinely engage in good practice to be willing to address practice structures that interfere with good actions. A further consequence is that, as a profession, nursing must continue to investigate what the characteristics of a good nurse are and then nurture these traits in the education and mentoring of nurses. A big question for the profession itself is whether all prospective nurses are capable of developing the characteristics of good nurses. If not, what is the profession's responsibility (assumed by its educators) to "weed out" those who are incapable of being good nurses?

Virtues of Nursing

Nursing practice and the fulfillment of nursing goals, then, can be understood as requiring the development of certain facilitative characteristics. Indeed, by exploring what is needed to provide good nursing care to patients—as outlined in the literature and in codes of ethics—relatively quickly, it becomes possible to compose a list of virtues that it would be good for nurses to cultivate. Additionally, nursing curricula should nurture these characteristics (Haggerty & Grace, 2008). Begley (2005) has composed such a list; it includes compassion, integrity, honesty, patience, tolerance, courage, imagination, perception, perseverance, self-reflection, and many more. For her dissertation, *Optimizing Stewardship: A Grounded Theory of Nurses as Moral Leader in the Intensive Care Unit*, Breakey (2006) studied characteristics of nurses who reportedly engaged successfully in end-of-life (EOL) decisions. Salient characteristics for this important nursing role included understanding the professional obligations of the role, the ability to empathize with others, and willingness to understand an issue in detail and to support others in their decision making using expertise and knowledge. The possession and exercise of any virtue within a nursing care setting will also rely on other interrelated virtues, the clinician's knowledge, and skills pertinent to the practice domain. Compassion for a cancer patient's suffering, for instance, without knowledge of how to mitigate it and/or the motivation to alleviate it is an empty virtue. However, theoretical knowledge of pain management without experience in patient assessment, planning, delivery, and evaluation or without understanding the meaning that suffering holds for the patient is also problematic.

Two studies of my own (currently in the publication stages), focused on understanding nurses' views of what are the characteristics of a "good" nurse, support these ideas. One study analyzed essays (N = 42) from a graduate nursing ethics class, and the other interviewed nurses from a variety of settings who had been identified by others as "good nurses" (N = 11). The major characteristics of "good" nurses are dependent on having a certain level of knowledge and expertise relevant to the setting. Roughly, they include perceptiveness, engagement, understanding of the nursing role as having obligations, good communication, the ability to collaborate, the ability to support others, and moral courage (the courage to act for the patient and/or family in the face of obstacles). Additionally, beginning data analyses from our CERN (Clinical Ethics Residency for Nurses) project, along with course discussions, support the assumption that being a "good" nurse requires nurses to understand and act on their obligations to patients, patients' families, and those they supervise. These studies are examples of descriptive ethics. *Descriptive ethics* portrays what people think are good actions and good characteristics. It is differentiated from *normative ethics*, which mandates certain types of behaviors. Where a code of ethics provides the normative aspects—that is, what nurses should do and how they should do it—descriptive ethics paints a picture of what is actually happening in practice or what nurses perceive as their obligation and appropriate action and what sorts of things get in the way of providing, or ensuring the provision of, "good" patient care. The two types of ethics taken together provide a bigger picture of what changes in education, environment, or policy may be necessary for good patient care.

For APNs, who are often required to supervise, mentor, or collaborate with others, virtues such as leadership, cooperation, and discernment of the different needs of those with whom they interact are important to cultivate in order to meet professional duties. Chapter 5 of this text discusses leadership characteristics in depth. The next section examines the idea that certain virtues are needed for interacting with patients who are faced with making decisions about their care. Patients give their consent to care, implicitly, verbally, or in written form, depending on the invasiveness or risk of the proposed action. APNs are in the privileged position of assisting with, or empowering the patient, to make healthcare decisions that by their nature have some sort of effect on that patient's life. With this privilege comes added responsibility.

Informed Consent

The principle of autonomy, as discussed in Chapter 1, underlies the idea of informed consent. Because human beings have the capacity to reason, decide, and act and because they might be presumed to know better than anyone else what their interests are, all things being equal, they have the right to make decisions concerning their health care. They should (barring any incapacitating factors) be free from the interference of others, at least as far as personal decision making is concerned. This translates into the right of patients to accept or refuse healthcare treatments, regardless of risk, given the possession of decision-making capacity and an adequate understanding of the risks of refusal and the potential benefits of treatment. This right was legislated in the United States under the Patient Self-Determination Act (PSDA), ratified in 1991 (as part of the Omnibus Budget Reconciliation Act [OBRA], 1990), which is discussed in more detail shortly. In the United Kingdom, the right to make autonomous care decisions is protected by the Mental Capacity Act (2005), and in several other countries the right is also legally protected. Regardless of whether or not there are legal protections for the healthcare professional in helping patients understand their human rights related to health care, understanding the generally accepted and fundamental right of persons to make their own decisions provides a strong foundation for advocating that patients' real needs are evaluated and met, including the need for information tailored to their level of understanding and preferences.

Types of Consent

People give three types of consent in permitting healthcare professionals to evaluate and act on their health needs. The first is implicit consent, the second is verbal consent, and the third is written consent. When a patient is unable to consent, as discussed later, then an informed proxy makes a decision on the patient's behalf and with the patient's best interests (where this is knowable) in mind. Informed consent, then, is the process of interaction between a healthcare provider and person in which necessary information is exchanged and an appropriate level of understanding is gained to enable that person to make a decision about acceptable care, treatment, interventions, or courses of action in light of his or her preexisting values, beliefs, and lifestyle. One critical message implicit in this idea is that consent is not a static concept. Evaluation of current circumstances, patient understanding, and continued willingness to participate or proceed requires that consent be, for the most part, an ongoing process. Advance care planning (ACP) for acceptable interventions in the event of incapacity is discussed in later chapters.

IMPLICIT CONSENT

In presenting to a healthcare delivery setting in search of assistance for health needs, a person is implicitly consenting, at minimum, to be evaluated for those needs. If the setting is an inpatient or institutional setting such as a hospital, the person might sign a form giving consent for certain routine evaluations. However, this form is general and does not detail all aspects of the evaluation, which may include tests and manual assessments such as a physical examination. Moreover, typically the admitting personnel charged with obtaining signatures have no or little medical or nursing knowledge. Thus, implicit consent is not usually very informed, and patients may well not understand what rights they have.

In primary care sites, those who present for care do not necessarily understand the customary routines of the practice site—nor are they required to accept them, although frequently both ancillary staff and clinic nurses do not act as if they understand this. For these reasons, nurses need to be ready to ascertain what the patient has understood, and what it would be helpful for him or her to know. If a patient objects to some aspects of routine care, nurses are responsible for discovering what underlies the objection, how important it is to gather the data in question, and whether acceptable alternatives may be offered. For example, a faculty colleague who is also a women's health NP reported that she was doing a breast exam on a patient as part of the patient's yearly checkup. She asked the woman if she did monthly breast exams on herself. The woman replied, "No, I don't like to touch my breasts, and for that matter I don't like anyone else to touch them either—not even my husband." At that point, my colleague realized both that she had not asked permission and had not sought to understand what, if any, meaning this particular act of assessment held for the woman. She apologized and the patient said she understood that it was part of the exam and had to be done. But my colleague wished she had thought to ask permission. She felt that this might have allowed the patient to discuss the issue with her, but the opportunity was lost. Touching someone without that person's permission is also a legal consideration and may subject a nurse to legal charges such as battery or assault.

The preceding scenario, which happened early in my colleague's professional life, made her more sensitive to the idea that patients can have good reasons for refusing even routine care and that they have a right to refuse it. However, nurses also have a responsibility to ensure that patients understand the implications of refusing evaluations, tests, or treatments and try to lessen any risks from this refusal by reformulating an acceptable plan of care. To illustrate this point, I give an example from my practice experience. A slightly overweight woman in her early twenties came to my primary care setting for treatment of a sore throat. It was her first visit. The office assistant, a nurse's aide, told her she had to be weighed as part of the "new patient" routine. The young woman refused. The aide tried to persuade her but to no avail.

I heard arguing in the hall, went to investigate, and saw a very upset young woman. I brought her right away into an empty room, acknowledged how upset she was, and asked her what happened. She said, "I really hate being weighed—I don't see why it is necessary—they used to do that at the other clinic." I explained that measuring a person's weight is in many cases a very useful assessment and had become a routine, but I realized from her reaction that we might need to rethink this policy. In the course of our interaction, and because she could see that I took her concern seriously, she confided that she used to be weighed weekly by her mother when she was a teenager and was physically punished for gaining weight. This opened an opportunity to help her further, and she eventually got counseling for unresolved issues with her mother.

After this, we changed our office policy and educated the medical assistants and aides about a patient's right to accept or refuse some of the routines that were not important for the given patient's care. If the routine was important, for example, weighing a patient with chronic heart failure, then rationale should be given. Alternatives, such as self-weighing and reporting significant changes, can be negotiated. Also, there are, of course, some cases when weighing a patient becomes crucial. For example, some drug dosages are calculated based on weight. In surgical operating areas, intensive care units, and pediatric settings, accurate weights may be crucial to avoid the harms (nonmaleficence) of over- or underdosing patients with essential therapeutics. In such cases nurses remain responsible for anticipating and minimizing any possible harms including psychological distress.

VERBAL CONSENT

Although for many patients a host of routines covered by implicit consent cause neither distress nor affect their care in any perceptible way, in the cases described earlier, informed consent to care was important both for the patients' immediate well-being and for determining whether follow-up care was necessary or desired. Gaining informed verbal consent permitted the nurse to understand what else might be required to provide good care. Sound clinical judgment, as described in Chapter 4, facilitates identification of the patient's particular needs, which in both cases proved to be more extensive than initially understood. Obtaining verbal consent to care—including evaluation, tests, therapeutics, and decisions about the best ways of managing chronic conditions—is synonymous with good APN practice in direct patient care and is dependent on establishing a nurse–patient relationship that is concerned with understanding the patient's vulnerability and needs and then addressing these.

WRITTEN CONSENT

The third type of informed consent is a written consent. Written consent "is intended to protect patients from . . . ethical or legal breaches and make formal their right to all relevant information, tailored specially to them" (Grace & McLaughlin, 2005, p. 79). Experienced nurses practicing in institutional settings are mostly familiar with *informed consent* as it relates to invasive medical procedures and perhaps to patients who are participating in research studies (see Chapter 6). In their definition of the term, Beauchamp and Childress (2009) acknowledge that "informed consent occurs if and only if a person or subject, with substantial understanding and in the absence of substantial control by others, intentionally authorizes a professional to do something" (p. 78). Although Beauchamp and Childress are explicitly discussing the necessary criteria for written and verbal informed consent rather than implicit consent, these criteria are also relevant for implicit consent.

In the case of proposed invasive procedures or surgery, the person responsible for carrying out or supervising the intervention is the one responsible for obtaining written consent. This is usually a physician, although increasingly it may be an APN. APNs who are qualified to carry out procedures or perform anesthesia are responsible for obtaining written consent. Staff nurses have responsibilities for ensuring that their patients are in a position to adequately understand what they are agreeing to. This has implications for the clinical nurse specialist (CNS) or nurse manager who serves as a floor resource, mentor, and educator and who sets the tone for the staff nurses on his or her unit.

Informed Consent: Ethical Problems

Informed consent, however, is a complex and tricky concept. For each person, the information needed for the person's consent to be "*substantially informed*" is different. For procedures or interventions that involve more than minimal risk (risk that is encountered in daily life), informing the patient should be viewed as a process because, for the most part, those faced with invasive procedures are already upset and anxious. Information processing under conditions of anxiety and stress is difficult, and studies have shown that patients do not retain information well under such conditions (Broadstock & Michie, 2000; Charles, Gafni, & Whelan, 1999; Kegley, 2002). The informing process involves understanding certain things about the patient. Nurses need to understand the patient's beliefs, including culturally based beliefs, values, and goals; the patient's ability to process information; and psychological, physiological, or environmental factors that might interfere with or facilitate processing of information.

Kegley (2002) notes that the "subjective substantial disclosure rule" (p. 461) is a standard that is starting to be used to understand what information is needed related to genetic testing and other complex decision-making scenarios. It "requires a substantial degree of knowledge about the patient, her context, and what is important to her" (p. 461). This represents a change from previous tests used in law to evaluate the adequacy of information given to a patient. The standards used in legal systems as a measure of adequacy either compared the knowledge possessed by the person in question against that of a knowledgeable group of physicians or against conceptions of what a reasonable person should know. Neither standard took into account the particular needs of a patient within the context of his or her life.

Patient-related psychological factors that can interfere with information processing are such things as psychological denial of a physical illness or diagnosis, loss of hope, unreasonable expectations of an intervention, a desire to please a provider or significant others, lack of energy to think through possible options and how they relate to goals, and cognitive problems. Physical factors include pain, sedation, fever, and poor cerebral perfusion, among others. Provider-related problems include inadequate knowledge about a procedure and its potential side effects (for example, a lack of understanding of the full range of implications related to genetic testing (discussed in the Women's Health chapter); an inability to connect with a particular person, which can interfere with the project of tailoring information to that person's specific needs and abilities; lack of understanding of the origins or meaning of any cultural factors; lack of knowledge about existing options or objections to providing the full range of options (for example, provider beliefs about the moral status of emergency contraception); and self-knowledge related to prejudice or bias. Additionally, certain situations are fraught with communication difficulties. Examples of such situations include language barriers, hearing impairments, and patients who are perceived as "difficult."

This discussion focuses on three important complicating factors related to appropriately informing patients: (1) the provider's appeal to conscience in not providing patients with the full range of options legally available, (2) cultural considerations in informing patients, and (3) the issue of difficult patients. Early identification of potential communication problems and attempts to anticipate and address these problems has been termed *preventive ethics*. One important professional problem is that of withholding information or not offering the available range of options for a patient's situation because it is against the provider's conscience. The next section addresses this issue.

CONSCIENCE AND PERSONAL INTEGRITY

The issue of healthcare professionals' refusal to provide patients with certain information and/or services has recently received publicity in the popular press in the United States. There are reports also from Europe of movements to protect healthcare providers who refuse care or limit information to patients based on conscience (Catholics for Choice, 2012). In 2010, the Parliamentary Assembly of the Council of Europe (PACE) debated the issue of the right of healthcare providers to conscientious objection (resolution #1763), urging states to provide patients timely access to legally permissible options (PACE, 2010). In opposition, the Swedish parliament has urged that their delegates work to change this resolution, reportedly because they overwhelmingly find it problematic that providers can withhold legally available options (Protection of Conscience Project, 2012). The ethical implications of refusing to disclose legally available options or to offer a full range of services have elicited renewed scrutiny on the part of moral philosophers, ethicists, and scholars in the various healthcare professions (Wicclair, 2011). Appeals to conscientious refusal to provide certain options are usually based on one of the following arguments: (1) although legally available, the healthcare provider finds the option morally objectionable based on religious grounds or on the basis of other personal beliefs; (2) the provider believes certain options to be congruent with his or her beliefs, and others are not, and there is no obligation to reveal this bias to the patient; or (3) the provider believes some available options are inferior or have too many side effects, and thus the provider is saving the patient from confusion.

As an example of the first argument, Jacobson (2005) highlights the case of registered nurse Andrea Nead, who did not want to "administer emergency contraception" (p. 27) as part of her role responsibilities. She claimed that she did not get a position she sought in a university health clinic because of her religious beliefs. Other examples (of the second and third arguments) from advanced practice settings include a colleague who referred patients in need of mental health services only to a Christian mental health facility, and another colleague who neglected to offer a variety of therapeutic options available for labor pains by encouraging patients to "have an epidural—it is a woman's best friend." In palliative care settings, refusal to provide adequate pain relief may result from providers' beliefs that they are contributing to a person's death.

The preservation of personal integrity is very important. It enables nurses to provide for a patient's good, sometimes against sturdy barriers and sometimes against the "generally accepted view" of what is permissible. Integrity means maintaining a sense of self as a whole. It is tied into ideas of personal identity (Benjamin, 1990). Loss of a sense of self and personal integrity has been associated with the experience of moral uncertainty and moral distress, as discussed in Chapter 1, especially when a nurse is unable to ensure that a patient receives the care that clinical judgment reveals is needed. These experiences can lessen an APN's confidence and resolve related to decision making. Provision 5 of the American Nurses Association's (ANA, 2001) *Code of Ethics for Nurses with Interpretive Statements* upholds nurses' needs to care for the self, asserting, "The nurse owes the same duties to self as to others, including the responsibility to preserve integrity and safety, to maintain competence, and to continue personal and professional growth." Additionally, many U.S. state laws (45 states) have conscience clauses that allow providers to refuse treatment or recuse themselves from participating in care based on philosophical or religious objection.

Charo (2005) notes that conscience clauses in U.S. state law result from "the abortion wars" in the United States (p. 2471). That is, conscience clauses are "laws that balance a physician's conscientious objection to perform an abortion with the profession's obligation to afford all patients non-discriminatory access to services" (Charo, 2005, p. 2471). These laws are often broad enough to protect other professionals from the legal consequences of conscientious objection to certain procedures or treatments.

However, legal protection is not a good reason for a person to impose his or her beliefs and values on someone else. In fact, refusing to provide care because of personal beliefs requires that the nurse carefully consider the situation and understand the implications of this refusal. This is especially important when the nurse is in a strong (powerful) position relative to the person who is seeking legally available information or treatment. A nurse's ethical responsibilities for good care may often include following the considered wishes of patients for something with which the nurse does not agree because it is not what the nurse herself would want, because the nurse does not think it is in the patient's best interests, or because the nurse thinks it is misguided. However, it is important to keep in mind that a healthcare decision should not be based on a provider's preferences; ideally decisions should be based on the lifestyle, culture, beliefs, and values of the person that they will most affect. Thus, nurses must understand whether they have the facts straight, to what extent they are likely to be affected by going against what they believe, and how enduring the insult to their sense of identity is likely to be. *Moral distress* is the feeling of disequilibrium experienced by nurses when they either cannot give the care needed or are asked to participate in care that they feel is wrong or harmful. The experience of moral distress and its residue (Webster & Baylis, 2000) can have long-lasting effects on nurses' practice. Some nurses leave the profession, whereas others may end up distancing themselves from certain patients because of repeated or serious experiences of emotional or ethical conflict. The question, then, is, "How do nurses preserve integrity while fulfilling their professional duties related to informed consent?" First, it is crucial to remember the almost inevitable inequality of any provider–patient relationship. Patients are vulnerable because of a lack of knowledge, skills, resources, or capacities in regard to meeting their health needs. They present to a provider trusting that their concerns will be taken seriously, the healthcare provider will be honest and transparent, and the healthcare provider will not either deliberately or unthinkingly hide available options or potential resources. In a sense, healthcare providers can be said to "hold the keys" to a wide variety of not easily available knowledge and have the necessary skills of interpretation for making distinctions clear. Such privileges should not be abused. The ANA (2006) position statement *Risk and Responsibility in Providing Nursing Care* provides important guidance. "The nurse who decides not to take part on the grounds of conscientious objection must communicate this decision in appropriate ways. Whenever possible, such refusal should be made known in advance and in time for alternate arrangements to be made for patient care." This position statement includes criteria for determining what level of personal risk is acceptable and what further responsibilities fall to the nurse involved. Magelssen (2012) has also provided a set of criteria for conscientious objection (see **Box 3-1**).

Several integrity-preserving options are open to APNs in difficult situations. First, self-reflection should reveal the source and strength of the objection and whether the APN has a thorough grasp of the state of the science involved. For example, many objections to emergency contraception are based on inaccurate information related to how it works. The APN's objection may stand even after researching the facts involved; nevertheless, fact gathering is a professional responsibility.

Box 3-1   Criteria for the Acceptance of Conscientious Objection

When the following criteria are met, conscientious objection ought to be accepted:

1. Providing health care would seriously damage the health professional's moral integrity by
   a) Constituting a serious violation...
   b) ... of a deeply held conviction
2. The objection has a plausible moral or religious rationale
3. The treatment is not considered an essential part of the health professional's work
4. The burdens to the patient are acceptable and small
   a) The patient's condition is not life-threatening
   b) Refusal does not lead to the patient not getting the treatment, or to unacceptable delay or expenses
   c) Measures have been taken to reduce the burdens to the patient
5. The burdens to colleagues and healthcare institutions are acceptable and small

In addition, the claim to conscientious objection is strengthened if:

6. The objection is founded in medicine's own values
7. The medical procedure is new or of uncertain moral status

Source: Courtesy of Magelssen, M. (2012). When should conscientious objection be accepted? *Journal of Medical Ethics*, 38, 18–21.

Second, the APN should answer the following questions: "If I needed information about a healthcare issue with which I was unfamiliar, what would I want from the specialist? How would I feel if I discovered the provider had selectively withheld options or information from me?" If the APN on answering these questions remains strongly opposed to participation in a legally available procedure or to providing certain types of information, the reason for not discussing options or not providing the requested care must be communicated to the patient. The patient should be enlightened about the fact that resources are available and/or referred to another provider who is willing to discuss the range of options or undertake the procedure (see Chapter 5 related to referral issues). APNs should clearly communicate that there are other options but that the APN's own beliefs do not permit him or her to discuss them.

Further, if the APN personally does not object to providing certain types of information or interventions but is restrained by the institution or practice (e.g., in a setting that is managed by a religiously based organization) from discussion of options or undertaking the procedure, this should be acknowledged and appropriate resources provided.

CULTURALLY BASED COMMUNICATION ISSUES

Other issues that serve as obstacles to obtaining substantially informed consent are related to culture differences and lack of fluency in the patient's language or the patient's lack of fluency in the language of the context. Although in Western cultures the idea of autonomy is valued, in many other cultures decision-making responsibility belongs to the head of the household or is a family affair. Trying to understand the beliefs and values of someone from another culture can be a perplexing and frustrating task. It can be difficult to separate issues of coercion and undue influence from the cultural norm. Additionally, the cultural norm in some cultures can be oppressive for one group such as women or, less commonly, may be age related.

What are the APN's responsibilities in such circumstances? There are no ready answers to such questions. It is an obligation of practice to learn more about a culture, if members of that culture are seen frequently in the APN's practice environment. In some cultures where there is evidence to show that certain practices are harmful, for example, female circumcision, the nurse can join with concerned others to understand more about the practice, the underlying assumptions of the practice, and what others have done to either change it or provide appropriate care for its subjects. Most important, maintaining a nonjudgmental but interested affect is probably the most helpful both in ascertaining a person's needs and providing assistance.

For language difficulties, certain considerations are important. Does the APN have a good interpreter? Are there ways to validate understanding and ensure that the interpreter has translated the intent of the APN's evaluation or information sharing? The following are some helpful hints synthesized from a variety of sources, including my own professional experiences.

In line with viewing informed consent as a process, time and patience are needed. More than one appointment or session may be required. It is helpful to speak in short units and have all parties take turns speaking—the nurse, the interpreter, and the patient. For exchanges involving complex information the nurse should request the interpreter to report what the patient understood the information to mean for him or herself in addition to conveying the patient's responses. This permits identification of areas of concern and facilitates patient understanding.

The nurse should look at the patient while speaking and be aware of the patient's body language and appearances of confusion or discomfort. The nurse must also validate with the patient if the nurse's perception is accurate and respond accordingly. Speaking directly to the patient is important, as in, "This will mean that you . . ." The interpreter will interpret everything, so the nurse should be careful not to say to the interpreter something that he or she does not want shared with the patient. Explanations should be supplemented with visual materials when possible. Practices may want to invest in video presentations in the patient's language as an adjunct, but this does not substitute for a fuller process of information gathering and giving. The focus should be on meeting the patient's needs, and not on any inconvenience or discomfort that the nurse feels.

It is best not to use family members for interpretation service (except for mundane matters such as what kind of food they like), especially not children. It can be a temptation to rely on a person's children because they may be more fluent in English (or the language of the provider) than their elders are, but interpreting is a heavy responsibility to place on them and inappropriately shifts family roles. A case study outlined in the Hastings Center Report (2004) describes the case of a 15-year-old daughter of a Chinese male immigrant. Her father was admitted with a cardiac problem. Circumstances were such that a Cantonese translator could not be found easily. The physician wondered if she should allow the daughter to translate for her father, among other things, the seriousness of his condition. This sketch is included at the end of the chapter, along with questions for discussion.

DIFFICULT PATIENTS

All nurses have encountered patients that they perceive as difficult in some way. Wolf and Robinson-Smith (2007) define difficult patients "as those whom nurses perceive consume greater periods of time than their condition suggests; they impede the work of the nursing staff with demands, complaints, and lack of co-operation" (p. 74). Sometimes it is not the patient so much as the patient's family that is perceived as difficult. Patients may seem or be difficult for a variety of reasons. Nurses may experience a dislike for them for unknown reasons. Perhaps the patient reminds the nurse of someone of his or her acquaintance with whom the nurse argues, or the patient questions the nurse's knowledge or expertise. Perhaps the patient is violent, abusive, or argumentative. Patients may be difficult because of the complexity of their issues or the perceived hopelessness of their situations. Additionally, certain patients may be stigmatized by their lifestyle, obesity, or disease.

Whatever the reason, APNs are still responsible for trying to meet these patients' needs. Wolf and Robinson-Smith's (2007) study investigates strategies that are used by CNSs in "difficult clinician–patient situations" (p. 74). Two frequently used strategies were demonstrating "respect for the patient" and "focusing on the issue at hand" (pp. 79–80). This includes avoiding labeling the patient and CNSs setting an example to others. Both of these strategies avoid bias and are aimed at trying to understand who the patient is and what underlies the patient's actions and affect in order to meet the patient's needs. In addition to the preceding problems related to assessing the patient's particular needs, the provider may also be subtly influenced to emphasize some aspects of information over others, as discussed next.

Other Influences on the Informing Process

CONFLICTS OF INTEREST

Ensuring that patients' decision making is adequately informed for their needs also requires nurses to reflect on which other factors may be subtly influential, such that they are not readily recognized. The ethos of the practice environment, economic or time constraints, the influence of drug company practices, and pressures from colleagues all have the potential to cause a subtle skewing of the information given to patients. Conflicts of interest (COI) are pervasive in healthcare practice, regardless of profession. A COI exists any time there is pressure or temptation to act in a way that a given patient's interests are not held as primary. COIs in professional nursing practice can be of several types: economic, for example the financial pressures on a clinic or healthcare institution can shift the primary focus off patient "good"; interpersonal, for example a battle between providers for control of a situation can cause loss of focus on mutual goals; environmental, for example others not noticing that there is a problem and putting pressure on nurses to go along with the status quo; appropriate resources/referring physicians are not available; in psychiatric and counseling practices, sexual or boundary-related issues can arise. Studies show, for example, that drug companies have been quite successful in influencing prescribing practices in the United States (Angell, 2004; Kassirer, 2005; Steinman, Harper, Chren, Landefeld, & Bero, 2007). An example from my experience is that of the drug company representative who provides dinner for the local APN association. He brings his samples to the office and urges us to try them with patients (Kassirer, 2005). Several studies have confirmed the suspicion that drug company gifts influence prescribing patterns (Coyle, 2002; Steinman et al., 2007; Wazana, 2000). Kassirer's book urges physicians to divorce themselves altogether from accepting drug company gifts. NP prescribing practices are perhaps not as amenable to study as physicians' are but probably would mirror those of physicians.

As discussed earlier, ensuring that patients are well informed is a difficult task that must not be taken for granted. Ongoing self-reflection and reflection on nursing practice are crucial, as is remaining aware that conflicts of interest are ever present and may result in subconscious biases that do not serve the patient well. Understanding the important elements of the process, as well as likely problem areas, necessitates vigilance. The other side of the problem has to do with the obstacles that exist for patients in apprehending and processing the information they need for decision making. The next section explores a concern related to informed consent, that of determining decision-making capacity. APNs in different roles and across specialties may be faced with the responsibility of determining whether a patient is reasonably capable of making an informed decision.

Decision-Making Capacity

How does an APN know when a patient is not able to make an informed decision? In some cases, the answer to the question is relatively easy. It is obvious, for example, that a comatose patient, a neonate, or a patient with an advanced dementing illness cannot process information or communicate his or her wishes directly to a provider. For such patients, an alternate decision maker is necessary. This person acts as a proxy either to convey what the person's wishes would probably have been, given knowledge of the person's beliefs, values, and life goals, or to ensure the patient's probable best interests where no knowledge is possible (neonates) or available. The issue of decision-making capacity is especially pervasive in mental health settings and is addressed in detail in another chapter.

In other cases, determinations of decision-making capacity may be more difficult. Buchanan and Brock (1989) note that decision making in healthcare settings is almost always for the purposes of accomplishing a task and occurs along a continuum. In the United States, the issue of decision-making capacity was explored in-depth by the President's Commission for the Study of Ethical Problems in Medicine and Biomedical and Behavioral Research, a group assembled by President Carter in 1978. This commission was formed in response to the increasing complexity of problems caused by biological and technological advances. Examples of such problems include how and when to determine death when it is possible to indefinitely prolong life artificially. What is the range of possible effects caused by the application of genetic innovations in health care? What can APNs do about health disparities? And, important for the purposes of this discussion, how do nurses ensure that patients are capable of making their own medical decisions and are not subject to undue interference by interested others who may or may not hold a person's best interests as primary? The commission's report (President's Commission for the Study of Ethical Behavior in Medicine and Biomedical and Behavioral Research, 1982) concluded that minimal capacities for decision making are "1. Possession of a set of values and goals, 2. the ability to communicate and to understand information, and 3. the ability to reason and deliberate about one's choices" (p. 57).

These criteria are made more stringent when the risks are high and the patient seems to be making a choice that is not in concert with his or her own values and goals. Beauchamp and Childress (2009) note that in cases where the risk of action or inaction is relatively high (the possibility of serious harm exists), it is also important to assess for the voluntariness of the decision. That is, nurses should evaluate whether some internal or external influence is pressuring the person to make a particular decision (see the section *Informed Consent: Ethical Problems* earlier in this chapter). The following case is provided as an example of considerations related to decision-making capacity.

CASE STUDY: JENNY

Jenny is a 33-year-old woman brought into the emergency room from a homeless shelter by shelter staff. She is evaluated by Pauline Hill, an emergency department NP, who, after evaluating Jenny, determines that Jenny's provisional diagnosis is pneumonia accompanied by dehydration. Jenny is also confused and keeps saying, "How did I get here?" The shelter staff person tells Pauline that Jenny completed detoxification for alcohol and unspecified drug abuse just 2 weeks ago, was staying sober, and had just gotten a job. Currently, she is febrile with a temperature of 103.5°F and RR 36. Pauline determines that intravenous fluids and antibiotics are necessary because Jenny is in danger of sepsis. Jenny refuses treatment; she says, "I am trying to stay clean. I want to get my kids back." Pauline talks to Jenny about her worries, tells her of the proposed plan, and reassures her that she is not receiving anything that will set her rehabilitation back. At first Jenny seems to understand and acquiesces, but when it is time to insert the cannula, Jenny starts crying and yelling, "No, I don't want it! I can't have it!" When questioned further, it becomes obvious that Jenny has not retained the information that Pauline discussed with her, nor does she see the connection between treatment and achieving her goals. Pauline realizes that Jenny is not capable of making this decision because she keeps misunderstanding what is proposed.

There is a lot more that could be said about this case, including responsibilities to try to improve Jenny's ability to process information (oxygen, or a respiratory treatment) or to consider alternative courses of action that might achieve the purpose of resolving Jenny's immediate physical needs without further distressing her. However, the purpose of Jenny's case is to illustrate a problem with decision-making capacity for the task at hand. The risks of not treating are high and do not serve Jenny's goals of becoming physically capable of having her children returned to her and being able to care for them. Therefore, the nurse does need to treat the pneumonia and dehydration because not to do so could result in Jenny's harm, perhaps even her death. Thus, the point is that, paradoxically, in treating her against her will, which could be seen as not honoring her autonomy, the nurse is actually facilitating autonomous future decision making. A person cannot exercise autonomy when she is not alive to do so.

Proxy Decision Making

Proxy decision making is the act of deciding what healthcare actions are permissible for someone who temporarily or permanently has lost decision-making capacity, never had decision-making capacity (profound cognitive deficits), or is not yet considered to have sufficient maturity to make health-care decisions (children). When children are involved, the proxy decision maker is usually a parent or guardian who makes decisions on the child's behalf. If developmentally appropriate, children may assent or dissent to a course of treatment. However, a child's dissent may be overruled by a parent or guardian when the risk of not treating is high. The issue of children and assent is discussed in more detail in Chapters 6, 8, and 13.

TYPES OF PROXY DECISION MAKING

In clinical ethics literature and practice a hierarchy of three levels of proxy decision making is used to determine appropriate treatment for those who are or have become incapacitated. The first level is based on the principle of autonomy and aims to reproduce as nearly as possible what an incapacitated person's wishes would have been. The person may have previously formulated a written directive (also known as a living will or advance directive[AD]) or may have appointed a person who could accurately represent those wishes. When these formal arrangements do not exist, the healthcare team may be able to discern what a patient's wishes would likely be by gathering information about the patient from family members and friends. The second level is often called the best interests standard. Beauchamp and Childress (2009) note that sometimes "the patient's relevant preferences cannot be known" (p. 138). In such cases a surrogate decision is made based on quality of life (QOL). Thus actions are favored if they are likely to provide the highest net benefits in terms of QOL. The best interest standard may permit overriding a surrogate decision maker's directions for treatment when the proposed treatment does not seem capable of benefiting the patient or may cause more harm than benefit. The third level is that of the reasonable person standard. It is used when neither level one nor two is applicable. For example, it is not possible to discern from neonates or profoundly cognitively disabled persons what they would want for themselves. In such cases a decision is made based upon what a 'reasonable' person would want. This third level is problematic because it is hard to determine who is 'reasonable' when there are a host of contextual factors involved in any decision-making process (Beauchamp & Childress, 2009; Grace, 2004b).

LEGAL ASPECTS

In the United States, what is accepted as legal surrogate decision making differs from state to state. This necessitates that APNs familiarize themselves with the laws of the state (or country) in which they practice. This section outlines some general issues associated with APNs' role in assisting their patients to be prepared for a variety of possibilities related to decision making.

Proxy decision making in health care may be needed for everyday healthcare decisions, for decisions related to an acute illness, and for EOL issues. Although many APNs do not work in a hospital setting, understanding a little about legislation related to EOL decision making, such as the PSDA (OBRA, 1990) in the United States, provides clarity about the reasons for such legislation and likely related issues. The PSDA applies to institutions that receive federal funding (almost all U.S. hospitals and long-term care facilities) and was meant to improve patient decision making especially around (although not limited to) EOL decisions. It was meant to improve providers' as well as patients' knowledge about patients' rights to accept or refuse therapeutics and interventions and providers' obligations to provide appropriate information. It was also hoped that providers would assist patients to think about what they would want in the event that they lost decision-making capacity.

ADVANCE DIRECTIVES

It is, of course, generally better for patients to have considered in advance what sort of care they would like and who might best serve as a good proxy decision maker on their behalf. Although such decisions may be made when patients are already critically ill, this is not optimal (Hiltunen, Medich, Chase, Peterson, & Forrow, 1999; Marshall, 1995; Wolf et al., 2001). Time, a low-pressure environment, and the assistance of a trusted health provider are probably the best conditions under which to process information. Thus, good APN practice means taking the opportunity to raise questions and provide necessary information related to the idea of proxy decision making if a patient appears receptive. Additionally, recent research (Parks et al., 2011) questioning prospective proxies and those for whom they were to make decisions found that "spousal proxies were more accurate in their substituted judgment than adult children, and proxies who perceive higher degree of family conflict [within their family] tended to be less accurate than those with lower family conflict" (p. 179). From my experiences in both critical care and primary care settings and from the research cited, it is very difficult to discuss such issues when a person is gravely ill, already receiving highly technical care, and in a noisy and hectic environment. Proxy decision making can be an arduous task at the best of times but is made even more difficult with the potential loss of a loved one looming and when the decision maker may already be overwhelmed with circumstances and lack of needed clinical knowledge. Preventive ethics strategies include providers making routine a practice of discussing patient preferences at primary care or regular provider visits; helping patients to select an appropriate surrogate—one who can separate personal desires and wishes from the preferences of the person in question; and encouraging patients to provide written instructions for their proxy. A reminder is needed that a proxy only makes healthcare decisions for another person in the event of that person's loss of decision-making capacity. When a proxy is obviously not making decisions that are in the patient's best interests, the proxy can legally be relieved of proxy duties.

Discussion about ADs need not be limited to the older population. McAliley, Hudson-Barr, Gunning, and Rowbottom (2000) studied adolescent attitudes toward living wills, or as they are alternatively known, ADs. Of the 107 participants in the study, the majority felt that it was "somewhat important" or "very important" for someone of their age to have a living will (p. 471). A study of young adults living with chronic illness also supported the idea that conversations about ACP are desirable (Wiener et al., 2008). The advent of ADs or living wills is relatively new. According to Clarke (1998), the term *living will* was invented in 1967 by Louis Kutner, a human rights lawyer and cofounder of Amnesty International, "in a law journal proposal" (p. 92). Kutner, having gone through a disturbing EOL scenario with a close friend, wanted to ensure the right of patients to determine how their last days should unfold in the event of a catastrophe.

THE PATIENT SELF-DETERMINATION ACT: INTERNATIONAL IMPLICATIONS

The PSDA in the United States (OBRA, 1990) was conceptualized as a result of several landmark right-to-die cases. It relies on state laws related to EOL care and "was designed to encourage communication about end-of-life issues" (Grace, 2004b, p. 310). It requires institutions that receive Medicare and Medicaid funds (U.S. government funds), which includes essentially all healthcare institutions in the United States, to inform patients in writing of their rights to accept or refuse care. It was meant to increase healthcare provider knowledge and thus affect current EOL problems arising in tertiary care institutions.

The PSDA has not been as effective as hoped, and there are many documented reasons for this. A large study undertaken to understand prognoses and preferences for outcomes and risks of treatment conducted over several years and initially involving observation but later adding interventions aimed at improving the communication of patients' wishes failed to show that patients' preferences were respected. Marshall (1995) and others have argued that this is because institutional hierarchies and power structures had not significantly changed as a result of the PSDA.

Others have noted a variety of concerns about ADs that might make some people reluctant to draft them and some healthcare providers reluctant to comply with them. The concerns include the idea that people do not like to imagine themselves experiencing serious illness or death. Accurately predicting what might be needed given a wide array of possibilities is difficult. Patients are afraid they might change their minds, but not in time to change their AD, or that not accepting certain interventions might lead to their abandonment by caregivers (Teno, Gruneir, Schwartz, Nanda, & Wetle, 2007; Wolf et al., 2001). Additionally, there are cultural and minority fears about the untrustworthiness of predominantly white middle-class healthcare professionals (Baker, 2002); see the next section for further discussion.

Regulations related to the use of ADs, whether in the written form or in the form of an appointed proxy, vary from country to country. Regardless of the existence of regulations enforcing or supporting patients' previously articulated wishes, it is a healthcare professional's responsibility to help patients and those close to them to think through what care and interventions they might wish for in the event of a loss of decision-making capacity. This permits advocacy and honors autonomy. Durbin, Fish, Backman, and Smith (2010) reviewed available research on the influence of educational interventions in improving AD completion. They found (perhaps not unsurprisingly) that a two-pronged approach—providing written and oral information—had the best effects on completion, but the results were not strongly compelling. More interventional research is needed.

Despite concerns about ADs, many professionals and ethicists who are involved in EOL care think that with time and custom more people will become involved in the process of advance planning for the event of lost decision making. The most effective plan is probably a two-part initiative:

the appointment of a trustworthy representative who may or may not be a relative, and written instructions to assist the proxy. Understanding both the benefits and criticisms of formal ADs allows APNs to assist patients in thinking about their specific advance planning wishes. In advanced practice, nurses are key to interpreting a variety of EOL scenarios in terms that are tailored to a particular patient's needs and level of understanding.

ADVANCED CARE PLANNING: MINORITY AND CULTURAL ISSUES

Although ACP is generally thought to be a good thing, facilitative of an individual's choices, there are historical and cultural reasons for certain groups to view ACP with uncertainty and fear. Indeed, such fears coupled with the ones noted earlier may be in part responsible for the slow progress made in preparing and educating the public about the potential benefits of ACP. Johnstone and Kanitsaki (2009) draw attention to the problem in the United States and Australia in particular; it is likely that in other multicultural societies certain groups feel disenfranchised by society as well. "Emerging international research suggests that in multicultural countries, such as Australia and the United States, there are significant disparities in end-of-life care planning and decision making by people of minority ethnic backgrounds compared with members of mainstream English-speaking background populations" (p. 405). Moreover, public policies in these countries are not always sensitive to this problem. Johnstone and Kanitsaki (2009) note that the few studies that have looked at differences between cultural majority and cultural or linguistic minority groups within a society related to ACP reveal several tendencies on the part of minority cultures: a smaller number complete ADs, family involvement in discussions about decision making is preferred, ADs are viewed as an intrusive and legalistic mechanism that has no place in health care, and aggressive treatment is preferred, especially when patients have experienced prior mistreatment or bias (Bito et al., 2007, p. 260). In ethical terms, these patients' prior experiences, distrust of the system, and fears about undertreatment can paradoxically lead to greater harms (a nonmaleficence problem) from overtreatment or treatment that is futile for the intended purpose and that causes unnecessary suffering. Strategies for APNs include engaging patients in dialogue about their cultural values, their prior experiences, and their fears. Planning for the future includes understanding what patients' goals are given a variety of scenarios and helping them to envision desirable courses of action.

Veracity and Transparency

Veracity is an ethical principle underlying the idea of trust and fiduciary relationships. "Veracity or truthfulness in giving patients information about their health-care needs facilitates autonomous choice and enhances patient decision making" (Grace, 2004b, p. 315). However, veracity is a more difficult concept to apply than it appears on the surface. It is fair to say that in ordinary life people are rarely completely truthful with friends, family, and strangers. People hold information back, either because they feel it could come back to haunt them or because to be completely truthful may well hurt another person. Yet "truthfulness has long been regarded as fundamental to the existence of trust" (Fry & Grace, 2007, p. 287), and as noted earlier, trust is fundamental to the nurse–patient relationship. Patients are vulnerable because of their healthcare needs and must rely on nurses to help them. If APNs are not able to gain a certain level of trust with patients, then their data-gathering activities are likely to be frustrated. This, in turn, lessens the likelihood that nurses will be able to give holistic care, which in turn means that nursing goals are not met.

However, being too honest or giving patients more information than necessary for their decision-making purposes can also frustrate the project of attending to their needs. Clinical judgment is required to make determinations about acceptable levels of information for a given patient; that is, what will permit the patient's participation in decision making. For example, to the family nurse practitioner (FNP) caring for Ms. Jones, a 60-year-old in a rural family practice clinic, it has become obvious that her patient needs to add an antihypertensive drug to her care plan. Although for several years Ms. Jones has, with the FNP's help, managed to control her blood pressure by increasing her exercise regimen, reducing stress, and being careful with her diet, her blood pressure is starting to show a pattern of persistent elevation above recommended levels. She does not want to start taking blood pressure pills, but the FNP has done a good job of educating her about long-term effects of poorly controlled hypertension, so she is willing to start taking them. What drug the FNP tries initially and how much information she gives Ms. Jones depends on what the FNP knows about Ms. Jones. Discussion of the side effects Ms. Jones is most likely to experience and how these match her lifestyle and preferences will facilitate a first choice. Explanation of likely side effects will also be tailored to her needs. However, transparency about the extensiveness of what is known related to the drug and the amount of information the FNP gives are also important. These are all clinical judgments based on knowledge of the patient and, like many clinical judgments, they have some element of uncertainty. With Ms. Jones, it might be beneficial to discuss major side effects, whether these effects are acceptable to her, and what she should report to the FNP. Additionally, the FNP should acknowledge that there are possible side effects that Ms. Jones may not experience and that the best way to deal with this is to remain accessible for questions Ms. Jones may have if she experiences unexpected changes.

In palliative care or EOL care settings, problems of veracity can occur when relatives pressure nurses and others to withhold the truth about a condition from patients. Veracity has some implications in the care of patients from cultures where the patient is traditionally protected from knowledge of the criticality of the condition. "Decision making about whether to honor [the demands] of veracity in such cases must take into consideration what is known about the culture, the particular patient, the strength of his or her personal and cultural beliefs, and whether there is evidence about what sort of things the patient would like to know" (Grace, 2004b, p. 316). If a patient is asking questions about his or her condition, then nurses need to respond accordingly. Nurses need to draw on what is known or has been discovered (evidence) related to a person's needs to come to terms with his or her condition and nearness to death. But nurses also may need to assist the family with their needs to fulfill cultural responsibilities. Resources may be found within the cultural community.

In pediatric settings, the issue of veracity is also complicated. Questions arise about how to communicate information in age- or developmentally appropriate ways. How do APNs interact with parents or guardians who seem overly protective or are working in ways that seem at odds with what is known about the child? This question is explored in-depth in later chapters.

Privacy and Confidentiality

The healthcare principles of privacy and confidentiality are also derivations of the ethical principle of autonomy. The terms *privacy* and *confidentiality* are often lumped together as if they mean the same thing. Privacy, however, is "the broader concept and includes the right to be free from the interference of others" (Grace, 2004a, p. 33) and freedom to grant or withhold access to information about oneself. Justification for the right to privacy, as noted by Beauchamp and Childress (2009), "flow[s] from fundamental rights to life, liberty, and property" (p. 295). Confidentiality is related more specifically to the protection of a person's information, particularly the person's health-care information. Beauchamp and Childress (2009) note that in healthcare settings, the right to privacy is most often a control right of sorts: it is the right to control both access to and distribution of information.

For Beauchamp and Childress (2009), a helpful distinction can be made between privacy and confidentiality in terms of the status of violations of these. Confidentiality is violated when one person discloses information about another person, whereas when privacy is violated, one person gains access to another person's personal data. Rights to privacy and confidentiality in healthcare settings are contemporary recognitions. The reason for recognition of these rights is that a person's healthcare information can be used in negative ways that cause harm. In nonhealthcare situations, the status of confidentiality is considered so important that it is protected by privilege and is "shielded from exposure by the legal system" (Grace, 2005, p. 114). For example, the clergy-supplicant privilege prevents courts from forcing clergy to reveal confidential information entrusted to them by congregants.

Limitations on the Right to Privacy

For healthcare providers, honoring privacy, which includes the maintenance of patient confidentiality, is important but does not supersede all other considerations. There may be occasions when an APN should break confidentiality to prevent serious harm to another person. The difficulty, however, lies in making the assessment of dangerousness—how imminent it is and how severe the likely consequences are.

The well-known *Tarasoff* case set a precedent in the United States related to limitations in provider–patient privilege. In October 1969, Prosenjit Poddar killed Tatiana Tarasoff. Poddar had been seeing a psychiatrist and told the therapist he was going to kill a woman, who was easily identifiable as Tatiana. At the time of Poddar's statement to his therapist, Tatiana was out of the country in Brazil. The therapist sought to have Poddar committed but was unsuccessful because Poddar appeared rational. No one warned Tatiana or her family of the threat, and on her return Poddar killed her. The courts, in this case, aligning against the idea that psychiatrist-patient privilege is absolute, concluded that "once a therapist does in fact determine, or under applicable professional standards reasonably should have determined, that a person poses a serious danger of violence to others, he bears a duty to exercise reasonable care to protect the foreseeable victim of that danger" (*Tarasoff v. Regents of University of California*, 1976).

Beauchamp and Childress (2009) note three main areas where limits on privacy might require a "balancing of privacy interests against other interests" (p. 297). These areas are "(1) screening and testing for HIV infection, (2) ensuring effective treatments for patients with active tuberculosis (TB), and (3) human genetics" (p. 297). Contemporary issues of dangerousness to others include the deliberate dissemination to, or careless exposure of, others by someone with a transmissible disease, such as HIV or TB. For example, recently there was a highly publicized case of a patient with extensively drug-resistant TB who traveled across the continent on public airliners.

The Meaning of Privacy in Health Care

The concept of privacy is important to the preceding discussion of informed consent, although this was not explicitly stated. Essentially, the privacy principle means two things: (1) patients should have a say in who is allowed access to their bodies or, for the purposes of evaluation and treatment, other information; and (2) unless the patient gives explicit permission, there is a proscription against healthcare personnel sharing information gained, except for the purposes of helping that patient. In contemporary society, privacy and confidentiality concerns are exacerbated by the pervasive nature of electronic media, as discussed in more detail shortly. The ease with which information, including photographs, can be transmitted via cell phones and other devices, and the ubiquitous use of social media such as Facebook, Twitter, and so on, can lead to the careless exposure of patient information. For example, a mother in the neonatal infant care unit takes a photo of her baby and posts it on Facebook; inadvertently she has included the baby in the next incubator and the visiting parents. The protection of a patient's privacy has a variety of implications, both in institutional settings and in primary care. It requires nurses to think carefully about their actions related to patients, including what they tell referral sources, how they transfer information, and what the implications of testing are related to privacy and protection. It is a reminder not to take privileged access to sensitive patient information for granted. Respecting a patient's right to privacy means that when a student APN interacts with a patient as part of gaining clinical expertise, the student status should be revealed. In patient rounds, persons in the rounding group should be clearly identified. Patients can waive this right but should be made aware of it.

The principle of privacy has other numerous implications; for the most part, concern for the delivery of good patient care will ensure that a patient's privacy is respected. For example, the privacy principle means that providers protect those who are not capable of protecting themselves from the intrusion of others, perhaps because they are not aware of the possibility that sharing personal information can affect such opportunities as job prospects and the ability to have health insurance. Providers in the United States should be aware of the so-called "Privacy Rule" and its impact on their practice. This rule is explored in more detail in the following section. It is impossible in this text to discuss the regulations surrounding privacy concerns in all countries that have such regulations; however, the implications of the privacy rule and ethical considerations concerning privacy and confidentiality are pertinent regardless of country of practice.

HIPAA and the Privacy Rule in the United States: History

According to Beauchamp and Childress (2009), "Privacy received little attention in the law or legal theory until the late 19th century" (p. 294), and then it was concerned with protecting family life, child-rearing practices, and other areas of personal choice. Confidentiality as a subcategory of privacy refers to patient rights to have their healthcare information safeguarded. The irony of confidentiality is that in order to receive care, highly personal information has to be revealed to those who will be providing that care. Those providing direct care may sometimes need to share patient information with others whose expertise is important in meeting patient needs. Thus, illness itself makes a person vulnerable, and in trying to address illness a person also becomes vulnerable, to those who have access to that personal information.

Prior to 1996, rights to privacy and confidentiality were protected by state or country laws, professional ethical codes, and ethical deliberation. The advent of large electronic databases for storing medical records, however, jeopardized providers' ability to protect their patients' records. Most who have been involved in health care in the United States, whether patients or providers, have become familiar with the Health Insurance Portability and Accountability Act (HIPAA); however, much confusion about this act remains (Anderson, 2007). HIPAA was enacted in 1996. Before HIPAA, if a person lost his or her job, they often also lost health insurance coverage, because health insurance in the United States for the most part is attached to a particular place of employment. HIPAA ensured that a person could continue coverage until regaining employment, at which point new coverage would begin with the work-associated health insurance company. HIPAA was also supposed to expand coverage. Another section of HIPAA, the "Privacy Rule," was meant to standardize the use of health information across the country while providing privacy protection. Suggestions had been made for the development of a mega database that could track almost everyone's health care in the United States from birth to death. Thus, HIPAA was supposed to accomplish two somewhat contradictory tasks: (1) allow for the flow of information that would enable research and access to patient care records for the purposes of improving care and public health, and (2) act as a brake on covered entities' free use of medical information enabled by such a database. A *covered entity* is a person, practice, clinic, pharmacy, or institution covered by HIPAA. Essentially, a covered entity is anyone providing patient care services or undertaking research on human subjects.

Subsequently, a privacy rule was attached to HIPAA (U.S. Department of Health and Human Services, 2003). The Privacy Rule specifically covers all individually identifiable information including written, oral, or computerized. This went into effect in 2003. An important point to note is that if state rules about privacy are more stringent than HIPAA, then the more stringent standard applies. That is, state regulations trump HIPAA if they are more rigorous than HIPAA standards.

The problem with the Privacy Rule, as noted earlier, and the problem with maintaining privacy and confidentiality based purely on ethical considerations (i.e., without such a rule) is that it is impossible to delineate all imaginable scenarios related to privacy infringements, so clinical judgment, including ethical reflection, is still needed for its interpretation in specific situations. "A rule of thumb for health care professionals related to sharing information with others is to disclose only as much information as is necessary to permit optimal care and only information that is pertinent to the situation" (Grace, 2005, p. 115). Additionally, prudence and mindfulness are required when other people's healthcare records are in the APN's hands.

Anderson (2007) provides tips for ensuring that patient information is not overheard or overseen. Importantly, care must be taken not to leave information lying around and not to discuss patients in public places, and the nurse must consider whether an outsider could identify the person being discussed if he or she overheard the conversation. In rural settings, maintaining confidentiality can be especially difficult. Providers are often members of the small communities in which they practice. It is not unusual for an APN to be asked about the status of a family member or friend's health in a grocery store or other local gathering place. Additionally, in rural settings office staff may have access to the records of family members or friends. Part of the APN's responsibilities in such settings is educating the staff about the implications of accessing information to which they neither have a need nor a right to access.

In a recent *American Journal of Nursing* article offered for continuing education credit, Anderson (2007), the privacy officer for her institution, provided and answered some questions that may be helpful in understanding the intent of the Privacy Rule; some of these suggestions also have utility outside of the Privacy Rule. Anderson posed some common questions to highlight confusions and to illustrate commonsense answers.

- Is it permissible to call or write to a community provider when referring a patient? *Yes, if the disclosure is for treatment purposes.*
- *Am I allowed to e-mail a diagnostic report to another provider for treatment or consultation purposes? Yes, but encryption is strongly encouraged.*
- May I videotape or photograph patients for teaching purposes? *Yes, but consent should be obtained or patients should be "de-identified."* (Anderson, 2007, p. 67)

Additional insights into experiences of APNs related to privacy and confidentiality are provided by Deshefy-Longhi, Dixon, Olsen, and Grey (2004). They conducted a series of studies aimed at describing the views of APNs and their patients related to the protection of healthcare data. Of nine issues identified in focus group explorations, six were identified by both patients and nurses. One of these mutual concerns was the issue of "breaches in privacy occurring through carelessness" (p. 387). Examples given included phone conversations that could be overheard, conversations about patient information that took place in public spaces, and patient information lying around or viewable on computer screens. Additionally, both groups worried that excessive regulation prevented needed information from being communicated to appropriate resources. Even the need to leave a telephone message for a patient at home posed concerns. Nurses wondered how much, if any, information to leave. Additional concerns of the APN group were abuses of privacy related to the use of computers and problems attending to the privacy concerns of adolescents.

Hidden Privacy and Confidentiality Hazards of Electronic and Social Media

A very contemporary threat to privacy and confidentiality is the widespread use of social media. A stable definition of social media is difficult because of the continual metamorphosis of the forms available. Boyd and Ellison (2007), information specialists, propose a tentative definition for a social networking site: "web-based services that allow individuals to (1) construct a public or semi-public profile within a bounded system, (2) articulate a list of other users with whom they share a connection, and (3) view and traverse their list of connections and those made by others within the system" (para. 4). Such sites facilitate information sharing that would otherwise be difficult or non-existent. Social media is very promising for healthcare professionals as a way of reaching more people with health information, assisting self-help health promotion groups, permitting patient access to results and records, enrolling research subjects, carrying out surveys, and so on. Additionally healthcare professionals use social media for personal reasons. The danger, as noted earlier, is that in the course of a healthcare professional's private discussions patient information might be revealed. Furthermore, unprofessional behavior that is publicly accessible can undermine public trust in an institution or in the profession. For example, a nursing student was conversing on Facebook with a medical student. They had both spent a couple of days in the same clinic as part of their unrelated clinical practices. They were making fun of a patient they had seen. What if the patient had been identified? Perhaps even more seriously, such behavior can undermine public trust in the professions. The ANA (2011) has provided tips for engaging with social media and for avoiding problems. They include guarding confidentiality, maintaining professional boundaries, remembering that postings are widely viewable, reporting unethical behavior of others, or calling it to the attention of the writer. Nurses can avoid problems by thinking through the possible ramifications of actions. Nurses can also help patients and visitors think about their actions before posting pictures or videos—Is anyone else inadvertently shown in the picture? is any confidential material being exposed? Questions to ask include, "Would I be ok if what I am posting appeared on the front page of the local newspaper? Could what I am saying be misconstrued as disrespectful or dehumanizing? Could what I am saying as a private citizen reflect on my professional standing? Should I be engaging with a patient this way? Does this cross professional boundaries?"

Summary

This chapter discusses characteristics that are important for good nursing care and good decision making in APN settings. It presents an argument for the APN to engage in ongoing professional and personal development in the interests of good patient care. The possession of certain nursing virtues is necessary both for facilitating patient decision making and protecting patient information. These virtues are not all or nothing—there are barriers to practicing well. Mindfulness allows the APN to maintain focus.

The discussion in this chapter reinforced the idea that professional nursing practice at the advanced level is still good nursing practice. All healthcare practice that involves individual human beings is ethical in nature because of professional goals. The broad importance of honoring the ethical principle of autonomy was the underlying assumption for the topics of this chapter. Patients have the right to make personal decisions both about what care will or will not be accepted and who may have access to personal information and for what purposes. The APN has responsibilities to help patients safeguard these rights.

Unfortunately, as hard as APNs work to secure information, insurance companies that are privy to the private information of their subscribers are not always so scrupulous. This issue will be discussed in more detail elsewhere in the text.

Discussion Questions

1. A case study outlined in the Hastings Center Report (2004) describes the case of a 15-year-old daughter of a Chinese immigrant man who was admitted with a cardiac problem. Circumstances were such that the physician could not get a Cantonese translator in the middle of the night, and he wanted the daughter to translate for her father, among other things, the seriousness of the man's condition.

   What are the implications of asking an adolescent to interpret for a family member?

   What information would an APN need to decide appropriateness? What risks are involved?

   How would you resolve this issue for the current situation? In the future?

2. Have you cared for a patient who you would describe as difficult? Explore the situation you encountered with classmates or colleagues. Identify assumptions that you made about the patient. What is the basis for these assumptions? Did you think the patient was responsible for the characteristic that made him or her difficult? In what ways was he or she responsible? How would you have liked the person to have acted? Have you ever been considered difficult or felt that you were misunderstood?

3. Joe, a 17-year-old patient, is scheduled for a sports physical at your clinic. After examining him, you decide to draw a complete blood count because he complains of feeling a bit "more than usually tired" after 30 minutes of shooting hoops. Joe asks you to tell his dad what you are doing because "he gets antsy when he has to wait." You bring Joe's dad into your office to talk to him, and he asks you to draw extra blood for drug testing and not to tell Joe what you are doing. He says, "I just know he is taking something."
   What is the main issue in this case?
   What are the APN's responsibilities?
   What are the implications of the Privacy Rule?
   Discuss with classmates or peers how this situation should be addressed.

4. What is the relevance of discussing ADs with your population of patients? (Neonatal intensive care unit nurses may have to imagine caring for another population.)
   Do you have an AD? Why or why not?
   What innovative approaches to educating patients about ADs might be used?
   What obstacles would you anticipate (e.g., personal, environmental, time-constraints, cultural)?

5. Have you seen unethical conversations about patients or practices on a social media site? As an APN and leader, how would you address such issues in your setting?

References

American Nurses Association. (2001). *Code of ethics for nurses with interpretive statements.* Washington, DC: Author.

American Nurses Association. (2006). *Risk and responsibility in providing nursing care.* Retrieved from http://www.nursingworld.org/MainMenuCategories/Policy-Advocacy

/Positions-and-Resolutions/ANAPositionStatements/Position-Statements-Alphabetically/RiskandResponsibility.pdf

American Nurses Association. (2011). *Principles for social networking and the nurse.* Silver Spring, MD: Nurse Books.

Anderson, F. (2007). Finding HIPAA in your soup: Decoding the Privacy Rule. *American Journal of Nursing, 107*(2), 66–71.

Angell, M. (2004). *The truth about drug companies: How they deceive us and what to do about it.* New York, NY: Random House.

Anscombe, G. E. M. (1958/1981). Modern moral philosophy. In *Ethics religion and politics: Collected Papers, Vol. 3* (pp. 1–19). Minneapolis, MN: University of Minnesota Press. Reprinted from *Philosophy, 33*(124), 1958.

Armstrong, A. E. (2006). Towards a strong virtue ethics for nursing practice. *Nursing Philosophy, 7,* 101–124.

Baker, M. (2002). Economic, political and ethnic influences on end-of-life decision-making: A decade in review. *Journal of Health and Social Policy, 14*(3), 27–39.

Beauchamp, T. L., & Childress, J. F. (2009). *Principles of biomedical ethics* (6th ed.). New York, NY: Oxford University Press.

Begley, A. M. (2005). Practising virtue: A challenge to the view that a virtue centered approach to ethics lack practical content. *Nursing Ethics, 12*(6), 622–637.

Benjamin, M. (1990). *Splitting the difference.* Lawrence, KS: Lawrence University Press.

Bito, S., Matsumura, S., Singer, M. K., Meredith, L. S., Fukuhara, S., & Wenger, N. S. (2007). Acculturation and end-of-life decision making: Comparison of Japanese and Japanese American focus groups. *Bioethics, 21,* 251–262.

Boyd, D. M., & Ellison, N. B. (2007). Social network sites: Definition, history, and scholarship. *Journal of Computer-Mediated Communication, 13*(1), Article 11. Retrieved from http://jcmc.indiana.edu/vol13/issue1/boyd.ellison.html

Breakey, S. (2006). Optimizing stewardship: A grounded theory of nurses as moral leaders in the ICU. Unpublished dissertation. Boston College, William F. Connell School of Nursing. Proquest document 3221256. Retrieved from http://search.proquest.com.proxy.bc.edu/docview/304913628/13D564FA2C2BC814F8/1?accountid=9673

Broadstock, M., & Michie, S. (2000). Processes of patient decision making: Theoretical and methodological issues. *Psychology and Health, 15,* 191–204.

Buchanan, A. E., & Brock, D. W. (1989). *Deciding for others: The ethics of surrogate decision making.* New York, NY: Cambridge University Press.

Catholics for Choice. (2012). In good conscience. Retrieved from http://www.catholicsforchoice.org/documents/InGoodConscience--Europe.pdf

Chambliss, D. F. (1996). *Beyond caring: Hospitals, nurses, and the social organization of ethics.* Chicago, IL: University of Chicago Press.

Charles, C., Gafni, A., & Whelan, T. (1999). Shared decision-making in the medical encounter: What does it mean? (or it takes at least two to tango). *Social Science and Medicine, 44,* 681–692.

Charo, R. A. (2005). The celestial fire of conscience—refusing to deliver medical care. *New England Journal of Medicine, 352*(24), 2471–2473.

Clarke, D. B. (1998). The patient self-determination act. In J. F. Monagle & D. C. Thomasma (Eds.), *Health care ethics for the 21st century* (pp. 92–116). Gaithersburg, MD: Aspen.

Coyle, S. L. (2002). Physician-industry relations. Part I: Individual physicians. *Annals of Internal Medicine, 136*(5), 396–402.

Deshefy-Longhi, T., Dixon, J. K., Olsen, D., & Grey, M. (2004). Privacy and confidentiality issues in primary care: Views of advanced practice nurses and their patients. *Nursing Ethics, 11*(4), 378–393.

Doris, J. M., & the Moral Psychology Research Group. (2010). *The moral psychology handbook.* New York, NY: Oxford University Press.

Durbin, C. R., Fish, A. F., Backman, J. A., & Smith, K. V. (2010). Systematic review of educational interventions for improving advance directive completion. *Journal of Nursing Scholarship, 14*(2), 234–241.

Feldman, F. (1978). *Introductory ethics.* Englewood Cliffs, NJ: Prentice Hall.

Fry, S. T., & Grace, P. J. (2007). Ethical dimensions of nursing and healthcare. In J. L. Creasia & B. J. Parker (Eds.), *Conceptual foundations: The bridge to professional practice* (4th ed., pp. 273–299). St. Louis: Mosby Elsevier.

Grace, P. J. (2004a). Ethical issues: Patient safety and the limits of confidentiality. *American Journal of Nursing, 104*(11), 33–37.

Grace, P. J. (2004b). Ethics in the clinical encounter. In S. K. Chase (Ed.), *Clinical judgment and communication in nurse practitioner practice* (pp. 295–332). Philadelphia, PA: F. A. Davis.

Grace, P. J. (2005). Ethical issues relevant to health promotion. In C. Edelman & C. L. Mandle (Eds.), *Health promotion throughout the lifespan (6th ed.)* (pp. 100–125) St. Louis: Elsevier/Mosby.

Grace, P. J., & McLaughlin, M. (2005). When consent isn't informed enough: What's the nurse's role when a patient has given consent but doesn't fully understand the risks? *American Journal of Nursing, 105*(4), 79–84.

Haggerty, L. A., & Grace, P. J. (2008). Clinical wisdom: Approximating the ends of individual and societal health. *Journal of Professional Nursing, 24*(4), 235–240.

Hanson, C. M., & Hamric, A. B. (2003). Reflections on the continuing evolution of advanced practice nursing. *Nursing Outlook, 51*(5), 203–211.

Hastings Center Report. (2004). A fifteen-year-old translator. *Hastings Center Report, 34*(3), 10–13.

Hiltunen, E. F., Medich, C., Chase, C., Peterson, L., & Forrow, L. (1999). Family decision making for end-of life-treatment: The SUPPORT nurse narratives. *Journal of Clinical Ethics, 10*(2), 126–134.

Hutchinson, D. S. (1995). Ethics. In J. Barnes (Ed.), *The Cambridge companion to Aristotle* (pp. 195–232). New York, NY: Cambridge University Press.

Jacobson, J. (2005). When providing care is a moral issue. *American Journal of Nursing, 105*(10), 27–28.

Johnstone, M. J., & Kanitsaki, O. (2009). Ethics and advance care planning in a culturally diverse society. *Journal of Transcultural Nursing, 20*(4), 405–416.

Kahnemann, D. (2011). *Thinking, fast and slow.* New York, NY: Farrar, Strauss and Giroux.

Kassirer, J. P. (2005). *On the take: How medicine's complicity with big business can endanger your health*. New York, NY: Oxford University Press.

Kegley, K. A. (2002). Genetics decision-making: A template for problems with informed consent. *Medicine and Law, 21,* 459–471.

Ketefian, S., Redman, R. W., Hanucharurnkul, S., Masterson, A., & Neves, E. P. (2001). The development of advanced practice roles: Implications in the international nursing community. *International Nursing Review, 48*(3), 152–163.

MacIntyre, A. (2007). *After virtue* (3rd ed.). Notre Dame, IN: Notre Dame University Press.

Magelssen, M. (2012). When should conscientious objection be accepted? *Journal of Medical Ethics, 38,* 18–21.

Marshall, P. A. (1995). The SUPPORT study: Who's talking? *Hastings Center Report, 25*(6), S9–S11.

McAliley, L. G., Hudson-Barr, D. C., Gunning, R. S., & Rowbottom, L. A. (2000). The use of advance directives with adolescents. *Pediatric Nursing, 26*(5), 471–482.

Mental Capacity Act of 2005. Retrieved from http://www.legislation.gov.uk/ukpga/2005/9 /contents

Nieminen, A. L., Mannevaara, B., & Fagerström, L. (2011). Advanced practice nurses' scope of practice: A qualitative study of advanced clinical competencies. *Scandinavian Journal of Caring Sciences, 25*(4), 661–670.

Omnibus Budget Reconciliation Act. (1990). PL 100-508, 42 U.S.C. § 4206.

Parks, S. M., Winter, L., Santana, A. J., Parker, B., Diamond, J. J., Rose, M., & Myers, R. E. (2011). Family factors in end-of-life decision-making: Family conflict and proxy relationship. *Journal of Palliative Medicine, 14*(2), 179–184.

Parliamentary Assembly of Councils of Europe. (2010). Women's access to lawful medical care: The problem of unregulated use of conscientious objection. Doc. 123. Rapporteur Ms. Christine McCafferty. Retrieved from http://eclj.org/pdf/EDOC12347doc20juillet .pdf

President's Commission for the Study of Ethical Behavior in Medicine and Biomedical and Behavioral Research. (1982). *Making health care decisions.* Washington, DC: U.S. Government Printing Office. PB 83236703.

Protection of Conscience Project. (2012). Homepage. Retrieved from http://www .consciencelaws.org/

Schober, M., & Affara, F. (2006). *International Council of Nurses: Advanced nursing practice.* Malden, MA: Blackwell.

Sellman, D. (2000). Alasdair MacIntyre and the professional practice of nursing. *Nursing Philosophy, 1*(1), 26–33.

Steinman, M. A., Harper, G. M., Chren, M. M., Landefeld, C. S., & Bero, L. A. (2007). Characteristics and impact of drug detailing for Gabapentin. *PLOS Medicine, 4*(5), e134. Retrieved from http://medicine.plosjournals.org/perlserv/?request=index-html&issn=1549-1676&ct=1

Tarasoff v. Regents of University of California. (1976, July 1). California Supreme Court 131. *California Reporter, 14.*

Teno, J. M., Gruneir, A., Schwartz, Z., Nanda, A., & Wetle, T. (2007). Association between advance directives and quality of end-of-life care: A national study. *Journal of the American Geriatrics Society, 55*(2), 189–194.

U.S. Department of Health and Human Services. Office for Civil Rights. (2003). *HIPAA fact sheet*. Retrieved from www.hhs.gov/ocr/privacy/hipaa/understanding/.../provider_ffg.pdf

Wazana, A. (2000). Physicians and the pharmaceutical industry: Is a gift ever just a gift? *Journal of the American Medical Association, 283*, 373–380.

Webster, G. C., & Baylis, F. (2000). Moral residue. In S. B. Rubin & L. Zoloth (Eds.), *Margin of error: The ethics of mistakes in the practice of medicine* (p. 208). Hagerstown, MD: University Publishing Group.

Wicclair, M. (2011). *Conscientious objection in healthcare: An ethical analysis*. New York, NY: Cambridge.

Wiener, L., Ballard, E., Brennan, T., Battles, H., Martinez, P., & Pao, M. (2008). How I wish to be remembered: The use of an advance care planning document in adolescent and young adult populations. *Journal of Palliative Medicine, 11*(10), 1309–1313.

Williams, B. (1985). *Ethics and the limits of philosophy*. London: Fontana.

Wolf, S. M., Boyle, P., Callahan, D., Fins, J., Jennings, B., Lindemann Nelson, J., . . . Emanual, L. (2001). Sources of concern about the Patient Self-Determination Act. In W. Teays & L. Purdy (Eds.), *Bioethics, justice and health care* (pp. 411–419). Belmont, CA: Wadsworth Thompson Learning. Reprinted from *New England Journal of Medicine, 325*(23), 1666–1671.

Wolf, Z. R., & Robinson-Smith, G. (2007). Strategies used by clinical nurse specialists in "difficult" clinician-patient situations. *Clinical Nurse Specialist, 21*(2), 74–84.

CHAPTER 4

Professional Responsibility, Social Justice, Human Rights, and Injustice

Pamela J. Grace

Where justice is denied, where poverty is enforced, where ignorance prevails, and where any one class is made to feel that society is an organized conspiracy to oppress, rob and degrade them, neither persons nor property will be safe.
—FREDERICK DOUGLASS, 1886

As long as justice and injustice have not terminated their ever renewing fight for ascendancy in the affairs of mankind, human beings must be willing, when need is, to do battle for the one against the other.
—JOHN STUART MILL, "The Contest in America," 1862

Introduction

This chapter explores the responsibilities of advanced practice nurses (APNs) for recognizing and addressing injustices that affect the health of persons. The APN's ethical responsibilities include "the prevention of illness, the alleviation of suffering, and the protection, promotion, and restoration of health" (American Nurses Association [ANA], 2001, preface). These are simply stated yet complex obligations. Fulfilling these goals may mean that APNs have to look for the antecedents of a patient's or population's problems in the value structure or politics of the larger community and that APNs take remedial actions either on their own or collaboratively with concerned others. Two important assumptions of professional nursing practice are (1) that each patient is equally worthy of attention and (2) the concerns of patients often cannot be effectively addressed without understanding the environment in which they live their daily lives. However, it can be very difficult to balance the needs of individuals within the APN's care with the needs of other patients or the larger population of patients. It is also difficult to know what social justice demands of nurses without understanding how ideas of social justice, including individual human rights, developed and why. This chapter first explores the nature of problems associated with asserting that attending to social justice is an obligation of the nurse. Second, solutions and strategies for nurse actions alone or in concert with others are proposed. Finally, underlying assumptions about the relationship of societal conditions and health are explored and illustrated with cases. The following provides a brief overview of these aspects of social justice and APN practice that are developed in more detail within the body of the chapter.

The Concept of Social Justice

Problems with the Concept of Social Justice

Both the International Council of Nurses (ICN) and the ANA posit that nurses should be concerned with addressing social justice issues that affect their populations, but neither entity defines social justice or what social justice demands of nurses. Various definitions and theories of social justice have been proposed, but all are subject to criticisms that they are inadequate to structure just societies for various reasons. Buettner-Schmidt and Lobo (2012) completed a concept analysis of social justice for the purpose of nursing work and settings. They drew on a broad array of related literature from different disciplines. Their definition captures many essential characteristics of the concept as it is generally, if somewhat vaguely, understood. No resulting framework for action is proposed, although the authors do note that one is needed to guide nursing actions. Grace and Willis (2012) propose a framework for remedying injustices in health care that draws on the ideas of Powers and Faden (2006). Their framework may not be applicable to all nursing situations, but it does provide a starting point, and modifications can be made in concert with ethical decision-making tools to address other situations.

Although it remains unclear what a good theory of social justice would look like, there is growing agreement among disparate cultures that justice demands, at a minimum, that each individual be treated as equally worthy of moral concern. This basically means that no individual can be treated as an object or the possession of another. The United Nations' (UN's) Universal Declaration of Human Rights affirms that "... recognition of the inherent dignity and of the equal and inalienable rights of all members of the human family is the foundation of freedom, justice and peace in the world"

(UN, 2012/1948). The UN consists of at least 192 member countries from all continents, cultures, and geographic regions, demonstrating that regardless of cultural ideology there is global recognition that respect for individuals is a worthy ideal. However, in balancing the needs of each person within the society against the needs of fellow citizens, some constraints on permissible individual actions are necessary. For example, a person cannot be free to cause another person serious harm. Additionally, balancing is needed in relation to the distribution of benefits and harms that occur as inevitable consequences of communal living. Societal values, nature, and powerful human interests all play a role in the distribution of individual benefits and harms; for this reason some inequities are difficult to avoid and the project of trying to remedy inequities is complex.

Many commentators have proposed that a just society should maintain a just healthcare system; support for this proposition is given later. However, a large body of literature critiques the U.S. healthcare system as being systematically unjust (Mechanic, 2006). The healthcare systems of many other countries, although not as inherently unjust, may well disadvantage or fail to appropriately serve the needs of certain populations. Even within a relatively just healthcare system that is accessible to all—that is, where all are able to get help with the resources needed for the protection or improvement of their health (within the boundaries determined by the society's political process)—nurses may face problems mediating between the needs of a particular patient and the needs of a patient population. Thus, gaining an understanding of the nuances associated with human rights and justice is important for all nurses, but especially APNs, who can be considered the profession's leaders, regardless of country of practice.

The general ideas behind social justice are that within a society everyone has a right to benefit from the collective skills and resources of its members and that any associated burdens should be fairly shared. Claims can be made against a society (via its political institutions) to ensure this right. However, the actualization of this ideal has proven problematic philosophically and politically, as explained in more detail shortly.

Social Justice Solutions

What does ambiguity about the concept of social justice and its warrants mean for APNs who encounter injustices then? Do they just throw up their hands, asking "If the philosophers and politicians can't agree on what a good theory of social justice is or how social institutions ought to be arranged to maximize fairness, then, how can we be expected to address injustices?" The answer is that there are actions that nurses can take (and as a profession have historically taken) to address particular injustices. APNs need not focus on this larger question of how societal institutions should be arranged and/or financed to ensure fairness (e.g., government, the legal system, education, health care, etc.), although they do need to understand the complexities of it. APNs have responsibilities to address injustices that affect their populations of concern. These responsibilities may include political action to influence inadequate local or national policies—indeed they may be the only observers of certain sorts of injustices (as discussed shortly). Problematic policies are those that negatively influence health or mistake the actual source of a problem. Additionally, there may be a lack of policies aimed at anticipating future health problems. In this context political action means activities—informed by nursing knowledge and clinical judgment (see **Table 4-1**)—undertaken by the nurse, often in collaboration with others and with the purpose of influencing necessary changes in policy at the institutional, local, or societal levels. At no time has it been more crucial for APNs to grasp the importance of this responsibility than now. Many countries are developing APN roles because of otherwise unmet health needs of populations (Ketefian, Redman, Hanucharurnku, Masterson, & Neves, 2001; Pulcini, Jelic, Gul, & Loke, 2010). As disciplinary leaders, APNs have crucial collaborative and integrative roles to play in addressing justice issues for their patients. The next chapter explores APN leadership responsibilities in more detail. The latter part of the chapter provides examples of different types of problems stemming from societal injustices and the nature of healthcare systems more broadly. APN responsibilities for addressing these problems at a multitude of different levels are delineated, and strategies are proposed for effective action, including, where necessary, political activism on behalf of the population served.

Social Justice Assumptions

Societies have formed both historically and contemporarily because no one individual is capable of providing for all of his or her own personal needs. Contemporary societies ostensibly exist to facilitate the lives of the individuals within them. Arguably, and as discussed shortly, not all societies deliberately intend to provide for the freedom or well-being of all persons who fall under their canopy. Historically, many societies have had a free class

■ Table 4-1   Clinical Judgment in Nursing

Clinical judgment in nursing is the nonlinear process of using knowledge, reasoning, tacit (experiential) skills, and interpersonal skills to determine—within the limits of available information—probable best actions given the inevitable existence of uncertainty about the possession of adequate knowledge and outcome of actions.

Components	Categories
Knowledge	Knowledge base of nursing: ■ Nature of the discipline ■ Purposes and goals ■ Nature of persons and environment ■ Characteristics of good practitioners ■ Scope and limits of practice Knowledge derived from other disciplines: philosophical (including ethical theory), physical, social, psychological, spiritual, biological Knowledge related to the situation: ■ Primary subject/who is involved ■ Subject's understanding of the situation, values, beliefs, and context ■ Goals
Experience	Previous experiences: ■ Personal ■ Professional
Characteristics and skills	Perceptual: ■ Grasp the nature and complexity of issues ■ Identify needed/potential resources ■ Envision resolution ■ Reflect on practice; engage in self-reflection ■ Be creative, articulate Relational: ■ Interpersonal ■ Collaborative ■ Mediation Motivation: ■ Professional responsibility ■ Emotional engagement

and an enslaved or indentured class. Nevertheless, contemporary democratic societies globally have as a guiding principle the idea that all citizens are equal under the law. As the UN Declaration of Human Rights, Article 7 reads, "[a]ll are equal before the law and are entitled without any discrimination to equal protection of the law. All are entitled to equal protection against any discrimination in violation of this Declaration and against any incitement to such discrimination" (2012/1948). That is, everyone is subject to the same freedoms and the same restrictions upon those freedoms that are needed for a fair distribution of the burdens and benefits of societal living. This is a starting place for justice and a helpful foundation for nurses in understanding their dual obligations to individuals and society.

The Historical Development of Ideas of Social Justice

The Social Contract: Hobbes

The mechanisms of many contemporary societies are rooted in some form of the idea of a social contract. This "is the view that persons' moral and/or political obligations are dependent upon a contract or agreement between them to form society" (Friend, 2006). Although traces of social contract theorizing are visible as far back as the time of the ancient Greeks, contemporary theorizing about the structure of a good society arguably begins with the writings and thoughts of Thomas Hobbes (1588–1679). Hobbes is well known in philosophical and other circles, both for his assertion that a social contract is necessary for an orderly and mutually beneficial society and for grounding this assertion in a graphic description of what life would be like for human beings without such a contract.

Like all philosophers, Hobbes' theorizing was influenced by his context. He lived in the turbulent times of the English civil war, a war fought between Royalists (supporters of the monarch) and Oliver Cromwell's supporters, who wanted parliamentary rule. His theory is based on a rather pessimistic view of human nature that does not take into account the possibility of human capacity for altruistic actions (action that is either not primarily or not wholly self-interested). Hobbes felt that an overall ruler, such as a monarch, was necessary to impose order. However, he did not believe that royalty derived its power directly from a supreme being. That is, he did not believe in the divine right of kings. Individuals comprising the potential society would elect a leader they felt could provide the most impartial leadership.

Once elected, the ruler would be entrusted with maintaining social order and permitted to do what was necessary for that end.

Hobbes's particular view of the social contract has been criticized on many levels. Most contemporary critics do not find his characterization of human beings accurate, nor do they agree with the structure he proposes. Nevertheless, his graphic description of life in a state of nature captures some of humanity's worst fears about how human life could be in the absence of some sort of societal structure and how these fears are exemplified currently by the terrible conditions that exist in certain parts of the world, where no identifiable or coherent social infrastructure seems to exist (for example, Haiti, Libya, Afghanistan, Iraq, and Sudan). Some have argued that even within so-called civilized societies, the conditions of certain marginalized groups of people are not so terribly far from Hobbes's conception of life without a social contract (Iceland, 2006; Papadimos, 2006; Rank, 2005).

The Social Contract After Hobbes

As noted, the structures and functioning of many modern societies are based on some conception of a social contract. Ideas about human nature and the social contract, however, have gone through several evolutions since the time of Hobbes. Contemporarily, many scholarly writers in bioethics and justice use John Rawls's (1971) ideas, detailed in *A Theory of Justice* (and explained in more detail in Chapter 1), to explore and/or critique the notion that justice is a particular view of fairness in the distribution of the benefits and burdens of living within a socially contracted society (a distributive justice theory). There are two important principles that emerged from his theorizing: (1) the *principle of equal liberty*, whereby each person has an equal right to the most extensive liberties compatible with similar liberties for all, and (2) the *difference principle*, which states that social and economic inequalities should be arranged so that they are both to the greatest benefit of the least advantaged persons and attached to offices and positions open to all under conditions of equality of opportunity (Rawls, 1971, p. 60).

As discussed, criticisms of these sorts of distributive justice theories derived from ideas of a social contract are varied. Feminists worry that the voices of women, the weak, and the vulnerable are muffled or muted by more powerful societal members, and thus their concerns are left out of the contract (metaphorically speaking). Additionally, the person at the center of the contract is generally conceived to be a self-sufficient, rational individual who is able to reason objectively. However, contemporary philosophers, feminists, and others have pointed out that in fact humans live in a web of relationships that inevitably are influential in complex ways that are not fully understood; therefore, the ideal of a rational person who can be divorced both from emotions and his or her relationships with others for the purposes of objective decision making is a myth. In view of this problem, the existence of a stable, just society is not possible. A more reasonable perspective is that there is an ongoing struggle to achieve justice within society. This struggle entails, among other things, a concerted effort to bring out and magnify the perspectives of the disempowered by those who are in a position to recognize the nature and origins of perceived injustices. It includes efforts to rein in the influence of the powerful or redirect such influences toward a just cause.

One other conception of justice that is sometimes used as a basis for discussions related to the allocation of scarce resources concerns the view that people should receive benefits in proportion to the contributions they have made or according to what they deserve (Pojman, 1999). Whether a person is considered deserving of special consideration or not depends on societal, community, or religious values, and these will be discernible from the supporting rationale. The problem for healthcare providers in relying on a conception of justice based on merit is that their knowledge base includes theoretical and empirical evidence that those who are privileged by supportive backgrounds and environments are often those who will appear more meritorious. It is easier to be meritorious if a person is not caught up in the struggle of merely surviving from day to day, for instance.

Powers and Faden on Social Justice in Public and Health Policy

Recently, Powers and Faden (2006) proposed a theory of justice that does not focus on trying to discover the best ways to distribute goods. Instead of focusing on discovering which conception of justice is correct—which they think is something of a futile quest—they wanted to focus on discovering "[w]hich inequalities matter most" (p. 3) and what is necessary for living a minimally decent life. For this, they concentrated on what they argue are essential dimensions of human living. A life missing, or "seriously deficient," in any one dimension will also have problems in all of the other dimensions because they are interrelated. These dimensions, they assert, are universally shared—people across cultures need a minimal level of each in order to have a meaningful quality of life, and they are not hierarchical. The essential aspects are roughly stated:

- Health—a common sense perspective of physical and psychological well-being or flourishing
- A sense of personal security—not living in constant fear and vigilance
- The ability to reason (theoretical as well as practical reasoning) — allows understanding of the world, helping individuals "make logical connections and detect logical errors . . . allowing [them] to navigate both the natural and the social world." (p. 20)
- Respect—self-respect, as well as respect for and from others
- Attachment—being able to form trusting relationships with others
- Self-determination—a person's ability to make his or her own choices, act on them, and be accountable for them

Powers and Faden were especially concerned with the effects of missing or inadequate dimensions in the lives of children, because effects on children tend to be pervasive and long term. Danny Willis's work exploring the experience of healing from childhood abuse exemplifies their point (currently prepublication). His study, which included only men who perceived themselves as healing subsequent to abuse, revealed that for most the healing process took decades. For many the main dimension affected could probably be pinpointed as a loss of sense of personal security—they reported persistent problems with physical and psychological health, inability to make and retain relationships, poor self-respect, and problems with reasoning and consequently self-determination (Grace & Willis, 2012). For the present purposes, then, Powers and Faden's (2006) ideas about social justice are helpful in many situations (although probably not all) that APNs face. Their main purpose was to determine "which inequities matter most" (p. 3). The next section provides a very abbreviated and simplified account of the evolution of contemporary democratic societies and the relationships of individuals to the societies in which they are members by virtue of location or abode. The purpose of this section is to highlight the nature and source of tensions that exist between individuals and society and, thus, implications for advanced practice in negotiating the levels of professional responsibility that exist.

Individuals and Society: Tensions

There are, of course, many different types of societies. The idea of a social contract is implied in some societies and not in others. Not all societies either historically or currently have held respect for individuals as a crucial value. In many societies, the interests of the group, or some other value, are considered by the society's rulers or traditions to be more important than respect for the individual. And, as noted earlier, even when consideration for the equal moral worth of each person is valued, some individuals are more powerful than others and thus more capable of ensuring that they are accorded respect.

The sinking of the Titanic provides a striking example of this point. The Titanic was a new type of oceangoing ship, touted as being indestructible. However, after a catastrophic encounter with an iceberg, many of the lower-class passengers traveling in steerage class were trapped below deck by gates meant to separate the classes. This meant that they could not easily reach the lifeboats (of which there were too few to accommodate everyone) as the ship was sinking. It was obvious that the lower classes were not treated as equally worthy of moral concern as the upper classes—their very lives were obviously deemed less important than those who had paid more for their passage. Although that event took place almost a century ago, disparities based on class and race continue.

For the purposes of this chapter, though, and because this text is written primarily for APNs in contemporary democratic societies such as the United States, the discussion assumes the existence of a society that (1) takes itself to be democratic, (2) values each citizen as being of equal consideration in the distribution of the benefits and burdens of community living, and (3) has developed implicit and explicit (moral and legal) rules for the conduct of its daily business. Another way of saying this is that within the society each citizen is considered the equal of any other citizen in influencing policy. Ideally all have a say in determining what goods and services are important and what restrictions on personal freedoms are necessary to achieve the desired ends. These assumptions, which represent values espoused in the Constitution of the United States of America and in the constitutional documents of many other countries, allow for critique of contemporary healthcare arrangements or policies that unfairly disadvantage people.

Democratic Societies, Cooperation, and Legal Protection

Democratic societies are to a certain extent cooperative, meaning that such things as goods and services are gained that would not otherwise be accessible to individuals, and such things as materials, time, labor, and money are given in exchange for needed goods and services. Cooperation permits efficiency in the production of goods and the delivery of services, but it also means that the actions of individuals within society necessarily have an impact on the lives of others with whom they interact or, even more broadly, on others in society. The impact may be positive in that mutual benefit occurs or negative in that someone's freedom is restricted or the expected or contracted service is not provided.

Tensions between the needs, desires, and freedom of individuals and what is perceived to be the good of the larger society are inevitable and often lead to political unrest. Not surprisingly, it is frequently those who are the most powerful or who have the most resources, natural and/or material, whose interests prevail. For societies to be successful in balancing individual interests with the interests of the larger group, effective rules and guidelines are needed to deal with inevitable tensions. These rules or guidelines are necessarily influenced by philosophical analysis and empirical evidence about problems, their antecedents, and promising remedies. Each democratic society, supposedly, develops its own system of justice based on the values of the society. "The provision of goods, when these are deemed by the society as vital for the well-being of individuals in the society . . . are safeguarded" (Grace, 1998, p. 98) by a system of laws. "The legislative system [of the society] determines in what manner, and to what extent, people will be legally protected from having their rights to these crucial goods violated" (Grace, 1998, p. 99). These, then, are the legal rights that a person within a society can claim as his or her due. Legal rights, however, are only one type of right. Moral rights also exist. The basis for moral rights may be the same as or different from those of legal rights depending on the underlying value systems of the society, that is, what sorts of belief systems are accorded legitimacy within the system and which values are deemed important enough to protect via formal sanctions.

Moral Rights

General Moral Rights

In addition to legal rights that are conceived within the society (and in democratic societies with the input of citizens) and for which impingements warrant formal sanctions of some kind, other conceptions of rights exist. So-called moral rights, Feinberg (1973) asserts, "exist prior to, or independently of, any legal or institutional rules" (p. 84). Moral rights may or may not be protected by laws. But what does the term *moral rights* mean? How do these rights differ from legal rights? As usual, in philosophy there is a variety of answers that can be given to these questions—as many answers as the different perspectives or theories that exist. Some of the important aspects of moral rights are sketched in the following paragraphs.

The idea that an individual has certain moral rights is centered on conceptions that some human goods are critically important and should be protected, preserved, or promoted. What is held to make these goods important may differ with varying religious and cultural beliefs, but there is a subset of goods that is universally important because without them people would not survive. These can be called *critical human goods*. The actions of protecting, preserving, or promoting critical human goods imply interactions taken by others on behalf of the subject. An evaluation of the proposed or actual actions is made on the basis of whether the action can or does actually serve its purpose. Moreover, some actions may be forbidden if they are likely to cause more harm than good.

In moral philosophy, the appraisal of actions usually falls into one of three categories. The action by the agent is required (obligatory), permissible (neutral), or forbidden. Although here the discussion is about action framed in positive terms, refraining from acting when action is needed to prevent harm or further a person's good is also subject to moral appraisal. The moral status of actions is generally linked to values espoused within a society—such as freedom of speech and equality of opportunity. These values may be based on a variety of moral theories (deontology, utilitarianism, virtue, and so on) or on a belief in divine rules. For example, say that a patient (an individual within a society) is conceived of as having a right to make his or her own decisions by virtue of societal values; no provider may interfere with that decision, all things being equal (in the absence of some reason to suppose that the person is incapable of acting independently). Admission to the hospital does not remove that right. This may seem rather obvious, but it is not always honored, and patient rights were frequently not respected historically. Physicians were often considered to know what was best for a patient whether or not the physician had a sense of the patient's own values. Moral rights are not always subject to legal enforcement, although they may be.

Although it is beyond the scope of this chapter to engage in, or even present, some of the many philosophical debates related to rights and obligations, it is perhaps helpful to note one differentiation that is sometimes made between a positive moral right—where a claim may be made against someone or some institution for assistance or for the provision of goods and services (often requires more government regulations)—and negative moral rights—or the right to be left alone and to be free from the interference of others or from the state (often implies limits on government interference or regulations). To make a claim that an individual has a right to health care is a positive right in this sense. Positive rights mean that a claim may be made against some entity to ensure a right—in this case the government of an individual's society. Claims about a right to health care are often made on the basis of human rights. Human rights are one type of important or critical moral right that are said to belong to humans regardless of the values held by their particular society. The belief that health care is a human right has implications for healthcare providers. The implications stem from the supposition that human beings all have the right to at least a minimally good life (Nickel, 2005; Powers & Faden, 2006).

Human Rights

HUMAN RIGHTS AS A CATEGORY OF MORAL RIGHTS: HISTORY

Human rights are a specific type of moral right that is no less important in healthcare settings than in wider contexts. But what are they? Where do they come from? And what is their force? In developed countries human rights are as natural as having legs or lungs: their existence is not questioned, and people believe that these rights are theirs to claim. People object to murder and torture whenever they occur and consider these acts violations of human rights. To take away a person's life puts an end to all of that person's potential future choices, aspirations, and actions. It ends their humanity.

Modern ideas about human rights trace their origins as far back as the Magna Carta of 11th-century England. Under pressure from his noblemen, King John was swayed to institute what was essentially a contract between the king and his subjects. It limited the power of the state to control its populace and delineated what individuals could lay claim to in the courts (British Bill of Rights, 1994). In essence, it served as the foundation for contemporary rules of law. This was an important development because prior to the Magna Carta the citizens of many societies were subject to the whims and desires of their leaders, often kings. Individual freedom was limited by the dictates of these rulers. The Magna Carta was pivotal for certain political changes but did not extend to all subjects, only to those who already had some power.

It was several centuries later during the Enlightenment when the issues of moral rights and human rights were taken seriously. The Enlightenment represents a period in American and European philosophy when the use of reasoning or analytic thought became valued as the main route to knowledge and was viewed as an essentially and uniquely human characteristic. Locke (1690/2003), for example, claimed that rights naturally flowed from the nature of humans as free and rational beings. Kant's ideas about the innate dignity of human beings served as his justification for the existence of human rights. According to Kant (1785/1967), human beings by virtue of their capacity for rational thought and for making moral rules are, and thus should be allowed to be, self-governing. For this reason, they should never be used purely as a means of serving someone else's advantage. Kant had a complicated argument for this but basically proposed that it is irrational to use an individual purely or primarily as a means to someone else's advantage. For example, if a person assented to this, that person would essentially be saying, "Everyone can treat anyone else as a means to an end" (this is Kant's Categorical Imperative roughly stated). But people would not want to be treated purely as a means to someone else's end; thus, it is irrational to treat someone else as a means to one's own end.

Moral rights, then, include such things as being free to make one's own choices and being free from the interference of the state in personal affairs. Human rights are a more fundamental category of rights. Whereas particular moral rights are based in theories of moral philosophy and may or may not hold depending on the values of a society, human rights are asserted to apply to every human simply by virtue of their humanity. Therefore, human rights apply to everyone regardless of the society to which they belong. Some human rights are considered to be inalienable, that is, they cannot be given away by the person. A classic example of an inalienable right is the right to be free. This means that a person cannot agree to be enslaved even if this would benefit his or her family in some way because it is the nature of humans to be free. It is important to note that there is no agreement about exactly what is the set of rights that are called human rights, although certain rights are generally agreed to be included.

HUMAN RIGHTS: CONTEMPORARY UNDERSTANDINGS

Following the Enlightenment period, attention to the issue of human rights waned temporarily. However, renewed interest emerged partly as a result of human abuses during World War II (1939–1945) as documented in Chapter 6, *Research Ethics: Advanced Practice Roles and Responsibilities*. This prompted a revisiting of the issue of human rights and attempts to further define what they are and why they should be honored. Fagan (2006) noted that contemporarily, "human rights have been defined as basic moral guarantees that people in all countries and cultures allegedly have simply because they are people." According to Nickel (2005), human rights "are concerned with ensuring the conditions . . . of a minimally good life" (p. 386) and, as noted earlier, Powers and Faden (2006) based their theory on this same premise. Fagan (2006), in his thoughtful discussion of human rights, noted that this idea of a minimally good life "has been enshrined in various declarations and legal conventions issued during the past fifty years, initiated by the Universal Declaration of Human Rights (1948) and perpetuated by, most importantly, the European Convention on Human Rights (1954) and the International Covenant on Civil and Economic Rights (1966)." Conceptions of a minimally good life are necessarily different depending on the society and its resources.

The idea behind an assertion that all human beings have rights simply by virtue of being human derives from the "philosophical claim: that there exists a rationally identifiable moral order, an order whose legitimacy precedes contingent social and historical conditions and applies to all human beings everywhere and at all times" (Fagan, 2006). This can be stated a little differently by saying either each human is equally worthy of moral consideration (viewed as important in his or her own right) or no one is. If no one is to be accorded moral consideration, then any person at any time might find their interests discarded on someone else's whim. Indeed, using Rawls's ideas about people in the original position deliberating behind "a veil of ignorance" (Rawls, 1971), it is imaginable that no one would feel secure about abolishing human rights for fear his or her position in society and assets might make them particularly vulnerable to the absence of such rights.

Human rights, however, are not bound to a particular society but are taken to apply across societal and national borders and political contexts. The declarations cited earlier allude to human rights as supporting such goods as a basic standard of living that includes education, provisions for health care, and protection from the effects of destitution. They prohibit torture, slavery, and exploitation. Unfortunately, the interpretation of these rights and how they should be applied in actual situations is a more difficult undertaking than asserting that they exist—as is enforcing them. Currently, in moral philosophy and bioethics circles there is debate about whether human rights imply the right to a certain basic level of health care that is consistent with the status of healthcare knowledge and societal resources.

Complicating things further is the absence of a definition of health that everyone can agree upon.

Is There a Right to Health Care?

This question has been raised by many scholars in the United States and elsewhere. It is an important problem to explore in this text because nurses assert, via the policies and position statements of their professional bodies (ANA, 2003; ICN, 2012) and the writings of scholars, that they exist to attend to the health needs of individuals and society in a nondiscriminatory manner (Ballou, 2000; Gaylord & Grace, 1995; Grace, 1998, 2001; Raphael, 1997; Spenceley, Reutter, & Allen, 2006). Thus, clarity about the influence of all of the following on health is important: universal human rights and their demands on societies, societal values implied (what people would tell you) versus actual (how societal institutions are set up), a person's social and/or economic standing, and the nature and accessibility of healthcare services. These factors are fundamental for understanding what actions are required to meet the health needs of an APN's population (where the definition of health depends both upon the patient's conception of this and insights from nursing knowledge development and the APN's specialty knowledge base).

Nurses, as Curtin (1979) and many other commentators have pointed out, are often the ones who "attend patients when distress is immediate . . . for sustained periods of time" (p. 4) and thus have the opportunity to experience patients in all of their humanity, including the struggle of the poor and otherwise disadvantaged for survival in an inequitable environment. Certain living conditions have been shown to contribute to or exacerbate health problems perhaps even more than a lack of access alone, although often persons living in substandard conditions also lack easy or adequate access to healthcare services. Thus, there are inextricable links among living conditions, social standing, economic status, and health (Danziger & Haveman, 2001; Iceland, 2006; Powers & Faden, 2006; Rank, 2005). For this reason, even if it can be agreed that there is a right to a basic level of health care, this will not ensure good health because even more fundamental justice problems arise within society that also require attention, such as needs for adequate nutrition, housing, and security, as discussed shortly.

Human Rights Arguments for Justice in Health Care

Before discussing professional advocacy for individual and societal health—which means comprehending the effects of poverty, socioeconomic standing, and abuse and neglect on persons' lives and their functioning and flourishing—it is important to gain an understanding of the relationship between human rights and rights to health care. Dernier (2005) notes when it is asserted that a right to health care exists, several related claims are essentially being made. A right to health care means that everyone encompassed by the society (regardless of status and perhaps even including so-called "illegal" immigrants), by virtue of being human, is entitled to a certain level of access to health care and society has a collective responsibility to ensure this. It is a strong societal obligation. This obligation should be reflected in policy debates, and failure to meet this obligation can be said to constitute an injustice.

As a profession, nursing takes the stance that providing basic healthcare services, including those that facilitate the prevention of illness, and the promotion and preservation of health for all members of society are a moral responsibility and should be treated as a human right (ICN, 2007). This is a starting place. A further question that is beyond the scope of this text to explore in detail is to ask, "What are the scope and limits of this right?" Buchanan (1984) noted in the 1980s that there was a growing belief in the idea that "the right to a decent minimum of health care" exists; indeed this is the title of his book. However, d'Oronzio (2001), along with many other philosophers, ethicists, healthcare professionals, and citizens, is concerned that viewing a basic minimum of health care as a human right is not compatible with the current U.S. healthcare financing arrangements. Although efforts to change the U.S. healthcare delivery system are in process, certain professional healthcare groups, notably the ANA (2008), have affirmed their belief that there is a right to health care and that this means the system must change. "The ANA endorses a single payer system as a way to integrate services and facilitate accessibility. ANA believes that health care is a basic human right . . . Thus, ANA reaffirms its support for a restructured health care system that assures universal access to a standard package of essential health care services for all citizens and residents" (ANA, 2008, p. 2).

The following section explores the scope and limits of an APN's responsibilities to patients and society. Role responsibilities are described as both narrow and broad. An argument is presented for understanding responsibilities in three areas: to individual patients, to influence societal conditions that affect groups of patients in terms of access to care or other influences on health, and to overcome obstacles to good care caused by the environment of practice.

Advanced Practice Nursing and Professional Advocacy

Professional Advocacy: A Broad Conception of Role Responsibilities

The term *advocacy* is commonly used in nursing circles as an ideal of practice. However, efforts are ongoing to define what this means in nursing contexts (Bu & Jezewski, 2007; Chafey, Rhea, Shannon, & Spencer, 1998; Grace, 1998, 2001; Mallik, 1997; Snowball, 1996; Spenceley et al., 2006). Consequently, the boundaries of nursing responsibilities related to advocacy are often not fully understood and shift depending on the definition of advocacy assumed. The term has various meanings to various people. I know this to be true both from available literature and from informal surveys of the many graduate and undergraduate students I have encountered over the years. Some say advocacy means defending patients' rights (Abrams, 1978; Curtin, 1982; Gadow, 1990; Jezewski, 1993; Miller, Mansen, & Lee, 1983; Pagana, 1987; Shirley, 2007; Zussman, 1982); some say it means ensuring that patients get their immediate needs met; still others might say that it is a role-related responsibility of nursing, meaning that any action taken by the nurse while acting in the role of a nurse is advocacy. Indeed, all of these definitions appear in the nursing and allied literature (ANA, 2001; Annas, 1974/1990; Bernal, 1992; Chafey et al., 1998; Gaylord & Grace, 1995; Grace, 2001; Hewitt, 2002; MacDonald, 2007; Mallik, 1997; O'Connor & Kelly, 2005; Snowball, 1996; Spenceley et al., 2006).

Elsewhere, I have examined the concept of advocacy in great detail (Grace, 1998, 2001); indeed, it was the topic of my doctoral dissertation. A colleague and I were initially stimulated to explore this topic by an article that appeared in the *Hastings Center Report* in 1992 by non-nurse ethicist Ellen Bernal. In the article, she chastised nursing for taking the stance that nurses are patient advocates. She argued that nursing uses advocacy to advance its autonomy as a discipline and thus improve its professional status. On closer reading, we realized she was using an interpretation of advocacy as meaning only a defense of patient rights and were moved to explore in more depth what nursing means by advocacy (Gaylord & Grace, 1995). This problem of ambiguity of meaning and thus expectations of the nurse became the impetus for a whole program of study related to professional responsibility.

Perhaps the most interesting insight gained during this investigation of advocacy concerned the roots of the term in legal settings. Advocacy as a practice ideal has its origins in the field of law. In law, it means the verbal act of arguing for a person's cause against the cause of an adversary. Lawyers, while advocating, have responsibilities only for that client (or group of clients) and the client's cause. If there are system injustices, these are dealt with outside of the immediate lawyer–client situation.

Nurses, however, do not have such limited responsibilities. In advocating for one patient to have his or her needs met, nurses may well cause disadvantage to another. For example, a primary care nurse practitioner (NP) in a busy clinic is told by one of her patients that she is being physically abused by her boyfriend. This is an urgent matter and the patient needs time and attention. But the nurse is in a practice with two physicians, who in response to economic pressures have limited the time allocated for nurse visits. The NP is the sole available provider this afternoon, and she has three other patients who are also waiting to be seen. She must make a decision that will affect somebody's care. An immediate decision must be made that balances the risk to the other patients against the likely benefit to the abused patient of spending more time with her. The NP has simultaneous responsibilities to more than one patient; thus, advocating for one to receive extra attention may well disadvantage others. Thus, her responsibilities cannot end with the immediate decision and ensuing action. The problem of inadequate visit time is recurring and results in part from a misunderstanding about the APN role, deliberate or inadvertent, on the part of the collaborating/supervising physicians.

Therefore, a different way of looking at the advocacy role of the APN is to view it as any action taken to further professional goals (ultimately related to promoting patient good). This permits nurses to see that their advocacy actions may be directed at different levels. "Professional advocacy, then, may be conceived both as actions taken to further nursing's purposes on behalf of individual patients and actions taken to expose and redress underlying problems that are inherent in the larger contexts of institutions, policymaking, and the health care delivery system" (Grace, 2001, p. 161). Many so-called advocacy situations "have their fundamental roots in such things as national health policy decisions, economic conflicts of interests, miscommunication, institutional barriers or a host of other grounds" (Grace, 2001, p. 152).

To provide some coherent structure to the exploration of advocacy viewed as professional responsibility to further nursing goals (responsibilities of the nursing role), the next section is divided into three parts. The first part describes advocacy viewed as the APN's professional responsibilities to individual patients encountered in practice settings. Second, advocacy is viewed as a responsibility to address the environment in which the APN practices. Finally, the APN's role in influencing social policy is explored. However, this is an artificial categorization because in many cases all three levels of responsibility coexist. When the APN is faced with a tension between trying to provide what is needed for a particular patient and the needs of others within the practice, clinical judgment is needed to prioritize action. Clinical judgment in this sense is synonymous with ethical or moral reasoning (see Table 4-1).

CASE STUDY: AN EXAMPLE OF COMMON ISSUES

This case appeared in the *Louisville Courier-Journal* (Coomes, 2007). It exemplifies the various levels of advocacy needed to ensure good care for this patient. Although this case might be considered peculiar to the United States, a review of associated international literature highlights similarities between Ms. Henley's situation and those in poverty in other countries. Research data from The Commonwealth Fund (2007) found that although the United States lags behind on many healthcare benchmarks, "experiences in all countries (Australia, Canada, Germany, The Netherlands, New Zealand, United Kingdom, United States) indicate the need for more integrated, patient-centered care 'systems.'" The object of the article was to point out that three simple things are all that is needed to improve health for many people. "They should stop smoking, eat better and exercise more" (Coombes, 2007). However, as the reporter noted, "Lack of access to health care providers, healthy foods and safe places to exercise can be roadblocks to healthier lives for those in rural areas and the poor across the state." Ms. Henley is just one example of a pervasive problem in healthcare settings. Healthcare providers know from empirical evidence what strategies are needed for health promotion or maintenance, but more than this is needed to keep people healthy. We need to know what the roadblocks are and help them negotiate these.

Additionally, Ms. Henley's predicament is familiar, one to which many nurses at all levels of practice can relate. "Portia Henley, a 50-year-old [African American] grandmother from Louisville [is] unable to keep a steady job. She has diabetes and struggles to pay for the better food and special drugs her condition requires; asthma inhibits her ability to exercise. 'I'm fighting a real battle,' said Henley. 'It's hard to stay on the straight and narrow in terms of what you eat when you don't have the income to handle the price of medicine, the price of going to doctors and the price of keeping a roof over your head, plus the cost of buying food for this one specific health problem.'"

Professional Advocacy for Individual Patients

THE NURSE–PATIENT RELATIONSHIP

The essence of nursing care is the individual nurse–patient relationship. This is a fiduciary relationship based on trust. Whether patients do or do not actually trust their nurses, in the sense of knowing who their nurses are and having confidence in their abilities, nevertheless, they are forced to trust that nurses have their patients' best interests in mind, know what they are doing, understand the limits of their knowledge and skills, and will steer patients in the right direction or put patients in touch with needed resources when they have reached the limits of their expertise. For this reason, transparency of purpose and affiliation is important. In some cases, especially in advanced practice settings, nursing's work is not directly aimed at patient benefit. Some examples are performing pre-employment wellness screenings or serving in the role of research nurse coordinator. In such cases, APNs have responsibilities to reveal their purpose and any existing conflicts of interest, to address misunderstandings, and to direct the involved person to a source of help as needed.

However, mostly the APN's role is to further patient good related to individual persons' actual or potential health needs. To further this good APNs use clinical judgment to determine appropriate actions. A definition of clinical judgment that was synthesized from extant literature in nursing, medicine, and the cognitive sciences appears in Table 4-1. Clinical judgment is needed to identify patients' needs, anticipate future needs, and facilitate care that is most likely to meet these needs. Because the goals of care involve understanding what is best for the patient whose life is necessarily contextual and nuanced, nurses need to engage with a patient (and with family members when this is indicated) to discover a patient's beliefs, values, and preferences so that the nurse's actions are tailored to that person's needs. Additionally, because nurses too are human and have their own beliefs, values, and biases, they must be careful to understand what these biases are and how such prejudices (prejudgments about the nature or attributes of a person) are likely to affect their clinical judgment in particular situations.

BIASES

Ms. Henley's case serves as an example of a possible bias (Doris & The Moral Psychology Research Group, 2010) that providers may exhibit related to poverty. Many people do not have a good understanding of the nature of poverty and its antecedents. Coryn (2002), in his literature review, noted that there are three distinct categories of attitudes people have related to poverty: these are "individualistic/internal, structural/external, and fatalistic." In the United States, the predominant attitude of the middle class is individualistic/internal, meaning the poor person is blamed for possessing a character flaw such as laziness or lack of ambition that has led to his or her present condition. Perhaps not surprisingly, among the poor themselves the predominant attitude is structural/external, meaning they attribute poverty to external circumstances (Coryn, 2002). Because most healthcare professionals are middle class, a bias against the poor can be anticipated (Crandall, 1990).

One way to avoid the effects of bias that arise from inexperience or ignorance is to try to understand what a person's life is like. What are the person's daily experiences and struggles like? Other biases or prejudices may exist because of negative past experiences with someone. For example, a nurse whose parent suffered from alcohol abuse may have a negative attitude toward patients she views as alcoholic. Advocacy, viewed as professional responsibility to further the goals of the profession for good care, obligates nurses to understand who patients are, what is needed for their care, and what obstacles exist to getting them the care they need.

IDENTIFYING AND ADDRESSING OBSTACLES

Obstacles to providing what the APN determines to be necessary for the good of an individual patient may take many shapes and forms. **Table 4-2** lays out the different levels at which obstacles may present and provides a synopsis of common problems. Strategies to address obstacles are presented shortly. The specialty chapters of this text provide strategies that are particular and pertinent to that specialty, but issues of poverty and disadvantages of various sorts are commonly encountered across settings. For Ms. Henley there are many obstacles to achieving optimal health even within the limits of her complex issues. Because some of these issues arise as a result of social inequities, addressing these requires influencing social policies, as addressed shortly.

In caring for Ms. Henley at the nurse–patient relationship level, the immediate concern is assisting with her current problems. Professional advocacy at this level means using an approach that is based in nursing's

■ Table 4-2   Categories of Obstacles to Ethical Nursing/Health Care

Category	Obstacles
Individual patient	1. Patient not viewed as unique: ■ Standardized patient care ■ Provider lacks understanding of the influence of important contextual details ■ Patient "labeled" by others 2. Prejudgment of patient (bias/prejudice) 3. Patient or family's need for knowledge not fully addressed (related to #2) 4. Interpersonal conflict: ■ Provider–patient ■ Patient–family ■ Provider–provider 5. Poor communication: ■ Provider–patient/family ■ Provider–provider 6. Power imbalances—coercion/silencing 7. Inadequate time—resources to evaluate and address needs (also a practice environment problem) 8. Patient's moral agency diminished (does not see self as having meaningful choices (Blacksher, 2002)
Practice environment	1. Lack of primary focus on patient good: ■ Economic conflicts of interest ■ Practice philosophy is to meet economic goals 2. Autonomous practice constrained: ■ Senior colleagues ■ Institutional mission ■ Managed care mandates 3. Unsupportive environment
Social injustices	1. Unjust aspects of the healthcare system: ■ Access ■ Financing ■ Priorities ■ Failure to attend to the real origins of certain health problems

(continues)

■ Table 4-2   Categories of Obstacles to Ethical Nursing/Health Care
(*continued*)

Category	Obstacles
	2. Socioeconomic disparities:
	■ Education
	■ Poverty
	■ Discrimination
	3. Lasting effects of violence, abuse, neglect
	4. Profit motive or business emphasis
	5. Fragmented services

philosophy of care and goals of practice. Although priority goals are to meet her immediate needs, it is still necessary to have an idea of who Ms. Henley is as a person. In the absence of a life-threatening emergency that would require immediate measures, it is not possible to adequately help meet her health needs if the nurse does not know more about her. The nurse needs to know, for example, how her maladies are affecting her, what she views as the priority issue, what she knows about her physical conditions, what resources are available to her, and what are her priorities. Advocacy at the level of nurse–patient relationship, then, means professional responsibility to ensure good patient care. This entails understanding what good actions are likely to be for this patient, working with her to determine what are good avenues of action from her point of view, and recognizing and accounting for potential and actual obstacles to good action.

Advocacy viewed as professional role responsibilities for good care presents the same obligations regardless of setting and is based in nursing's philosophy of care and disciplinary goals. Thus, Ms. Henley could have presented for care at any number of different specialty practices—primary care adult health, family practice, women's health primary care, emergency room, as a preanesthesia workup, in a diabetes or asthma clinic, and so on. The time required to address all of her issues may be different in different settings because some aspects of her care may well be beyond the knowledge and skills of the clinician, who will then need to refer Ms. Henley to others for care of those aspects. Nevertheless, the APN's responsibilities include evaluating the quality and appropriateness of the referral made.

Advocacy, as described earlier, can be seen as an onerous and unrealistic responsibility given current environments of practice with their inevitable time constraints and pressures. This view is not uncommon and may be true in many settings. Nevertheless, the APN's role responsibilities include understanding and influencing the context of care so that nursing goals can be met. In those situations where the APN finds intractable differences between his or her philosophy of care and those of her practice colleagues, it is the nurse's responsibility to consider whether a different type of setting might be more fitting.

Nurses see firsthand the effects of unaddressed or poorly addressed problems upon their population of patients. They may be the first or only ones to understand both what those effects are and what changes are needed. Therefore, nurses' responsibilities do not end when the presenting patient's priority needs are met, especially when it is recognized that the practice environment may actually be working against nursing goals of providing care for the patient as a person.

Professional Advocacy and Practice Environments

The varied environments in which APNs work and care for patients also give rise to problems that can interfere with optimal care for a given patient (see Table 4-2). Role responsibilities exist so that nurses can understand how a particular setting and its values are impinging on ethical patient care. The problem may involve a particular patient or may be seen as recurrent. In the case of Ms. Henley, a practice focus of constricted time slots or on managing only the acute presentation would lead to fragmented care, is at odds with nursing goals that include anticipation and prevention of future problems, and would affect many of the patients within the practice. As another example, in correctional settings the facility's goal of prisoner behavior control may interfere with a nursing emphasis on providing for an individual prisoner's well-being. In yet other settings, unit, institutional, or practice policies, conventions, or expediencies may raise barriers to good patient care. Like other healthcare providers in primary care settings especially, constraints related to financing arrangements, reimbursement issues, and managed care practices pose some of the most troubling, difficult, and time-consuming problems for NPs (Creel & Robinson, 2010; Johnson, 2005; Ulrich et al., 2006; Ulrich & Soeken, 2005).

Professional Advocacy and Social Injustices

At the broadest level, APNs in concert with other nurses, physicians, and allied health professionals have a collective interest in addressing social injustice. This is because the goals of almost all healthcare professions have to do with improving the health of individuals. Improving the health of individuals often requires addressing injustice that is deeply rooted in a society. It is not expected that most APNs will be capable of single-handedly tackling an issue; however, their knowledge and experiences place them in the ideal situation to join with colleagues or collaborate with other professionals to inform policy debates.

Nurses, both because they provide direct care and have a perspective and approach that permits hearing patients' health and illness stories within the contexts of patients' daily lives, may be the first or only ones to recognize existing and developing patterns of injustice or disparity. Nurses, along with other healthcare providers, see firsthand the end results of poor access to health care or poor health maintenance. Thus, viewing advocacy as a broader responsibility to further professional goals at both the individual and societal level highlights the range of knowledge, skills, and actions that may be needed. In addition to the fact that taking a broad view of nursing responsibilities is needed for meeting nursing goals, positive action at a level different from the immediate situation is also a way of mitigating the moral distress or unease felt when APNs are unable to provide the care needed for a particular patient because of environmental or other obstacles (Arthur, 1995; Corley, 1995; Corley, Minick, Elswick, & Jacobs, 2005; Erlen & Sereika, 1997; Fowler, 1989).

HEALTH DISPARITIES AND POVERTY

Although health disparities are by no means the only nursing care issues that require professional advocacy at the societal level, the issue of poverty internationally and its pervasive influence on health provides an important exemplar and argument for APNs to take seriously their ethical responsibilities to advocate for health policy changes. Poverty affects people in a variety of ways that are not always easily discernible but that have been well documented in the literature and supported by empirical studies (Danziger & Haveman, 2001; Iceland, 2006; Rank, 2005). Patients like Portia Henley, for whom daily life is an ongoing struggle to make ends meet, may delay seeking care until their problems are out of control. They may have inadequate insurance, transportation difficulties, lack of family support, be the primary caretaker for others whose needs they put first, or have any number of other obstacles to getting the assistance they need. As a diabetes clinical nurse specialist (CNS) or APN, my immediate goal would be to assess Ms. Henley's priority needs for knowledge, self-care, nursing, and other necessary therapeutics, which would include understanding her values and priorities. Next steps would be to help her obtain the resources and supports she needs to achieve a level of health that she desires and that is realistic in the context of her life. Finally, what is really needed is an exploration of the environmental and economic conditions that resulted in her current status.

The next section briefly presents some ideas for influencing change in the broader healthcare environment. Nursing has a rich history of activism to improve health care, starting with the efforts of Florence Nightingale (1820–1910). Nightingale used evidence and influence to change the way wounded soldiers were treated during the Crimean War, and she used her knowledge, skills, and influence to ensure that a patient's environment would be conducive to his or her healing.

Professional Advocacy: Influential Strategies

APNs are uniquely positioned to research and articulate the likely consequences of problematic practices to those in charge of policy decisions, whether this is at the institutional, local, and/or societal levels. The current healthcare climate necessitates the political action of nurses individually, collectively, and in collaboration with others and is exceptionally open to the input of nurses because "physicians have lost much of their influence and control to corporate medicine in recent years" (Mechanic & Reinhard, 2002, p. 7). Although not all nurses can, as Malone (2005) notes, "become policy experts . . . in addition to providing direct patient care . . . all nurses can assess, identify, and articulate for [or on behalf of] patients" on certain problematic issues and "provide information to patients on options for impacting policy; and work to effect policy change through professional and advocacy organizations" (p. 136).

Nurses can (and should) include in their nursing assessments possible "policy factors that may have preventive, etiological, or therapeutic significance" (Malone, 2005, p. 136). This may sound complicated but is actually elementary. For example, it means asking why certain poor patients with diabetes are not managing their diet and medicines well. Is the reason that they are unaware of resources (the system is not allowing for adequate patient education), cannot afford the medicines (health insurance problems), have access problems, or some other issue? One effective strategy is for an APN to join forces with other nurses, physicians, and allied professionals whose concerns mirror their own. As a group they can publicize the problem, provide convincing rationale, and outline probable consequences.

Individual patient narratives as exemplars of a larger problem can be very powerful. Blacksher (2002), a philosopher, documented the life of her mother (only on reading the acknowledgments does the reader discover that Sally is her mother). Sally was born into extreme and unremitting poverty. She had no opportunities to develop a sense of self. She was periodically abused by others—beaten by her mother and then her husband. This affected her health, development of a sense of self as worthwhile, and ability to rise above. Blacksher's vivid portrayal is of a woman who was "stuck." She was unable to develop and exercise moral agency, that is, to choose actions that would benefit either herself and others. In fact, she did not see herself as having choices. "Chronic socioeconomic deprivation can create environments that undermine the development of self and capacities constitutive to moral agency—i.e., the capacity for self-determination and crafting a life of one's own" (pp. 455–456). What nursing can do in such cases on an individual level is to provide a "key" to unlock a person's potential and facilitate the development of a sense of self as worthwhile. Nursing actions include treating patients with respect, providing resources and referral, and empowering—this is a process. But it is also important to examine the particular aspects of the environment that served to perpetuate the patient's situation. In Sally's case, years of neglect from health care and social systems alike had an impact.

Providing a submission to the op-ed page of a newspaper or a letter to the editor often gets public attention and raises questions for discussion in a more public forum. Membership in relevant institutional or local committees is another good strategy and can serve as an important forum for educating other committee members about nursing concerns. For example, acute care CNSs or NPs can provide a valuable voice for patients when they sit on hospital ethics committees and patient care committees.

APNs can be instrumental in educating and providing information for grassroots patient organizations. They should recognize that the information they have about patient situations is valuable and can be articulated in a variety of arenas and forums to inform needed changes. For example, family nurse practitioner (FNP) students joined with their mentors and a specialty organization to change the practice of one managed care company related to antihistamine prescriptions. The formulary allowed only diphenhydramine for seasonal allergy treatments, but this was making many of the children drowsy. A letter-writing and publicity campaign managed to change the practice and make better options available to these children. Another example of effective nursing political activity was given by Murphy, Canales, Norton, and DeFilippis (2005) and is related to improved pain control. "Through regulatory policy advocated for by nurses and many others in the political arena, optimal pain control is now part of standard practice" (p. 22). Nurses are urged to join with colleagues and/or collaborate with allied professionals to publicize a problem. This can also be done via letters to the editor of local papers, or by emailing, calling, or writing to local or state representatives.

Conclusion

Professional advocacy is synonymous with the idea that all nursing actions have ethical implications. This is because all nursing actions have the ultimate purpose of furthering the goals of nursing related to patient well-being. The goals of nursing involve providing health and well-being for individuals who are inextricably a part of the larger society in which they reside. Consequently, patients are susceptible to inequities occurring as a result of societal arrangements. Good patient care often requires attention to the underlying circumstances that have given rise to the need for nursing's services, including poverty and other disparities that leave patients especially vulnerable to their healthcare needs.

Summary

This chapter provides an essential background for understanding the breadth of APN responsibilities to attend to the health needs of both individuals and society. An argument is provided for the importance of balancing the needs of individuals with societal needs related to health and health care. To fulfill professional goals, APNs need to engage with individual patients, taking into account their patients' unique needs and addressing obstacles that prevent meeting these needs. Additionally, APNs may need to engage in political activity at a variety of levels, either singly or in collaboration with others.

Discussion Questions

1. All nurses have patients or types of patients who we find ourselves avoiding. This is human nature. The person reminds us of someone in the past, perhaps, who treated us badly or at whose hands we suffered, the person may just be difficult to please, or their problems may seem intractable, as in the case of Blacksher's mother, Sally. Other intractable problems might be a person with an addiction whose problem seems overwhelming or who exhibits drug-seeking behavior. In the United States there are a set of patients, often homeless, who are labeled "frequent flyers" because of their repeated visits to the emergency department. In light of the discussion of advocacy, explore ways in which you might make a connection with a difficult patient. What are a nurse's responsibilities related to different levels of advocacy?

   To what extent do you see such problems as ones of human rights, moral rights, and social justice?

2. In your practice or from your nursing experience, identify the common barriers/obstacles that make it difficult for you to give the care that in your clinical judgment is required. How should such problems be addressed?

3. You are one of the two APNs in a group practice. You and your colleague are being pressured to assume the same approach to practice as your physician colleagues and the physician's assistant. Your colleagues are receptive to your input and you have a collegial relationship. How would you explain to them that your nursing perspective requires a different approach?

4. What does it mean to be self-reflective? How does one know when you have been genuinely self-reflective (versus justifying your values)?

5. Do you think that everyone should have access to the same basic level of health care? What would this include?

References

Abrams, N. (1978). A contrary view of the nurse as patient advocate. *Nursing Forum, 17,* 258–267.

American Nurses Association. (2001). *Code of ethics for nurses with interpretive statements.* Washington, DC: Author.

American Nurses Association. (2003). *Social policy statement*. Washington, DC: Author.

American Nurses Association. (2008). *Health system reform agenda*. Retrieved from http://ana.nursingworld.org/MainMenuCategories/HealthcareandPolicyIssues/HealthSystemReform/Agenda.aspx

Annas, G. J. (1974/1990). The patient rights advocate: Can nurses effectively fill the role? In T. Pence & J. Cantrall (Eds.), *Ethics in nursing: An anthology* (pp. 83–86). New York, NY: National League for Nursing Publication.

Arthur, E. (1995). Coping with moral distress. *Minnesota Nursing Accent, 67*(3), 5.

Ballou, K. A. (2000). A historical-philosophical analysis of the professional nurse obligation to participate in sociopolitical activities. *Policy, Politics, & Nursing Practice, 1*(3), 172–184.

Bernal, E. W. (1992). The nurse as patient advocate. *Hastings Center Report, 22*(4), 18–23.

Blacksher, E. (2002). On being poor and feeling poor: Low socio-economic status and the moral self. *Theoretical medicine and bioethics, 23*(6), 455–470.

British Bill of Rights. (1994). *The Magna Carta*. Retrieved from http://www.hrweb.org/legal/otherdoc.html

Bu, X., & Jezewski, M. A. (2007). Developing a mid-range theory of advocacy through concept analysis. *Journal of Advanced Nursing, 57*(1), 101–110.

Buchanan, A. (1984). The right to a decent minimum of health care. *Philosophy and Public Affairs, 13*(1), 55–78.

Buettner-Schmitt, K., & Lobo, M. L. (2012). Social justice: A concept analysis. *Journal of Advanced Nursing, 68*(4), 948–958.

Chafey, K., Rhea, M., Shannon, A. M., & Spencer, S. (1998). Characterizations of advocacy by practicing nurses. *Journal of Professional Nursing, 14*(1), 43–52.

Commonwealth Fund. (2007). International health policy survey in several countries. Retrieved from http://www.commonwealthfund.org/Surveys/2007/2007-International-Health-Policy-Survey-in-Seven-Countries.aspx

Coomes, M. (2007, May 11). Kentucky's health: Critical condition. *Louisville Courier-Journal*. Retrieved from http://www.courier-journal.com/apps/pbcs.dll/article?AID=/20051214/NEWS01/512140410&template=printart

Corley, M. C. (1995). Moral distress of critical care nurses. *American Journal of Critical Care, 4*, 280–285.

Corley, M. C., Minick, P., Elswick, R. K., & Jacobs, M. S. O. (2005). Nurse moral distress and ethical work environment. *Nursing Ethics, 12*(4), 381–390.

Coryn, C. (2002). Antecedents of attitudes towards the poor. Unpublished paper. Retrieved from http://www.iusb.edu/~journal/2002/coryn/coryn.html

Crandall, L. A. (1990). Advocacy of just health policies as professional duty: Cultural biases and ethical responsibility. *Business and Professional Ethics Journal, 9*(3&4), 41–53.

Creel, E. L., & Robinson, J. C. (2010). Ethics in independent nurse consulting: Strategies for avoiding ethical quicksand. *Nursing Ethics, 17*(6), 769–776.

Curtin, L. (1979). The nurse as advocate: A philosophical foundation for nursing. *Advances in Nursing Science, 1*(3), 1–10.

Curtin, L. L. (1982). What are human rights? In L. L. Curtin & M. J. Flaherty (Eds.), *Nursing ethics: Theories and pragmatics* (pp. 3–16). Bowie, MD: Brady Communications.

Danziger, S. H., & Haveman, R. H. (2001). *Understanding poverty*. Cambridge, MA: Harvard University Press.

Dernier, Y. (2005). On personal responsibility and the human right to healthcare. *Cambridge Quarterly of Healthcare Ethics, 14,* 224–234.

d'Oronzio, J. C. (2001). A human right to health care access: Returning to the origins of the patients rights movement. *Cambridge Quarterly of Healthcare Ethics, 10,* 285–298.

Doris, J. M., & The Moral Psychology Research Group. (2010). *The moral psychology handbook.* New York, NY: Oxford University Press.

Douglass, F. (1982). U.S. abolitionist. In J. W. Blassingame (Ed.), *The Frederick Douglass Papers.* New Haven, CT: Yale University Press. Original speech April 1886, Washington, DC.

Erlen, J. A., & Sereika, S. M. (1997). Critical care nurses, ethical decision-making and stress. *Journal of Advanced Nursing, 26,* 953–961.

Fagan, A. (2006). Human rights. *The Internet encyclopedia of philosophy.* Retrieved from http://www.iep.utm.edu/hum-rts/

Feinberg, J. (1973). *Social philosophy.* Englewood Cliffs, NJ: Prentice Hall.

Fowler, M. D. M. (1989). Moral distress and the shortage of critical care nurses. *Heart and Lung, 18,* 314–315.

Friend, C. (2006). Social contract theory. *The Internet encyclopedia of philosophy.* Retrieved from http://www.iep.utm.edu/s/soc-cont.htm

Gadow, S. (1990). Existential advocacy: Philosophical foundations of nursing. In T. Pence & J. Cantrall (Eds.), *Ethics in nursing: An anthology* (pp. 40–51). New York, NY: National League for Nursing. Reprinted from *Nursing Images and Ideals,* 1980, pp. 79–101.

Gaylord, N., & Grace, P. (1995). Nursing advocacy: An ethic of practice. *Nursing Ethics, 2*(1), 11–18.

Grace, P. J. (1998). *A philosophical analysis of the concept "advocacy": Implications for professional–patient relationships.* Unpublished Dissertation. University of Tennessee, Knoxville. Retrieved from http://proquest.umi.com. Publication No. AAT9923287, Proquest Document ID No. 734421751.

Grace, P. J. (2001). Professional advocacy: Widening the scope of accountability. *Nursing Philosophy, 2*(2), 151–162.

Grace, P. J., & Willis, D. G. (2012). Social justice and professional responsibilities: An analysis in support of disciplinary goals. *Nursing Outlook, 60,* 198–207.

Hewitt, J. (2002). A critical review of the arguments debating the role of the nurse advocate. *Journal of Advanced Nursing, 37*(5), 439–445.

Hobbes, T. (1967/1651). Leviathon. In A. I. Melden (Ed.), *Ethical theories: A book of readings* (2nd ed., pp. 218–231). Englewood Cliffs, NJ: Prentice Hall. Original work published in 1651.

Iceland, J. (2006). *Poverty in America* (2nd ed.). Berkeley, CA: University of California.

International Council of Nurses. (2007). ICN Position statement: Nursing and development. Geneva, Switzerland: Author. Retrieved from http://www.icn.ch/publications/position-statements/

International Council of Nurses. (2012). Code of ethics for nurses. Geneva, Switzerland: Author. Retrieved from http://www.icn.ch/about-icn/code-of-ethics-for-nurses/

Jezewski, M. A. (1993). Culture brokering as a model for advocacy. *Nursing and Health Care, 14,* 78–85.

Johnson, R. (2005). Shifting patterns of practice: Nurse practitioners in a managed care environment. *Research and Theory for Nursing Practice, 19*(4), 323–340.

Kant, I. (1967). Foundations of the metaphysics of morals. In A. I. Melden (Ed.), *Ethical theories: A book of readings* (pp. 317–366). Englewood Cliffs, NJ: Prentice Hall. Original work published in 1785.

Ketefian, S., Redman, R. W., Hanucharurnku, S., Masterson, A., & Neves, E. P. (2001). The development of advanced practice roles: Implications in the international nursing community. *International Nursing Review, 48,* 152–163.

Locke, J. (2003). *Two treatises of government and a letter concerning toleration.* I. Shapiro (Ed.). Binghamton, NY: Vail-Ballou Press. Original work published in 1690.

MacDonald, H. (2007). Relational ethics and advocacy in nursing: Literature review. *Journal of Advanced Nursing, 57*(2), 119–126.

Mallik, M. (1997). Advocacy in nursing—a review of the literature. *Journal of Advanced Nursing, 25,* 130–138.

Malone, R. E. (2005). Assessing the policy environment. *Policy, Politics, & Nursing Practice, 6*(2), 135–143.

Mechanic, D. (2006). *The truth about health care: Why reform is not working in America.* Piscataway, NJ: Rutgers University Press.

Mechanic, D., & Reinhard, S. C. (2002). Contributions of nurses to health policy: Challenges and opportunities. *Nursing and Health Policy Review, 1*(1), 7–15.

Mill, J. S. (1862). The contest in America. *Harper's New Monthly Magazine, 24*(143), 683–684.

Miller, B. K., Mansen, T. J., & Lee, H. (1983). Patient advocacy: Do nurses have the power and authority to act as patient advocates? *Nursing Leadership, 6*(6), 56–60.

Murphy, N., Canales, M. K., Norton, S. A., & DeFilippis, J. (2005). Striving for congruence: The interconnection between values, practice, and political action. *Politics, Policy, & Nursing Practice, 6*(1), 20–29.

Nickel, J. (2005). Poverty and rights. *Philosophical Quarterly, 55,* 385–402.

O'Connor, T., & Kelly, B. (2005). Bridging the gap: A study of general nurses' perceptions of patient advocacy in Ireland. *Nursing Ethics, 12*(5), 53–67.

Pagana, K. D. (1987). Let's stop calling ourselves "patient advocates." *Nursing, 17,* 51.

Papadimos, T. J. (2006). Charles Dickens hard times and the academic health center: A tale of the urban working poor and the violation of a covert covenant, an American perspective. *Online Journal of Health Ethics, 1*(2), 71–72.

Pojman, L. (1999). Merit: Why do we value it? *Journal of Social Philosophy, 30*(1), 83–102.

Powers, M., & Faden, R. (2006). *Social justice.* New York, NY: Oxford University Press.

Pulcini, J., Jelic, M., Gul, R., & Loke, A. Y. (2010). An international survey on advanced practice nursing education, practice, and regulation. *Journal of Nursing Scholarship, 42*(1), 31–39.

Rank, M. R. (2005). *One nation underprivileged: Why American poverty affects us all.* New York, NY: Oxford University Press.

Raphael, A. R. (1997). Advocacy oral history: A research methodology for social activism in nursing. *Advances in Nursing Science, 20*(2), 32–43.

Rawls, J. (1971). *A theory of justice.* Cambridge, MA: Belknap/Harvard University Press.

Shirley, J. L. (2007). The limits of autonomy in nursing's moral discourse. *Advances in Nursing Science, 30*(1), 14–25.

Snowball, J. (1996). Asking nurses about advocating for patients: Reactive and proactive accounts. *Journal of Advanced Nursing, 24,* 67–75.

Spenceley, S. N., Reutter, L., & Allen, M. N. (2006). The road less traveled: Nursing advocacy at the policy level. *Policy, Politics, & Nursing Practice, 7*(3), 180–194.

Ulrich, C. M., Danis, M., Ratcliffe, S. J., Garrett-Mayer, E., Koziol, D., Soeken, K. L., & Grady, C. (2006). Ethical conflict in nurse practitioners and physician assistants in managed care. *Nursing Research, 55*(6), 391–401.

Ulrich, C., & Soeken, K. L. (2005). A path analytic model of ethical conflict in practice and autonomy in a sample of nurse practitioners. *Nursing Ethics, 12*(3), 305–316.

United Nations. (2012). The universal declaration of human rights. Retrieved from http://www.un.org/en/documents/udhr/index.shtml

Zussman, J. (1982). Want some good advice? Think twice about being a patient advocate. *Nursing Life, 2*(6), 46–50.

CHAPTER 5

Ethical Leadership by Advanced Practice Nurses

Nan Gaylord and Pamela J. Grace

> *May I stress the need for courageous, intelligent, and dedicated leadership...Leaders of sound integrity. Leaders not in love with publicity, but in love with justice. Leaders not in love with money, but in love with humanity. Leaders who can subject their particular egos to the greatness of the cause.*
> —Dr. Martin Luther King, Jr., "Challenge of a New Age," Speech on the Prayer Pilgrimage for Freedom in Washington, DC, May 17, 1956

Introduction

Nurses have responsibilities for individual and societal health. These responsibilities are to further the profession's goals of promoting, protecting, and restoring health. Nursing has a central unifying focus on these goals that is evident in the discipline's collective and historical literature (Willis, Grace, & Roy, 2008). This focus is primarily on humanization in the context of a person's health needs throughout his or her lifespan. Nurses over the decades and across nations have been concerned with advancing the health of their societies in the face of tremendous obstacles. These obstacles include the lack of respect accorded to women, racism, dehumanization of the poor, expediencies of war, and ignorance of (or disregard for) the roots of ill health in societal conditions. Pioneering nurses recognized the deeply entrenched nature of many healthcare problems in the organization of society and the special interests of those in power and were concerned enough to marshal political support for change using formal and informal knowledge, skills, and political savvy. Many of these nurses exhibited a courage that put them at risk.

The fact that that almost all of these leaders were women at a time when women's views were not taken seriously makes their successes even more remarkable. How did they do it? What motivated them? And most importantly, what can be learned from their leadership, as well as from new understandings and philosophies of leadership, in order to empower modern day advanced practice nurses (APNs) in their desire to enable good practice? Nursing is no longer essentially a female profession; males, including APNs, are becoming nurses in increasing numbers (United States Census Bureau, 2011), contributing to the diversity of the profession. Nevertheless, furthering nursing's purposes in contemporary healthcare environments requires constant efforts and solid leadership skills. APNs should not necessarily subject themselves to the sorts of serious risks that some of their predecessors did; however, among other things, the APN role is a leadership role. APNs can envision and address needed changes in the immediate context of care or in broader environments including the healthcare delivery system, and calculating acceptable levels of risk is an inevitable part of their decision-making process.

This chapter provides some definitions of leadership that are pertinent for meeting the professional responsibilities of APNs regardless of their role (direct or indirect patient care). It discusses characteristics needed for facilitating nursing goals, including skills of collaboration, communication, mediation, and where necessary, referral. Several types of leadership are explored and related to the essentials of advanced practice, as delineated specifically in the United States (American Association of Colleges of Nursing [AACN], 2011; Zaccagnini & White, 2011), and explicitly as well as implicitly in other countries where the APN role has been developed (Pulcini, Jelic, Gul, & Loke, 2010). Although advanced practice roles are relatively new in terms of the broader nursing profession's development, evidence supports the increasing need for nurses who are well educated, skillful, knowledgeable, and motivated to meet the healthcare needs of their populations (Aiken, Clarke, Cheung, Sloane, & Silber, 2003; Benner, Sutphen, Leonard, & Day, 2009; Institute of Medicine [IOM], 2010; International Council of Nurses [ICN], 2010). Finally, because it is critical that APNs advocate for justice in health care and in healthcare access and that they influence policies that negatively impact their populations, some past and current projects of pioneer APNs are highlighted and useful leadership strategies are discussed.

Leadership Defined

Leadership has been defined as moving a group of persons toward a common goal. Leaders establish a direction and influence others to follow that direction; they motivate people toward a shared goal (Curtis, de Vreis & Sheerin,

2011; Sullivan & Garland, 2010; Weihrich & Koontz, 2005). This ideal of movement toward common goals is, in a sense, what distinguishes leadership from management. A review of studies on the psychology of leadership defines leadership as "a process of social influence in which one person is able to enlist the aid and support of others in the accomplishment of a task or objective" and characteristics of effective leadership as requiring that "the person in the leadership role establish trust and credibility to enlist the support of followers; build relationships with those followers that motivate them to contribute their energy and resources to the collective effort; and manage, direct, and apply those collective resources to accomplish the group's mission or task" (Chemers, 2001, p. 8580).

Many types of leadership have been described in the literature. Two major types derived from studies are transactional and transformational leadership, and there are elements of overlap between the two. Different leadership styles may be successful depending on whether there is a specific task that needs to be completed or an ongoing process of change. For example, elements of transactional leadership may be needed to achieve a task within a process of transformational leadership for change.

Transactional Leadership

Transactional leadership is perhaps most reflective of many contemporary institutional management practices. It can be conceptualized as a bartering system where one person has more power in the process than others. There are three discernible styles of transactional leadership as discussed by Howell and Avolio (1993). In one scenario, the leader rewards participants for a job well done—contingent leaders. In a second, the leader sets the terms and rules and takes to task those who do not perform well—active leadership. In a third, the leader does not set the rules but expects certain outcomes, passively watches what is going on, then when things go wrong takes remedial actions. Criticisms of transactional leadership include the idea that it is task oriented rather than visionary (Howell & Avolio, 1993; Murphy, 2005).

Transformational Leadership

Transformational leadership is aimed at change. The leader has a vision or mission to achieve certain goals. To reach those goals the assistance of others is needed. Initially these others are followers in the sense that they are persuaded that the leader's goals are both worthwhile and of interest. "Such leaders energize and motivate their followers to achieve their goals, share their visions, and embrace empowerment" (Grimm, 2010, p. 76). Several characteristics have been noted as important for effective transformational leadership: (1) Transformational leaders have charisma—others are fascinated by them and inclined toward their ideas; (2) they are self-motivated in relation to their goals (internal locus of control) and inspire others accordingly; (3) they are intellectually curious and willing to challenge assumptions or be challenged; and (4) their attention is individualized and focused on the needs of followers. They act as mentors and coaches (Chemers, 2001; Grimm, 2010; Judge & Piccolo, 2004; Murphy, 2005).

Characteristics of Effective Leadership

There are certain leadership traits that are found in many good leaders. Kirkpatrick and Locke (1991) identified six core characteristics that the majority of effective leaders possess:

1. **Drive**—Leaders are ambitious and take initiative.
2. **Motivation**—Leaders want to lead and are willing to take charge.
3. **Honesty and integrity**—Leaders are truthful and do what they say they will do.
4. **Self-confidence**—Leaders are assertive and decisive and enjoy taking risks. They admit mistakes and foster trust and commitment to a vision. Leaders are emotionally stable rather than recklessly adventurous.
5. **Cognitive ability**—Leaders are intelligent, perceptive, and conceptually skilled but are not necessarily geniuses. They show analytical ability, good judgment, and the capacity to think strategically.
6. **Business knowledge**—Leaders tend to have technical expertise in their businesses.

In addition to these characteristics, the nature of the APN role inevitably also requires well-honed communication and mediation skills. Communication skills are needed for the comprehensive and appropriate exchange of information, and mediation skills are needed to offset conflicts caused by individual personality and perspectival differences within a group, especially a multidisciplinary group. Interdisciplinary collaborative efforts require that all members of a working group have their perspectives and ideas heard. This means drawing out the voices of the reticent and restraining the input of the overly insistent in a respectful and dignity-preserving way. This facilitates collaborative efforts that are egalitarian (Grace, Willis, & Jurchak, 2007). Other commentators (Grimm, 2010; Lachman, 2007) on leadership for nursing purposes have added the characteristic of moral courage. Moral courage is a necessary characteristic of nurse leaders who "hold true to their beliefs and convictions" (Grimm, 2010, p. 75) even when it is risky to do so. However, the risks taken are calculated and rational. Moreover, leaders have "ethical fitness." Ethical fitness means they reflect on the values and beliefs that underlie their own thoughts and actions with the intent of understanding prejudices and biases and accounting for them.

The Goals of Nursing: Advanced Practice Leadership

Throughout this text, the responsibilities of APNs are described as firmly grounded in the idea that first and foremost an APN is a member of the nursing profession and bound by the code of ethics of the profession. Codes of ethics are developed by the profession as public articulations of the services provided and the expected conduct of nurses in the course of their nursing work. Although the nursing bodies of many countries have developed their own country-specific codes of ethics, the nursing organizations of these countries also had input in and affirm the ICN's code of ethics (ICN, 2012). The internationally specified goals of nursing are to promote health, prevent illness, restore health, and alleviate suffering (ICN, 2012). Meeting these goals for individuals and groups may require anticipatory proactivity (analyzing the status quo or proposed policy changes for their likely effects), ethical perception or discernment (that things are not right and why), and moral agency (actions toward change). Every nursing action taken should be aimed at furthering one of these nursing goals for an individual, a particular society, or sometimes on an international level (as in nurses involved with global issues). When working conditions, the environment, or other influences block the ability to further these goals, nurses have further obligations (Grace, 2001). At the APN level, these responsibilities include ethical leadership for change. Ethical leadership by the APN means that he or she uses knowledge, skills, and influence to lead a group of persons (perhaps other nurses or perhaps an interdisciplinary group) toward a shared goal of improving an aspect of health care or healthcare delivery. Many experienced and thoughtful nurses without advanced preparation have proven themselves as effective leaders—changing practice and environments, and influencing health policy—but APNs are especially well prepared to serve as leaders. The ICN's nurse practitioner/advanced practice nursing network has recognized some unifying aspects of the role internationally:

> Integrates research, education, practice and management,
> High degree of professional autonomy and independent practice,
> Case Management/own case load,
> Advanced health assessment skills, decision-making skills and diagnostic reasoning skills,
> Recognized advanced clinical competencies,
> Provision of consultant services to other health providers,
> Plans, implements and evaluates programs,
> Recognized first point of contact for clients. (ICN, 2009)

Although not listed explicitly, these role expectations clearly depend on leadership abilities. Advanced education is widely recognized as critical for the APN role.

The Doctor of Nursing Practice

In the United States, there has been a recent drive to educate APNs at a higher level. Initially the goal was that all master's degree programs would convert to the Doctor of Nursing Practice (DNP) degree by 2015. The DNP degree is distinguished from a research doctorate in that it is aimed at preparing practitioners to provide institutional leadership and also serve as educators rather than researchers, although they may still be involved in research. Since the DNP was formally approved by the AACN in 2004, well over 90 programs have been launched (Edwardson, 2011). The focus of the practice doctorate is to improve outcomes "for individuals or populations, including the direct care of individual patients, management of care for individuals and populations, administration of nursing and healthcare organizations, and the development and implementation of health policy" (AACN, 2004, p. 1).

The DNP degree is controversial, having both critics and supporters. The "pro" positions assert that added education helps nurses fill certain gaps or shortcomings in healthcare provision. Magyary, Whitney, and Brown (2006) assert that the existence of a DNP degree is very important in that it will equip nursing leaders and managers with the wherewithal to critically question practice status quo and underlying assumptions in order to influence future practices. To this end, the degree includes additional courses in leadership, management, financing, health informatics, and policy (AACN, 2006). A major focus is on improving health outcomes and engaging in practice improvement projects. Additionally, DNPs are able to fill clinical faculty positions. In the United States, there is a serious shortage of qualified faculty (AACN, 2012). Moreover, it is thought that this advanced education will remove barriers to autonomous practice for nurses with advanced knowledge and skills. One other argument is that nursing master's degrees are already very course heavy beyond that of almost any other academic master's degree because of curricular and clinical practice requirements; thus it is not a very big step to add a few more courses that would put the DNP in line with other professional practice doctorates such as pharmacy and physical therapy.

The "con" arguments are from various sources both within and outside of the discipline. The medical community has been fairly vocal in its opposition in the media and in academic journals. There are worries that the DNP role will increase confusion for patients as nurses' roles and physicians' roles are more closely interactive than those of other professions (Miller, 2008). Additionally, nurse scholars worry that these APNs will lose their focus on nursing goals. Concerns about interprofessional conflicts include the deleterious effects on patient care and collaborative relationships, which are essential for projects that require both nursing and medical knowledge for their success (Miller, 2008).

While it is important for U.S. APNs to understand the issues related to the DNP so that they can discuss them in interdisciplinary forums, the most important point for any nurse who is working in an APN role is to stay mindful of the fact that it is a nursing rather than a medical role and, as such, be guided by nursing's perspectives and goals regarding human health. Moreover, the leadership responsibilities that accompany these roles mean that APNs may need to help and collaborate with others in order to envision good practice and work toward good outcomes. In the inevitably interdisciplinary settings where advanced nursing is practiced, staying focused on nursing goals and perspectives may be the most difficult task. There will be many distracting influences. Another difficult task is articulating to others what it is that nurses bring to patient care and policy discussions that is different from, and complementary to, the contributions of allied health professionals and physicians (Grace et al., 2007).

The Institute of Medicine's Report

In the United States, a recent exploration of the status of nursing commissioned by the IOM, an independent, nonprofit, multidisciplinary organization, resulted in the report, *The Future of Nursing: Leading Change, Advancing*

Health (IOM, 2011). The report emphasizes the importance of the profession to the nation's health. In the preface it is asserted "[W]e believe nurses have key roles to play as team members and leaders for a reformed and better-integrated, patient-centered health care system" (IOM, 2011, p. xii). A summary of the report (IOM, 2010) outlines four key messages; two of them are especially focused on advanced practice. Key Message #1 contends that nurses should be able to practice to the full extent of their education and training. Over a quarter of a million nurses are now educated at an advanced level. Thus legal restrictions placed on nursing practice by individual states should be questioned. Leaders in nursing are called upon to advocate and lobby for state boards of nursing and legislatures to remove practice restrictions imposed by other health professionals. Key Message #3 argues that nurses should be considered full partners with physicians and other health professionals in redesigning health care in the United States. Full partnership implies equality of voice and influence. That is, nursing's perspective on the health of persons should receive parity of expression and consideration in multidisciplinary assemblages. As discussed earlier, the DNP is one movement aimed at enhancing nursing practice and making visible the particular perspective and expertise of nurses.

Enhancing APN Leadership

There are ongoing questions about who is or can be a leader. Some people are obvious leaders; some might even say they are "born leaders." But the question remains if leadership is possible for all APNs. The answer has to be yes. Leadership is possible for all, but the level of leadership may differ depending on setting and goals. Earlier a reminder was given of the nature and extent of APNs' responsibilities for individual and societal health. This is what makes all leadership ethical. APNs must have some capacity for taking the lead in furthering these goals. Otherwise they cannot be said to have ethical responsibilities. In order to be held ethically responsible, choices in action must exist. Many, many books have described leadership models and leader characteristics or traits. Seminars to develop leaders are offered within institutions, outside institutions, sometimes even by employers or contracted by employers for their employees. Nurses should avail themselves of opportunities to develop and refine their own leadership skills and behaviors. Arguments about whether leadership skills can be learned or whether natural personal traits are required for leadership continue; however, leadership behaviors that are regularly practiced can become well-honed skills, just like other skills developed for nursing practice. Case examples of leadership behaviors and the education and skills underlying them are given shortly.

APN Leadership Expectations

This next part of the discussion assumes that leadership by APNs is both an expectation and an ethical activity. For nursing, all leadership activities have ethical content. They are directed toward the ultimate goals of protecting and promoting health and relieving suffering using nursing's perspectives, whether at the individual level or at unit, clinic, or health-policy levels. The Canadian Nurse Practitioner Core Competency Framework (Canadian Nurses Association [CAN], 2010, p. 10) is directed at the nurse practitioner (NP) role but exemplifies (with the exception of the NP-specific criteria) leadership expectations for APNs in general. They include: effective "management of clinical care and [serves as] a resource person, educator and role model". The NP mentors other nurses, peers, and interdisciplinary team members. He or she should be able to explain the nuances and benefits of advanced practice roles to others including allied "health-care providers, social and public service sectors, the public, legislators and policy-makers". As an essential aspect of the role, the NP "[A]dvocates for and participates in creating an organizational environment that supports safe client care, collaborative practice and professional growth" and "provides leadership in the development and implementation of standards, practice guidelines, quality assurance, and education and research initiatives". At the public and health policy level the NP is responsible for activities that inform and influence decision-making.

To insist to the new APN graduate that leadership is an expected responsibility within the role may be unrealistic initially. The new graduate in a direct patient care role is orienting to a new clinical environment, with many processes and expectations to master. One antecedent of good leadership is an understanding of the environment. However, once an APN is in the role for a period of time, clinical or policy concerns become evident. It is at this time that leadership skills are needed to implement the needed changes. One of the assumptions reinforcing this reality is stated in the Canadian

Nurse Practitioner Core Competency Framework (CAN, 2010, p. 7, #10): "Newly graduated nurse practitioners gain proficiency in the breadth and depth of their practice over time, with support from employers, mentors and health-care team members." Sherman (2013), however, encourages younger nurses to seek leadership opportunities and describes a competency model used for nursing leadership development. The Nurse Manager Leadership Partnership's (NMLP) Learning Domain Framework was developed by the American Organization of Nurse Executives, the Association of periOperative Registered Nurses, and the American Association of Critical-Care Nurses. The model's key domains include the science and art of leadership and the development of the "leader within." Shirey's (2007) discussion accords with Sherman's argument. She likens leadership development to that found in Benner's work on the development of nurses from novice to expert that occurs over time. However, Shirey's leadership development model maintains that the successful attainment of leadership competencies is more important than years of experience. Leadership abilities are developed on the same continuum from novice to expert, and leaders are frequently in roles where they have no particular leadership competencies. To progress to competence, these leaders need access to leadership learning opportunities or to identify mentors who can guide them. The American Nurses Association (2013) is building a cadre of nurse leaders through its Leadership Institute, which offers a series of five webinars (interactive conferences). This institute covers five key areas: strategic thinking, results-oriented leadership, leading people, personal leadership, and unleashing innovation and creativity. Implied qualities or skills underlying the key areas are those of making connections with others, communicating well (skills of listening and articulation), mediating conflicts, and motivating others.

Models of Leadership Useful for Nursing

EMPOWERMENT

In the past, the nursing profession and its members have sometimes been, or have seen themselves as being, disempowered for a variety of reasons including that nursing is a predominantly female profession (Manojlovich, 2007; Matheson and Bobay, 2007). Thus, an empowerment model of leadership make sense to use when educating nurses to be leaders. The theoretical basis for the empowerment model is found in Paulo Freire's critical pedagogy of the oppressed. Freire's contention is that the oppressed must be made aware of their position and the reasons they are oppressed in order to be able to transcend the oppression. The oppressed must be willing to rethink their way of life and to examine their own role in oppression if true liberation is to occur. This insight allows the oppressed to regain a sense of dignity and become empowered to act (Freire, 1970). Freire was interested in liberating oppressed members of a society to enhance their situation. The nursing profession has two related tasks in regard to empowerment; (1) it must facilitate the empowerment of it members, (2) so that they can provide needed and promised (via codes of ethics) services. A nursing study (MacPhee, Skelton-Green, Bouthillette, & Suryaprakash, 2011) from Canada describes a nursing leadership intervention with a theoretical empowerment framework. This framework was chosen because, according to the author's research, structural and psychological empowerment resulted in safer work environments. This model was effective in developing nurse leaders by demonstrating how to remove organizational (structural) barriers and instill confidence (psychological) that the nurses had control and influence over their work environments. Empowered nurses can empower others. The outcome of the study was that nurse leaders reported "increased self-confidence with respect to carrying out their roles and responsibilities, positive changes in their leadership styles, and increased recognition of staff for positive stylistic changes" (p. 159).

EMANCIPATORY

Emancipatory leadership is another model of leadership utilized in nursing. Emancipatory leadership involves integrated knowing being brought to bear on an environment to transform it. This model of leadership draws on Carper's ways of knowing and extends them to include socio-political knowledge as described by White (1995). From Barbara Carper's (1978) extensive review of the nursing literature, she identified four interrelated patterns of knowing that nurses use to achieve nursing purposes. The ways of knowing are empirics (the science of nursing knowledge of facts and evidence), esthetics (the art of nursing), ethics (what are good actions), and personal (self-knowledge). Chinn and Kramer (2008) argued that integrated knowledge permits nurses (as well as others) to free themselves from situations that limit ethical actions (see **Figure 5-1**).

Jackson, Clements, Averill, and Zimbro (2009) proposed that each of the areas of knowing could also be considered knowledge required for nursing

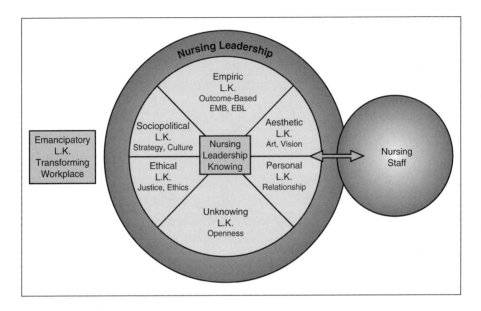

■ Figure 5-1   Nursing Leadership Knowing (N.L.K.) Model

Source: Jackson, J., Clements, P., Averill, J., & Zimbro, K. (2009). Patterns of knowing: A theory for nursing leadership. *Nursing Economics, 27*(3), 149–159.

leadership. Empirical knowing facilitates appropriate and comprehensive data collection, analysis, and evaluation. Esthetic knowing can be considered the art of leadership and includes empathic understanding of others and what might motivate them. Personal knowing is essential for ethical leadership. It is the ability to know one's self and be authentic; it is the cultivation of reflectiveness to listen and evaluate one's presence as a leader. Ethical knowing supports the core values of nursing and the conduct that supports those values. The leader is responsible for the moral environment in which nursing is practiced. This includes respect for patients and colleagues. Arries (2009) found that student nurses judged their interactions with other nurses as unjust in terms of fairness and quality of the interpersonal treatment in comparison to another person or standard. Ethical leadership requires intervention when unethical behaviors occur in the workplace. Leadership is needed for the promotion of justice, fairness, and respect for persons in the workplace and other environments in which nursing is influential. Nursing leaders, however, are also frequently required to intervene beyond their immediate area of concern or comfort. Their contributions may be needed to impact an institutional or political system where laws and healthcare justifications are made. Effective nurse leaders are knowledgeable about rules, regulations, and policies governing nursing practice, and they collaborate with others to modify them as needed. This is socio-political knowing. There are times when the leader does not know the answer or the direction in which to move, and acknowledgment of knowledge limits is a characteristic of the good leader. These integrated ways of knowing are possessed by effective nursing leaders and used to transform the workplace. Transformation of problem practice environments and healthcare policies requires emancipatory leadership.

Levels of Leadership

Gallagher and Tschudin (2010)—the current and former editors of the international *Nursing Ethics* journal, respectively—delineate levels of nursing's ethical leadership into the following:

> the micro-level—where nurses provide leadership as role models in their work with individuals and teams
>
> the meso-level—where nurses contribute to organisational discussions and policy development; and
>
> the macro-level—where nurses engage politically, lobbying politicians and ensuring that their voice is heard in national and international forums (Gallagher & Tschudin, 2010, p. 225).

How leadership plays out at each of these levels is exemplified by real life cases shortly. Importantly, Gallagher and Tschudin argue that "the meaning of ethical leadership begins with self (personal) knowledge especially of one's emotional and practical boundaries" (p. 225). They also highlight the reality that nurses who understand their professional responsibilities and when necessary assume a leadership role may sometimes opt to "follow" and support another who they wisely recognize as better able to achieve a mutually shared purpose. Thus leaders are sometimes followers. "Life is a constant stream of responses in conversations and to events, and how we respond to people with whom we talk, or to items of personal or media-generated news, depends largely on values that have been acquired through upbringing, culture, training, or deliberate choice. These are not static aspirations, however, and to remain ethically alive, change is necessary in order to make the fitting response in a given situation" (p. 225).

Facilitators of and Barriers to Ethical Leadership in Nursing Practice

Barriers to ethical leadership are environments that do not support nursing's goals for the good of the patient. In those environments, there are frequently no leaders who are role models for addressing the issues or barriers to good care. Nurses in these environments do not feel as though they have the ability to control their own practice or workplace. When leaders arise from these environments, it is from their own intrinsic motivation that they act and make a difference. However, nurses and even APNs may feel inadequately prepared educationally to take on a leadership role (Curtis et al., 2011).

Facilitators of ethical leadership in nursing practice are the same as those that support ethical nursing practice or environments that have the patient's, group's, or perhaps society's good as the motivator of every action. These include supportive unit or clinic structures, strong collegial and collaborative relationships, adequate preparation, and strong mentors. Other facilitators mentioned previously include leadership development academies or educational opportunities for nurse leadership. Contemporarily, there are many examples of all levels of nursing leadership, although the public visibility of such leaders may not always be as high as deserved. Nevertheless, the difference made in peoples' lives is real and often profound.

Cognitive Processes Underlying Nursing Leadership

Ethical leadership for nurses in advanced practice roles means taking action to meet nursing goals for patients, patient groups, and society and engaging and motivating necessary others in the interest of a successful outcome. The leadership process in turn can be described in terms of Rest's cognitive processes. Rest (1982) derived a model of the cognitive processes needed for ethical action—as described or exhibited by the individuals studied—from research literature. Rest is clear that this process is not a guarantee of ethically correct action, but rather is a description of what happens in the brain of a person who is motivated to do the right thing. The processes are as follows: first, a problem that has ethical aspects is perceived and interpreted; second, pertinent knowledge and analytic skills are mobilized to determine what possible appropriate courses of action exist; third, actions are planned and initiated; and finally, the person perseveres even in the face of adversity to achieve desired goals.

Historical and Contemporary Nursing Leaders

Each nursing leader listed in this section exhibited the qualities that are needed for ethical leadership. However, their environments were such that these early leaders sometimes had to be more autocratic than egalitarian in their leadership actions. All perceived a problem that interfered with human well-being—an ethical problem—and determined that the problem had to be addressed. They used knowledge, skills, and decision-making processes to determine what possible courses of action were appropriate. They carefully planned their actions, enlisting the assistance of powerful and/or influential others as needed. Finally, they persevered until nursing goals were actualized.

Leadership at the Macro or Health-Policy Level

Florence Nightingale saw that soldiers from the Crimean War were dying of typhus and cholera in far greater numbers than soldiers who were dying of wounds. She understood that these were needless deaths and also what was needed to lessen the death toll. But she met resistance from the military doctors and leaders. She used data, influence, and persuasion in order to be allowed to change the situation. She and her nurses travelled to the front lines, where they activated sanitation measures that were successful in reducing the death rate by two-thirds (Lee, Clark, & Thompson, 2013).

Mary Breckenridge was born to a wealthy Kentucky family. She was aware of the terrible deprivations suffered by the poor people in the Appalachian states, especially the high infant mortality rate. Having suffered many losses herself and having been exposed to the work of the British nurse-midwives in France during World War I, she was determined to get the education she needed to change the situation. Using a model of care she had witnessed during her nursing education in Scotland and funding it out of her own money-raising efforts, she set up a decentralized system of clinics staffed by nurse-midwives from the United Kingdom who went out to the homes of patients to give primary health and midwifery care. Eventually as the U.K. nurses left for home, she set up a school in Kentucky to educate the first U.S. nurse-midwives (American Society of Registered Nurses, 2007).

Other examples of nurse leaders in the United States can be found at the American Academy of Nursing website, *Raise the Voice. Edge Runners.* All of these APN nurses "are the practical innovators who have led the way in bringing new thinking and new methods to a wide range of healthcare challenges. Edge Runners have developed care models and interventions that demonstrate significant, sustained clinical and financial outcomes. Many of the stories underscore the courage and fighting spirit of nurse leaders who have persevered despite institutional inertia or resistance" (American Academy of Nursing, n.d.). Additionally, scattered throughout the IOM's report, *The Future of Nursing: Leading Change, Advancing Health*, are more examples of leadership, almost exclusively demonstrated by APNs (IOM, 2011).

Leadership at the Meso Level: Contributions to Organization Discussion and Policy

Two APNs with whom the second author of the chapter (Grace) has collaborated on ethics-related projects—Ellen Robinson, Clinical Nurse Specialist in Ethics at Massachusetts General (MGH) and Martha Jurchak, Executive Director of the Ethics Service at Brigham and Women's Hospital (BWH) in Boston, Massachusetts—are exemplars of transformational leadership at the institutional level. In the necessarily interdisciplinary settings of their institutions, they provide ethics leadership that is aimed at including consideration of all relevant perspectives. In addition, both have been instrumental in mentoring other staff and APNs to institute interdisciplinary ethics rounds and ethics on their units in the interests of good care. Finally, Robinson, Jurchak, Grace, and MGH Chaplain Angelika Zollfrank, with funding from a U.S. Government Health Resources and Services Grant, were able to develop and put into practice a model of ethics education that enhances the confidence of point-of-care nurses and APNs in their ethical decision making and advocacy. This endeavor is called the Clinical Ethics Residency for Nurses (CERN).

On a recent visit to Switzerland, Grace met several APNs who had also exhibited leadership at the meso level. Hansruedi Stoll is a master's prepared oncology nurse and educator at the Universitätsspital Basel. His interest in informed consent issues led him to develop an outpatient program to help people interpret what they want from their lives. He notes, "this question also lies at the core of an advance directive . . . when asking a patient about his/her values, the plans and the question what makes my life worth living. Ultimately this all leads to the question what is my life worth to me.

This cannot be answered by a certain mg of an anticancer drug." Hansruedi also models this philosophy and approach with colleagues and students. Monica Fliedner is a master's prepared oncology/palliative care nurse at the University Hospital in Bern, Switzerland. Along with colleagues, she recognized the need for a dedicated palliative care unit in her hospital and was instrumental in proposing and collaboratively developing an inpatient palliative care unit in her institution where members of different disciplines work together to plan and provide the best care possible for patients.

Leadership at the Micro Level: APNs as Role Models in Their Work with Individuals and Teams

Ursi Barandun Schäfer is a clinical nurse specialist for the surgical intensive care unit at the Universitätsspital Basel. One of her many leadership activities involves using a model of ethical decision making developed by an interdisciplinary team, of which she was a member. This model guides unit nurses in their early identification of emerging ethical problems, analysis of the issues, and ways of collaboratively addressing the problem. In this sense, it serves as a preventive ethics strategy. Additionally, the authors of this chapter believe that APN educators have an obligation to mentor their students in leadership roles. Case analyses, group discussions, and role playing can all help to develop APN leadership characteristics. Such activities can be considered leadership at the micro level.

Summary

The nursing profession should encourage all nurses, particularly APNs, to be leaders. The content of APN education varies internationally, but the same critical skills are needed for leadership in health policy and public health, in addition to the clinical skills for direct care, in order to meet nursing's goals. Where any of these foci are not included in curricula, nurse educators need to lead the way in advocating for their inclusion. APN graduates are encouraged to seek additional opportunities for leadership development commensurate with their practice setting and associated leadership needs. As all leadership in nursing must be aimed at improving individual and societal health, an ethical nurse leader is one who takes this charge seriously, identifies deficits in the environment, and works for change that serves the needs of the population, whether it is an individual patient, group, society, or global concern. Nurses have unique perspectives on health care and the care needed for health. They should continue to involve themselves in contemporary healthcare debates and equip themselves to provide leadership for change.

Discussion Questions

1. Who are the nurse leaders in your country or state at the macro level? What are their characteristics? How did they achieve change?

2. Who are the effective leaders in your area of practice at the meso and micro levels? What are their characteristics? How did they achieve change?

3. What are the areas of knowledge needed contemporarily to provide leadership in the clinic environment or at the bedside?

4. Upon reflection, what do you feel you need to become a more confident, empowered leader? What skills/education is needed? How will you access those opportunities?

5. Thinking about your current context, what is one concern that needs to be addressed? Suggest several appropriate plans of action that may be instituted. Describe your motivation for the action and how you will persevere through adversity.

References

Aiken, L. H., Clarke, S. P., Cheung, R. B., Sloane, D. M., & Silber, J. H. (2003). Educational levels of hospital nurses and surgical patient mortality. *Journal of the American Medical Association, 290*, 1617–1623.

American Academy of Nursing. (n.d.). Raise the voice. Edge Runners. Retrieved from http://www.aannet.org/edgerunners

American Association of Colleges of Nursing. (2004). AACN position statement on the practice doctorate in nursing. Retrieved from http://www.aacn.nche.edu/publications/position/DNPpositionstatement.pdf

American Association of Colleges of Nursing. (2006). The essentials of doctoral education for advanced nursing practice. Retrieved from http:// www.aacn.nche.edu/publications/position/DNPEssentials.pdf

American Association of Colleges of Nursing. (2011). The essentials of master's education in nursing. Retrieved from www.aacn.nche.edu/education-resources/MastersEssentials11.pdf

American Association of Colleges of Nursing. (2012). Nursing faculty shortage fact sheet. Retrieved from http://www.aacn.nche.edu/media-relations/fact-sheets/nursing-faculty-shortage

American Nurses Association. (2013, March/April). Building a pipeline of nurse leaders. *The American Nurse*, 4.

American Society of Registered Nurses. (2007, November 1). Chronicle of nursing: Mary Breckenridge. Retrieved from http://www.asrn.org/journal-chronicle-nursing/206-mary-breckenridge.html

Arries, E. J. (2009). Interactional justice in student-staff nurse encounters. *Nursing Ethics, 16*, 147–160.

Benner, P., Sutphen, M., Leonard, V., & Day, L. (2009). *Educating nurses: A call for radical transformation*. Carnegie Foundation for the Advancement of Teaching. San Francisco, CA: Jossey-Bass.

Canadian Nurses Association. (2010). Canadian nurse practitioner core competency framework. Retrieved from http://rnantnu.ca/Portals/0/Competency_Framework_2010_e.pdf

Carper, B. (1978). Fundamental patterns of knowing in nursing. *Advances in Nursing Science, 1*(1), 13–23.

Chemers, M. M. (2001). The psychology of leadership. In N. J. Smelser & P. B. Baltes (Eds.), *International encyclopedia of the social and behavioral sciences* (pp. 8580–8583). Burlington, MA: Elsevier.

Chinn, P. L., & Kramer, M. K. (2008). *Integrated knowledge development in nursing* (7th ed.). St. Louis, MO: Elsevier-Mosby.

Curtis, E. A., de Vries, J., & Sheerin, F. K. (2011). Developing leadership in nursing: Exploring core factors. *British Journal of Nursing, 20*(5), 306–309.

Edwardson, S. R. (2011). Imagining the DNP role. In M. E. Zaccagnini & K. W. White (Eds.), *The doctor of nursing practice essentials: A new model for advanced nursing practice*. Sudbury, MA: Jones & Bartlett Learning.

Freire, P. (1970). *Pedagogy of the oppressed*. New York, NY: Herder and Herder.

Gallagher, A., & Tschudin, V. (2010). Educating for ethical leadership. *Nurse Education Today, 30*, 224–227.

Grace, P. J. (2001). Professional advocacy: Widening the scope of accountability. *Nursing Philosophy, 2*(2), 151–162.

Grace, P. J., Willis, D. G., & Jurchak, M. (2007). Good patient care: Egalitarian inter-professional collaboration as a moral imperative. *American Society of Bioethics and Humanities. Exchange, 10*(1), 8–9.

Grimm, J. W. (2010). Effective leadership: Making the difference. *Journal of Emergency Nursing, 36*(1), 74–77.

Howell, J. M., & Avolio, B. J. (1993). Transformational leadership, transactional leadership, locus of control, and support for innovation: Key predictors of consolidated business-unit performance. *Journal of Applied Psychology, 78*, 891–902.

Institute of Medicine. (2010). Report brief: The future of nursing: Leading change, advancing health. Retrieved from http://www.iom.edu/Reports/2010/The-Future-of-Nursing-Leading-Change-Advancing-Health/Report-Brief.aspx?page=2

Institute of Medicine. (2011). *The future of nursing: Leading change, advancing health*. Washington, DC: National Academies Press. Retrieved from http://www.nap.edu/openbook.php?record_id=12956&page=R12

International Council of Nurses. (2009). *Nursing matters. Nurse practitioner/advanced practice nurse: Definition and characteristics.* Geneva, Switzerland: Author. Retrieved from http://www.icn.ch/publications/advanced-practice/

International Council of Nurses. (2010). Leadership for change. Geneva, Switzerland: Author. Retrieved from http://www.icn.ch/pillarsprograms/leadership-for-change/

International Council of Nurses. (2012). *International Council of Nurses code of ethics for nurses.* Geneva, Switzerland: Author.

Jackson, J., Clements, P., Averill, J., & Zimbro, K. (2009). Patterns of knowing: A theory for nursing leadership. *Nursing Economics, 27*(3), 149–159.

Judge, T. R., & Piccolo, A. F. (2004). Transformational and transactional leadership: A meta-analytic test of their relative validity. *Journal of Applied Psychology, 89*(5), 755–768.

Kirkpatrick, S. A., & Locke, E. A. (1991). Leadership: Do traits really matter? *Academy of Management Executive, 5*(2), 48–60.

Lachman, V. D. (2007). Moral courage: A virtue in need of development? *MEDSURG Nursing, 16*(2), 131–133.

Lee, G., Clark, A. M., & Thompson, D. R. (2013). Florence Nightingale: Never more relevant than today. *Journal of Advanced Nursing, 69*(2), 245–246.

MacPhee, M., Skelton-Green, J., Bouthillette, F., & Suryaprakash, N. (2012). An empowerment framework for nursing leadership development: Supporting evidence. *Journal of Advanced Nursing, 68*(1), 159–169.

Magyary, D., Whitney, J. D., & Brown, M. A. (2006). Advancing practice inquiry: Research foundations of the practice doctorate in nursing. *Nursing Outlook, 54,* 139–151.

Manojlovich, M. (2007). Power and empowerment in nursing: Looking backward to inform the future. *Online Journal of Issues in Nursing, 12*(1). Retrieved from http://www.nursingworld.org/MainMenuCategories/ANAMarketplace/ANAPeriodicals/OJIN/TableofContents/Volume122007/No1Jan07/LookingBackwardtoInformtheFuture.asp

Matheson, L. K., & Bobay, K. (2007). Validation of oppressed group behaviors in nursing. *Journal of Professional Nursing, 23*(4), 226–234.

Miller, J. (2008). The doctor of nursing practice: Recognizing a need or graying the line between doctors and nurses? *The Medscape Journal of Medicine, 10*(11), 253. Retrieved from http://www.ncbi.nlm.nih.gov/pmc/articles/PMC2605113/?report=printable

Murphy, L. (2005). Transformational leadership: A cascading chain reaction. *Journal of Nursing Management, 13,* 128–136.

Pulcini, J., Jelic, M., Gul, R., & Loke, A. Y. (2010). An international survey on advanced practice nursing education, practice, and regulation. *Journal of Nursing Scholarship, 42,* 1, 31–39.

Rest, J. R. (1982). A psychologist looks at the teaching of ethics. *Hastings Center Report, 12*(1), 29–36.

Sherman, R. O. (2013). Too young to be a nurse leader? *American Nurse Today, 8*(1), 34–37.

Shirey, M. (2007). Competencies and tips for effective leadership: From novice to expert. *Journal of Nursing Administration, 37*(4), 167–170.

Sullivan, E. J., & Garland, G. (2010). *Practical leadership and management in nursing.* Harlow, UK: Pearson Education Limited.

United States Census Bureau, Department of Commerce. (2011). American community survey. Retrieved from http://www.census.gov/acs/www/

Weihrich, H., & Koontz, H. (2005). *Management: A global perspective* (11th ed.). Singapore: McGraw-Hill.

White, J. (1995). Patterns of knowing: Review, critique, and update. *Advances in Nursing Science, 17*(4), 73–86.

Willis, D. B., Grace, P. J., & Roy, C. (2008). A central unifying focus for the discipline: Facilitating humanization, meaning, choice, quality of life and healing in living and dying. *Advances in Nursing Science, 31*(1), E28–E40.

Zaccagnini, M. E., & White, K. W. (2011). *The doctor of nursing practice essentials: A new model for advanced practice nursing.* Sudbury, MA: Jones & Bartlett Learning.

CHAPTER 6

Research Ethics: Advanced Practice Roles and Responsibilities

Pamela J. Grace

Science has given to this generation the means of unlimited disaster or of unlimited progress. There will remain the greater task of directing knowledge lastingly toward the purpose of peace and human good.
—SIR WINSTON CHURCHILL, speech, New Delhi, January 3, 1944

Man who lives in a world of hazards is compelled to seek for security.
—JOHN DEWEY, The Quest for Certainty, 1980

Introduction

The Aims of Research

The preceding quote is from Dewey's (1929/1980) set of lectures entitled *The Quest for Certainty*. Dewey, a philosopher of the American Pragmatist School, observed that it is characteristic of human nature to seek control over, and thus stability in, the experienced world. This inherent drive has produced philosophers and empirical scientists. *Empirical* means planned and structured observations of experiences and nature. Philosophers try to make logical sense of the world and discover meaning via reasoning (thought), and scientists have tried both to make sense of the world through formal methods of study and experimentation (action) and more recently to control aspects of the world using their discoveries. The distinction between science and philosophy is somewhat artificial because many philosophers have also engaged in practical experiments, philosophical inquiry is important in challenging the underlying assumptions of an empirical endeavor and in conceptualizing important questions that can be studied empirically, and philosophically derived theories often provide the foundation for empirical studies. As Dewey (1929/1980) noted, "The problem of philosophy concerns the *interaction* of our judgments about ends to be sought with knowledge of the means for achieving them. Just as in science the question of the advance of knowledge is the question of *what to do*, what experiments to perform, what apparatus to invent and use. . . . [T]he problem of practice is what do we need to *know*, how shall we obtain that knowledge and how shall we apply it?" (p. 37), and these are philosophical questions.

Records show that the human quest for knowledge of both kinds—theoretical and practical—dates back to as early as the era of the pre-Socratic Greek philosophers, that is, from roughly the sixth and fifth centuries B.C. (Wheelwright, 1988). The human ability to satisfy this drive has been increasing in sophistication over the past two and a half millennia. Over the past few centuries, the human ability to study the natural world has accelerated rapidly as a result of technological and biological knowledge development. Often innovations occur so rapidly that they outpace society's ability to come to terms with the philosophical and ethical implications of them. Philosophical inquiry historically involves asking questions about observed events, phenomena, and human characteristics. It attempts to analyze their elements to discover relationships and causes. Wheelwright (1988) argues that there are three fundamental human drives underlying philosophical inquiries. He concludes this from a review and synthesis of historical philosophical writings. One of the drives is the religious drive to discover what is "greater and more excellent" (p. 2) than man. Explorations and questions that result from this drive constitute the study of metaphysics or attempts to understand what, if anything, underlies or transcends the physical world. For example, questions about whether there is a creator or overseer of the universe are metaphysical questions not directly observable in nature. The second drive is the scientific quest to understand physical matter, measurement (for example, how to divide property and how to quantify things), and the relationship of the stars and solar system to earth. Thus, philosophy and research are intimately related and can be seen as different sides of the same coin. A third drive can also be identified in historical as well as contemporary literature, and that is the human quest for self-understanding.

Contemporary researchers have built upon previous knowledge developments and/or used their imaginations, undoubtedly fed by prior experiences, to derive new questions and ideas that can then be tested for soundness or validity. They have used increasingly sophisticated tools to carry out in-depth explorations of the nature of the world and of human beings. The results of these explorations include innovations that, although they have the capacity to do much good, also possess the power to do harm. Risks are exacerbated when innovations are used without deliberative forethought or mindfulness of their possible impact on individuals, society, and in some cases the world. This is the status of research generally, and of human subjects research, particularly. The results of research endeavors have greatly improved the human potential for living a good life, but unethical research has caused immeasurable suffering. Moreover, evidence suggests that abuses are ongoing and it requires constant vigilance by the research community, ethicists, and involved healthcare professionals to anticipate problems and maintain both research integrity and the safety and well-being of subjects.

The Aims of Research Involving Human Subjects

In human subjects research, the temptation and tendency of researchers to lose sight of the ultimate goals of research—the promotion of human good—have been well documented (Emanuel & Miller, 2007; Swazey, Anderson, & Louis, 1993; illustrative examples are given later). Research aimed at developing knowledge about and for human beings logically derives its focus from the idea that facilitating the human good is a worthy goal. The research community, professionals who design studies or use research findings, and society—via its philosophers, activists, and citizens—all bear responsibility for ensuring that the focus on human good is maintained. Vigilance and mindfulness of the ease with which a research goal can become perverted are needed to prevent the true aims of human subjects research from fading in the course of the research process. Additionally, it does not make sense to ignore or discount a given individual participant's needs so that a greater societal good can be achieved, because individual human beings make up the greater society, and without individuals society would not exist. If consideration for any given individual is not of strong concern, what are the grounds for asserting that the ends of research are best aimed at a societal good? Moreover, a lack of focus on individual good in societal arrangements, research, or healthcare practice makes all members of society more than ordinarily vulnerable to the vagaries of life (Sellman, 2005).

Ironically, perhaps, research completed in the cognitive, psychological, and social sciences has supported the idea that the motivation and disposition of human beings to good action can be influenced both by internal factors and situational aspects (Doris and The Moral Psychology Research Group, 2011; Zimbardo, 2005). (This will be discussed in more detail later in the chapter.) Knowledge developments in these and other disciplines, stimulated in part by the long history of the abuse of human beings by others in their species, support the idea that it is easy for human beings either not to recognize the moral components of human interaction or to stray from the moral path related to treatment of their fellow human beings. Arguably, the most difficult task for those in human services professions or engaged in human subjects research is that of staying true to the purpose of the work. There are many circumstances or situations that can cause a loss of focus on the ultimate aim of research on human beings.

Research-Related Roles of the Advanced Practice Nurse

As healthcare professionals, advanced practice nurses (APNs) may be involved in all aspects of human subjects research, from study design to the use of the knowledge gained in practice settings. APNs may contribute unanswered questions that arise from practice experiences. They may assist in research studies or oversee the clinical aspects of them. Their patients may be subjects of research or request advice about whether enrolling in a given study is prudent in light of their health concerns. APNs may even be the designers and principal investigators for a study. As APNs working in nursing roles, the profession's goals provide the foundation for all actions and take priority over all other concerns when conflicts occur. The profession's goals give nurses a point of view from which to advocate for the patient/subject's or healthy subject's safety and ongoing informed consent to participate. APNs who work in clinical research settings are not subject to different rules or responsibilities. Responsibilities relate to individual good as well as societal good and are not to be subverted by the goals of scientists and other professionals, whether serving as researchers or otherwise (American Nurses Association [ANA], 1994; International Council of Nurses, [ICN], 2011). Further, nurses do a majority of the work in human subjects research settings. As a result of their study of research nurses working in diverse settings and areas of the United States, DeBruin, Liaschenko, and Fisher (2011) argued that there is a "need to refine the oversight system for trials to reflect an understanding of [the] day-to-day work" (p. 121), much of which falls to nurses. Nurses may be the only ones who see the day-to-day problems in carrying out research safely in the face of many confounding factors. Over the past few years serving as an ethics advisor for the nurses working in the clinical research center of a major Boston hospital, the critical advocacy role of research nurses has become clear to me.

The next section explores the history of human subjects research, high-lighting the source and nature of benefits and abuses. It traces regulatory efforts to overcome the ethical issues inherent in human subjects research settings. Finally, the chapter uses cases and examples to illustrate issues that APNs may face in their various roles related to the conception and conduct of research and the use of research findings in practice. The cases serve as a springboard for discussion and clarification. Some strategies for dealing with unethical conduct in the context of human subjects research are proposed.

Background: Human Subjects Research

Definition of Research

Although most professionals in healthcare settings probably feel that they have a good grasp of the meaning of human subjects research based on their experiences with research protocols and from reading research findings, what constitutes human subjects research is not always clear cut. Some studies that do not seem to involve a risk to persons, perhaps because they do not involve a direct interaction with a human being, may nevertheless present some danger—perhaps the data gathered can be misused and add to a person's vulnerability. For example, revealing genetic information or the probability of developing a disease may jeopardize a person's ability to obtain work, or health or life insurance depending on country of residence and types of protective regulations in effect. It may create psychological burdens and subject persons to bias and prejudice. Genetic information gained about one person also may carry implications for another person's privacy. For further discussion of ethical problems associated with genetic information see Chapter 9 on women's health. APNs' professional goals, as discussed throughout this text, have to do with providing a good for individuals, and in so doing APNs must also be careful to minimize the possible harms that could come from their actions. Thus the APN's inter-ests in research endeavors are necessarily focused on the impact, negative or positive, of the given research on the well-being of persons. This requires diligence, vigilance, and rigor in uncovering the hidden implications—long term and short term—of innovations for the lives of individual human beings and for society. The next section provides information about the history of human research and its abuses as a foundation for developing confidence in decision making when research issues are an aspect of the practice environment.

In the United States, research is defined by the federal government in the Code of Federal Regulations (CFR) as a "systematic investigation, including research development, testing and evaluation, designed to develop or contribute to generalizable knowledge" (National Institutes of Health, Office for Human Research Protections, 2004). This definition is broad and not confined to human subjects research. A more particular definition given in the CFR demarcates a human subject as "a living individual about whom an investigator (whether professional or student) conducting research obtains (1) Data through intervention or interaction with the individual, or (2) Identifiable private information" (National Institutes of Health, Office for Human Research Protections, 2004).

The term *intervention* includes both physical procedures by which data are gathered (e.g., venipuncture) and manipulations of a subject or a subject's environment that are performed for research purposes. *Interaction* includes communication or interpersonal contact between an investigator and a subject. *Private information* includes information about behavior that occurs in a context in which an individual can reasonably expect that no observation or recording is taking place, and information that has been provided for specific purposes by an individual and that the individual can reasonably expect will not be made public (e.g., a medical record). Private information must be individually identifiable (i.e., the identity of the subject is or may readily be ascertained by the investigator or associated with the information) in order to obtain the information to constitute research involving human subjects. (National Institutes of Health, Office for Human Research Protections, 2004)

Together these two definitions delineate what is meant by human subjects research. This definition is supported in principle by the research governing bodies of other countries and implicitly by the World Medical Association (WMA, 2008). The ensuing discussion uses this description, along with the APN's professional responsibilities as discussed in earlier chapters, to explore the history of human subjects research, its uses and abuses, as well as contemporary implications for advanced nursing practice.

The Historical Development of Research Ethics

Human Subjects Research: Researcher Motivations

Evidence suggests that human vivisection took place in ancient Rome with the probable aim of understanding more about the human body. Vivisection is the dissection or cutting up of live beings. The literature extensively supports the idea that since ancient times research efforts have been viewed as important, and the development of research methods and tools has continued through the ages. There is, however, also a long history of what is currently referred to as human subject abuses. These abuses are indicative of several attitudes: (1) the predisposition on the part of researchers toward furthering the social good even when this may be risky for individual participants; (2) a disposition to gain knowledge by whatever means necessary (human subjects are not a significant moral concern); (3) the belief that certain classes of persons (slaves, minorities, lower classes) are not as worthy of concern as are others; (4) the perspective that some groups of persons are disposable and thus expedient objects of research (e.g., the Nazi experiments); or (5) a desire/pressure to fulfill personal/professional ambition.

There are areas of overlap among these attitudes, and the following general categories of disregard for human subjects may evidence more than one of them. Grasping this point is important for APNs in considering the source of problems with research integrity.

1. *Society versus individuals.* Public health or societal interests in healthy people have often provided the impetus for research endeavors that involve populations. These studies try to understand how to prevent, attenuate, or cure diseases that are either serious or pervasive in the population (e.g., cardiovascular diseases) or affect large numbers of people (e.g., infectious diseases). History has shown that sometimes in the urgency to resolve pressing societal problems, the interests of individuals have been trampled. Katz (1992) documents the comments of a Swedish investigator who used young children as subjects in a variola vaccine experiment: "[P]erhaps I should have first experimented upon animals, but calves—most suitable for these purposes—were difficult to obtain because of their cost and their keep" (p. 230). This attitude signifies a fairly common theme in research aimed at stopping the ravages or spread of communicable diseases; vaccines have often been developed and tested on healthy persons, frequently children. Testing has not always involved knowledgeable consent. Indeed, many of these studies involved healthy children who were not of an age where they could be considered developmentally capable of processing the information necessary for understanding. These efforts have been termed "challenge studies" (Hope & McMillan, 2004). Perhaps the most well-known of these studies is Jenner's inoculation with cowpox (a mild form of smallpox discovered in cows) of an 8-year-old boy,

James Phipps. This took place in 1796. When Phipps recovered from the cowpox, he was then inoculated with smallpox without ill effect. It had been noted that milkmaids who had had cowpox did not seem to succumb to smallpox—a much deadlier disease.

2. *Knowledge for its own sake.* Some scientists have been interested in seeing if their theories are right regardless of, or perhaps despite, their ability to further human good or cause harm. Although most scientists involved in human subjects research would probably deny that they have any but the most altruistic motives for their research, historically knowledge developments related to the human psyche point to the possibility of other motives, whether these are conscious and/or subconscious. The most infamous example of research carried out without any intention of benefit to its subjects is the Nazi's experimentation on concentration camp inmates. Experiments included grafting bone and muscle tissue from one person to another to study nerve regeneration, immersion in freezing water to track the limits of human endurance, the effects of poison, and more (Jewish Virtual Library, 2008). In fact, many such studies were aimed at helping the war effort by understanding the effects of adverse conditions upon the armed forces.

3. *Inequality of moral concern and perceived disposability.* Some segments of society have historically been more susceptible to research abuses related to their subservient status or vulnerability to the whims or design of others. Savitt (2001) notes that, especially in the old South, slaves "were considered more available and more accessible [for experimentation purposes] . . . they were rendered physically visible by their skin color but were legally invisible because of their slave status" (p. 215). Axelsen (2001) describes Dr. Marion Sims (1813–1883), the "father of gynecology," as having shown a "shocking disregard for the personhood of African-American women" (p. 225), on whom he practiced experimental surgeries. The infamous Tuskegee study, which lasted several decades (until 1972), studied untreated syphilis in African American men. Even when treatment did become available, it was withheld from them. At the Willowbrook State School for mentally disabled children, a study was conducted ostensibly to see the effects of gammaglobulin inoculation. However, children were deliberately infected with hepatitis and treatment was often withheld (Ramsey, 2001). In 1966, Beecher published an article in *The New England Journal of Medicine* detailing 22 cases of ethically suspect

research that had appeared in the medical literature, including the Willowbrook study. More recently, some research initiatives carried out in developing countries by researchers from developed countries have been criticized as unethical for a variety of reasons, including that accepted ethical principles and standards of care were not upheld (Häyry, Takala, & Herissone-Kelly, 2007).

4. *Personal/professional ambition.* It is widely recognized that humans are susceptible to favoring personal gain, material or psychological, over benevolent actions toward others when they perceive (consciously or subconsciously) that providing for someone else's needs disadvantages them in some way. This susceptibility is stronger for some than for others and depends for its strength on a variety of factors related to an individual's background, experiences, and the current circumstances. The susceptibility may be consciously experienced and result in "cognitive dissonance" (Festinger, 1957) or subconscious and not noted by the agent (Doris and The Moral Psychology Research Group, 2010; Eagleman, 2011; Kahneman, 2011; Verplaetse, de Schrijver, Vanneste, & Braeckman, 2009). This is not to discount the idea that humans are also capable of altruism (Nagel, 1991) but rather to make the point that no matter how objective researchers think they are being, they can never be completely free from a variety of influence. Research and theoretical work in cognitive, motivational, and social psychology, and moral development have increased understanding of the influence of bias, prejudice, and self-interest on action. The human predisposition to rationalize behavior is extensively documented (Bandura, 1986, 1999; Tavris & Aronson, 2007; Weiner, 1992; Weston, 2005). Rationalizing behavior means using reasoning ability to justify the preferred action over an alternative that is just as reasonable or even more so or offering justification as an explanation for behavior that has occurred. Rationalizations do not usually hold up under objective scrutiny. Thus, for example, a nurse who was complicit in the Nazi euthanasia experiments might claim that she had no option but to follow orders. Yet it is known from other nurses who objected that this choice existed (Benedict & Kuhla, 1999).

HUMAN MALLEABILITY

One further problem associated with ethical research, and related to the situations just described, has to do with the human predisposition to act in accordance with situational conditions. People can feel powerless to affect a bad situation and become numb or immune to a problem and/or continue to participate in a bad situation, thus perpetuating an unethical practice. Additionally, a subtle shift in perspective can occur, causing a person to believe what others are saying (Bandura, 1999; Chambliss, 1996; Mohr & Mahon, 1996). The possibility of situationally influenced perspective shifts was illustrated in the Stanford Prison Experiment, conceived and executed in 1971 by psychologist Philip Zimbardo. The experiment's aim was to explore the effects of prison on individuals. It used college student volunteers and a simulated prison environment to study the ways in which people react or behave under those types of conditions. The experiment was supposed to have lasted 2 weeks but was terminated after 6 days (in response to criticism from a person of importance to the researcher). There was no disinterested oversight of the research, and the researchers themselves admitted to failing to notice the seriousness of the psychological impact of the study upon the participants, both prisoners and guards. Although the experiment has been criticized as unethical, findings from the study support the idea that human beings can be influenced by situational factors to behave badly toward one another. As Zimbardo (2005) stated of the study, the "power of social situations to distort personal identities and long cherished values and morality as students internalized situated identities in their roles as prisoners and guards" was striking. The experiment randomly assigned volunteers to one of two groups, prisoners and guards. The prisoners were subjected to dehumanizing and demoralizing routines, and the guards were reminded of the inferior nature of the prisoners. Both groups came to assume the characteristics of the roles assigned to them. "Within a few days the role dominated the person," Zimbardo noted (Alexander, 2001).

The Development of Human Subjects Research Regulations

In the United States and in many other countries, contemporarily it has been recognized that there must be independent oversight of research processes to lessen the likelihood that participants in biological or behavioral research will be wittingly or unwittingly abused. There is wide recognition that certain ethical principles should underlie all aspects of the research process, from the conceptualization of a question to be studied to the use of findings. The Nuremberg Code (U.S. Department of Health and Human

Services, 1949), which was formulated as a result of the Nazi Doctors Trial after World War II, stresses the importance of the voluntary participation of subjects. It provides support for the "judgment of the Nuremberg Tribunal that the Nazi physician-scientists had been guilty of perpetrating deeds of agony, torture, degradation and death on human beings in the name of medical science" (Katz, 1992, p. 228).

Katz wrote that, interestingly, the only antecedent to the Nuremberg Code was promulgated in 1931 in Germany. This document, entitled "Regulations on New Therapy and Human Experimentation," was issued by the Reichsminister of the Interior and in many ways mirrored the eventual prescriptions for ethical research laid out in the Nuremberg Code, including the need for voluntary informed consent of participants. Vollman and Winau (1996) noted that the need for ethical rules to guide research had been discussed in Prussia for several decades before the edict from the Reichsminister. The 1931 document also makes a distinction between "therapeutic . . . and nontherapeutic research . . . and set out strict precautions" (p. 1446) to be followed.

So-called "therapeutic research" involves testing potential new treatments or therapies for their ability to provide benefit to those suffering from an ailment. Using the term "therapeutic" is a little misleading, because it has not been determined that these interventions are actually effective for the purpose designed—they may or may not actually have therapeutic value. Thus therapeutic effects are still in question. Nontherapeutic research is experimentation on healthy subjects or without the aim of possible subject benefit. (The significance of this distinction is discussed in more detail toward the end of the chapter.) The prescriptions of the Nuremberg Code were soon realized by the international medical community to be too stringent and in some cases involved injustice. Requiring voluntary informed consent left several groups of people out of consideration for studies that might have led to benefit for them or their cohort. This realization led to the formulation of the Declaration of Helsinki with its ongoing revisions (World Medical Organization, 1964/2008). Subsequent to the Declaration of Helsinki and in response to ongoing research abuses, *The Belmont Report* was issued in the United States. (All of these documents and their implications are discussed briefly in the following sections.) More recently the Council for International Organizations of Medical Sciences (CIOMS, 2012) formed a working group from various countries to revisit international research ethics guidelines in response to emerging ethical challenges in research.

THE NUREMBERG CODE

The Nuremberg Code (U.S. Department of Health and Human Services, 1949) was conceptualized and formulated as an attempt to protect human rights. It is best viewed in the context of its development over the course of the Nazi Doctors Trial and subsequent deliberations about the atrocities perpetuated on the captive populations of the Nazi concentration camps. Its priority tenet, a reaction to the involuntary nature of the manipulation of human subjects that occurred, states that "[T]he voluntary consent of the human subject is absolutely essential" (cited in Katz, 1992, p. 227) in research endeavors. Although many of its other guidelines have been incorporated into contemporary documents on the protection of human subjects, the first principle of the code was soon realized to be problematic. If only voluntary participation is allowed, those who might benefit from research, such as the cognitively challenged and children, would be left out of research endeavors, yet such studies might be necessary to address their particular types of health problems. As Munson affirmed, "[F]ew people [actually] doubt the need for research involving human subjects" (2008, p. 7). The results of research studies have provided significant improvements in the human life experience. Thus, to leave out of research endeavors those who might benefit or whose cohort might eventually benefit is a justice issue, as discussed shortly.

Additionally, many researchers outside of the Nazi context saw the Nuremberg Code as not pertinent to them and their research efforts. The Nazi's actions were seen as aberrations. Such blatant disregard by researchers and physicians of their obligations to do no harm was generally and naïvely taken to be unlikely in the research and medical communities. Yet innumerable cases in which human rights were discounted and subjects of research misused have subsequently been documented.

THE DECLARATION OF HELSINKI—1964 AND LATER REVISIONS

The World Medical Association (WMA) is an international body that represents physicians. It was founded in 1947 in response to the events of World War II that resulted in the Nuremberg Tribunals. Initially, 27 countries had representatives in the WMA. The purpose of the WMA was "to ensure the independence of physicians, and to work for the highest possible standards of ethical behavior and care by physicians, at all times" (WMA, 2012). The Declaration, which has been revised several times since it was first adopted in 1964 (most recently in 2008), introduced the idea of proxy consent. As noted earlier, the Nuremberg Code's proscription of any but voluntary participation gave rise to another set of ethical issues related to justice. (This topic is discussed later under ethical principles.) Proxy consent permits a responsible person, chosen in light of certain criteria, to enroll another individual who does not have decision-making capacity in a research study. (The criteria and considerations for enrollment are discussed in a later section.) Additionally, the distinction between therapeutic and nontherapeutic research was articulated more clearly, with rationale provided.

EVENTS LEADING TO FORMALIZATION OF RESEARCH ETHICS REGULATIONS IN THE UNITED STATES AND INTERNATIONALLY

During this same time frame in the United States and elsewhere (1945–1960s), there was scant independent oversight of research endeavors. Physicians and other researchers continued to be largely responsible for policing themselves. Rothman (1991) described the tremendous upsurge in research endeavors that followed World War II, resulting in part from the availability of federal and national funding initiatives. The existence of funding changed the nature of research endeavors from small independent initiatives to, in many cases, much larger enterprises that were more difficult to design and more complex to oversee. Although the importance of informed consent was acknowledged, many studies nevertheless proceeded without the participants or participant proxies being informed of important aspects of the study or in the absence of careful scrutiny of the possible deleterious effects on individual subjects. This occurred despite the fact that the Nuremberg Tribunal had codified these as crucial considerations. One explanation for this, as noted earlier, is that researchers did not identify with the Nazi researchers, believing the Nazi atrocities to be the acts of especially wicked persons and somewhat of an anomaly (Faden, Lederer, & Moreno, 2003). Important safeguards and guidelines from the Nuremberg Code related to research design, conduct, and human subjects' protections included the advice that research results should be likely to benefit humanity in some way, influence or coercion of subjects to participate is forbidden, in certain cases prior research on animals should be completed, likely results should justify any risks, and risks should be minimized including mental or physical suffering, which are not permissible. As previously mentioned, in 1966, after several rejections and a severe pruning of examples, Henry Beecher, a Boston physician, published an article in *The New England Journal of Medicine* detailing problems in the ethical conduct of research. Although he had gathered from the medical literature many more than the 22 examples he described in his article, what he presented was a "devastating indictment of research ethics" (Rothman, 1991, p. 15). The research studies had taken place in a wide variety of settings, so they could not be ignored as aberrances—the problem was apparently widespread. Even Beecher's exposé, however, was not enough to radically change the status quo in the United States.

On July 26, 1972, a journalist brought to the public's attention a study that had been carried out on black men to explore the effects of untreated syphilis. The study had been ongoing over a period of 40 years, and many publications had been issued from it—thus, the study was not carried out in secret. Not only was the informed consent of the men not sought, but in addition, deceptive practices were used to keep them from seeking effective treatment even after it became available. The widespread exposure of the Tuskegee Experiment, as it was called after the location of its study population, finally mobilized a change in the oversight, regulation, and ethical conduct of research and led to the National Research Act of 1974. It is important to note that although most unethical research involved or involves biomedical research, research in the social sciences also came under fire. The Stanford Prison Experiment described earlier and the Milgram (1974) experiment, which was designed to explore obedience to authority and involved subject deception and psychological distress, are just two of many such examples.

THE U.S. NATIONAL RESEARCH ACT OF 1974

In 1974, the National Research Act (NRA) was passed in the United States. This act led to the creation of the National Commission for the Protection of Human Subjects of Biomedical and Behavioral Research.

One of the charges of the Commission was to identify the basic ethical principles that should underlie the conduct of biomedical and behavioral research involving human subjects and to develop guidelines that should be followed to ensure that such research is conducted in accordance with those principles. In carrying out this task, the Commission was directed to consider: (1) the boundaries between biomedical and behavioral research and the accepted and routine practice of medicine, (2) the role of assessment of risk–benefit criteria in the determination of the appropriateness of research involving human subjects, (3) appropriate guidelines for the selection of human subjects for participation in such research, and (4) the nature and definition of informed consent in various research settings (National Institutes of Health, Office of Human Subjects Research, 1979).

One outcome of the NRA was *The Belmont Report*, which identified three crucial ethical principles that should frame the research process as it applies to researchers in the United States and U.S. government–funded research studies conducted abroad. These principles are respect for persons, beneficence, and justice. (A more specific discussion of them as they relate to the human subjects research process occurs later in this chapter.) *The Belmont Report* led to 1981 regulations entered into the CFR under Title 45 (Public Welfare), Part 46 (Protection of Human Subjects). A further result of *The Belmont Report* was the inception of institutional review boards (IRBs), sometimes called human subjects review boards or committees (discussed further later in the chapter). In 1991, 17 different federal departments and agencies agreed to be governed by these regulations, and the regulations became known as the Common Rule relating to research or the use of innovative techniques and technology on human subjects (Dunn & Chadwick, 2001). Outside of the United States, the Council for International Organizations of Medical Sciences (CIOMS), in collaboration with the World Health Organization (WHO), in 2002 issued *International Ethical Guidelines for Biomedical Research Involving Human Subjects* (CIOMS, 2012). These guidelines are under revision currently. Guideline 2 articulates the necessity of review board oversight. Review boards may be at different levels from local to international depending on the study but importantly will provide independent review of "scientific merit and ethical acceptability."

In the United States, any institution carrying out research and receiving government funds must have an IRB that will provide ethical oversight of human subjects research proposals and studies. IRBs function in accord with the CFR to ensure the ethical conduct of research within a given institution. The purpose of IRBs is to discern unethical aspects of a research project including the rigor, soundness, and integrity of the design; ability to answer the question posed; the safety of participants; and the voluntariness of subject participation. All federally supported research projects at an institution, academic, or healthcare delivery system must be approved by an IRB prior to commencing. Additionally, ongoing protocols are reviewed annually. CIOMS recommendations for Research Ethics Committees are similar to those of the CFR related to IRBs.

One major problem with formal regulatory oversight is that it tends to occur at a specific point in the process and when there are serious adverse events, but ethical compromise can be subtle and occur anywhere within the research process. Everyday issues are not necessarily noted or understood, as DeBruin and colleagues (2011) in their study of clinical research nurses report. APNs working within their own countries and who have patients on research protocols are advised to understand how their Research Ethics Review committees work and what resources are available. Such committees can generally provide advice about how to proceed when unethical research practices are occurring.

In the United States, once a proposed research protocol has received approval, subsequent changes to it must also be submitted for IRB approval as an amendment. Amendments are reviewed either by individual committee members or the full committee, depending on the nature of the amendment. Initial protocol reviews may be one of three types: full review, expedited, or exempt. Expedited reviews undertaken by one or more IRB members may be carried out for research involving minimal risk. Minimal risks are those that might be encountered in daily life. What is a minimal risk for one person might be more than a minimal risk for another. For example, a diabetic may need to monitor blood sugars several times a day via needle puncture. The diabetic's minimal risk would be different than that of someone who did not have to experience needle punctures. Protocols that are exempt from review fit in one of six categories where there are no identifiable risks (U.S. Department of Health and Human Services, 2005). The makeup of IRBs varies by institution. **Box 6-1** explains the minimum criteria set by the Office for Human Research Protections (OHRP). Some studies that can be considered under an expedited review when conducted on adults might nevertheless require full board review when conducted on children. For example, an interview with a child could inadvertently reveal information about the family that could jeopardize the family.

Research Ethics: Guiding Principles

Chapter 1 provides an in-depth discussion of ethical principles used in healthcare decision making. The philosophical origins and implications of those principles are pertinent in research settings and should be reviewed if necessary. Both the CIOMS guidelines and *The Belmont Report* in the United States rely on the same ethical principles for guiding researchers and healthcare professionals as they strive to protect research subjects or research participants. APNs work in a variety of practice settings where they may be required to advise patients about research protocols or may

Box 6-1 Makeup of Institutional Review Boards: Minimum Membership

- There should be a minimum of five members with varied backgrounds, some with expertise in the types of protocols typically reviewed
- Professional members should be experienced and qualified
- Members should include persons from more than one profession
- At least one member whose concern is primarily scientific and one whose concerns are not scientific should be included
- At least one member who is not affiliated with the institution should be included; citizen members represent the population served or have specialist expertise
- For protocols involving a vulnerable group, including a member of that group or someone who is knowledgeable about the group is advisable
- When protocols involve information that is beyond the expertise of the committee, an expert can be invited to assist, but this individual will not have voting privileges unless accepted to ongoing membership

Source: Data adapted from U.S. Department of Health and Human Services. (2005). DHHS, 2005 Title 45, Part 46, Subpart D, Section 46.402. Additional protections for children involved as subjects in research. Retrieved from http://www.hhs.gov/ohrp/humansubjects/guidance/45cfr46.htm#subpartd

serve in a research-related role. Familiarity with the principles of research ethics and what they entail is crucial for APNs' advocacy and advisory roles. Additionally, these principles provide nurses with the language and rationale for questioning suspect research practices. External oversight and regulation of research are necessary but not sufficient to protect human subjects. Those involved in the research process have to remain vigilant. They may have dual roles. First and foremost they must protect the individual, but they are often also in the position of responsibility for preserving study integrity. Sometimes these two responsibilities conflict with each other. Participants or potential participants in research studies are not necessarily aware of the complexity of the research process, nor of all the ways that they could be harmed, as exemplified in the Gelsinger and TGN1412 cases discussed later. Additionally—and it is easy for participants to forget or discount this idea—the motives behind a research endeavor are not primarily to promote the given individual's well-being; the goals of research are different than clinical goals, but subjects do not always understand this. This misunderstanding has been termed "therapeutic misconception" (Applebaum, Roth, & Lidz, 1982; Glannon, 2006; Kimmelman, 2007). Basically therapeutic misconception means that the research subject thinks the aim of the study is to benefit him or her. Potential subjects may need assistance in the decision-making process and require an advocate or interpreter to help them understand what participation in the research means for them and how it is, or is not, likely to further their particular goals.

The meaning and implications of each of the research ethics principles set out in *The Belmont Report* (National Institutes of Health, Office of Human Subjects Research, 1979) and reflected in the CIOMS guidelines are discussed separately in the following paragraphs; in many ways the principles are related or overlapping. As previously mentioned, the principles include respect for persons, beneficence, and justice. They have their basis in the idea that all human beings are equally worthy of moral consideration and concern and no one individual should be used as a means to achieve another person's or society's goals. For such reasons, Miller and Wertheimer (2007) have argued that it is important to understand that although paternalism (beneficence) is pervasive in contemporary human research endeavors, it is not necessarily incompatible with respect for persons. That is, there is a need and an obligation on the part of researchers and others to protect subjects from study harms that would be impossible for them to anticipate.

Paternalism means acting in a patient's best interest and preventing a patient from coming to harm when he or she is unable, for a variety of reasons (including a knowledge deficit), to protect himself or herself. Paternalism may or may not be in accord with a given patient's autonomous choice—that is, a person's right to make his or her own decisions. However, when a nurse grasps that a patient is not in possession of appropriate information to make a decision in his or her own interests, paternalism may well be justified and respectful of the individual as a person.

CASE STUDY: MRS. JONES

Mrs. Jones wishes to be involved in a trial with a principal investigator she knows and trusts, Dr. Green. The study is aimed at testing the safety and efficacy of a new anti-hypertensive drug. Her blood pressure is well controlled with the drug she is currently taking, which has minimal side effects. However, Mrs. Jones is sure that Dr. Green would not offer to enroll her if the doctor did not think the research would benefit her, so she is willing to follow Dr. Green's advice that she participate. This willingness hints at Mrs. Jones's misunderstanding of the goals of research and calls into question how informed she is. To respect Mrs. Jones as a person is to understand what is required for her autonomous decision making and to facilitate this. In line with the discussions in Chapters 1 and 3, this problem demonstrates a failure of the informed consent process. Dr. Green's responsibility is to ensure that Mrs. Jones understands the distinction between the primary goals of the healthcare provider and of the researcher. If she does not understand this, Mrs. Jones should not be permitted to enroll. Moreover, if Mrs. Jones eventually enrolls because she becomes more fully informed, her best interests are more likely to be served by having a separate primary care provider.

In addition to the regulatory aspects guiding human research in a given country, clinical judgment is required to ascertain what the patient or subject needs to know to make an informed decision about what is acceptable. As Miller and Wertheimer (2007) have pointed out, "[T]he question arises . . . whether standard protections for research subjects are inherently paternalistic" (p. 24) and how this paternalism coexists with the "primacy of informed consent."

When is paternalism justified and when is it not? IRBs, for example, do not approve protocols when the language is not clear or the description of the study is not well articulated because a subject entering is unlikely to be adequately informed, and a subject cannot enroll until the study is approved. This paternalism both protects the subject and shows respect for persons.

The Ethical Principle of Respect for Persons

AUTONOMY AND ITS LIMITS

The principle of respect for persons has its philosophical roots in the ethical principle of autonomy. As noted in *The Belmont Report* (National Institutes of Health, Office of Human Subjects Research, 1979), "[R]espect for persons incorporates at least two ethical convictions: first, that individuals should be treated as autonomous agents, and second, that persons with diminished autonomy are entitled to protection" (Principle 1). As in general healthcare practice, this principle serves both as the foundation for obtaining informed consent from those with decision-making capacity and places responsibilities on the researcher or patient advocate, including APNs, to ensure that a proxy decision maker is appropriate and able to make an informed and uncoerced decision for the person with diminished autonomy. It also means understanding under what other circumstances a person's autonomy might be constrained.

Vulnerability

Vulnerability to coercion or persuasion limits a person's capacity for autonomous decision making. For example, a prisoner may be influenced to enter a research trial because of fear of retribution from prison officials or in the hopes that participation will facilitate an early release. Thus, the principle of respect for persons also takes into account inordinate vulnerability. Another way of looking at this principle is to see that the particularities of a person, including context and influences, are important aspects of respecting that person.

All of the following groups have been viewed as vulnerable: those with impaired cognition (congenital, developmental, or organic), prisoners, pregnant women (because of the implications for both the woman and her fetus), and children.

The fact of vulnerability does not mean that these groups cannot be enrolled as subjects. Indeed, as discussed later, justice requires that they are not left out of studies that might benefit them and that special consideration be given to the study of their particular issues. "The particular needs of the economically and medically disadvantaged must be recognized" (WMA Declaration of Helsinki, 2008, Section A8). Rather, the issue of vulnerability means that special precautions must be taken to ensure that consent is informed, that the research does not pose inordinate risks, that the potential benefits of the research outweigh the risks to the subject, and where benefit to the subject is not possible, that any likely benefits will accrue to the subject's cohort. For example, in the case of prisoner research, the results of the research are aimed at benefiting other prisoners in similar circumstances. Research on prisoners remains controversial (Parascandola, 2007). APNs working with especially vulnerable populations need to familiarize themselves with the literature about ethical issues and research implications for their populations and area of practice.

Another example of vulnerability concerns the situation of immigrant communities and populations. In such cases, persons may not be proficient in the English language and/or the local culture and values. In such cases, researchers must first consider whether it is just (discussed later) to leave such populations out of consideration as potential subjects. If it is decided that immigrant populations should be offered the opportunity to participate, the question of what special accommodations are needed must be addressed. Knowledge of the culture, language, and other aspects of their situation is crucial. For nurses, there is the additional question of whether there is a professional responsibility to ensure that they learn about the particular needs of such groups to best serve them. Many studies initiated by doctorally prepared nurses or predoctoral nursing scholars have focused on understanding the very nature of a population's vulnerability with the aim of designing interventions; thus, being aware of ethical issues involved in studying such populations is a professional responsibility.

Altruism

One further implication of respect for persons, viewed as a person's right to make his or her own choices, is that a person has the right to participate in research for altruistic purposes even if that choice is highly risky.

CASE STUDY: MRS. BROWN

Ms. Brown has a genetic form of a chronic lung disease that is in its advanced stages. She has two sons and a daughter. A research study aimed at preventing the progress of this disease has been approved by the IRB at the institution where Ms. Brown is an outpatient. It is under way and enrolling participants. She meets the criteria for participation. As the clinical nurse specialist (CNS) in the pulmonary clinic, Ms. Darrowby is asked by Ms. Brown about the study. Her son read about it on the Internet. Ms. Darrowby is familiar with the study, although not involved directly in it. Because several of her patients have asked for more information about the study, she talked with the researcher about it and has familiarized herself with the protocol. She discusses what she knows with Ms. Brown and helps her to understand that because of her advanced disease, personal benefit is either extremely unlikely or not possible and that there are serious risks involved, including the risk of death. Ms. Brown insists that she would like to participate. She is able to articulate her understanding of the purposes of the study and its implications for her. She views her participation as a legacy for her children and others like them. It is a meaningful and considered request. Ms. Darrowby refers Ms. Brown to the principal investigator for further information, assuring Ms. Brown that she will continue to provide her care and help her process information about the study as necessary. If all other aspects of the study are sound, and ongoing protections are in place, Ms. Brown would be permitted to enroll. Ms. Darrowby's professional responsibilities would be to monitor her, provide care that is in line with the protocol criteria, and ensure that Ms. Brown knows she can withdraw later if she wishes and still receive appropriate care.

Adequately Informed

In the case of Ms. Brown, the nurse made a determination after much exploration and discussion that she was making an informed, uncoerced, and voluntary decision to participate. Although her caregivers may not agree with her choice, it is hers to make and they can continue to support her. However, in many cases an individual's decision-making process and the influences upon it are not so transparent. In such cases, determining what is needed for informed consent is more difficult. What does it mean to say that a person who is deemed to have decision-making capacity and who is not more than usually vulnerable (all people are all somewhat vulnerable to the unpredictable nature of daily life) can give or has given informed consent?

There is no one reliable answer to this question, even though a great deal of attention has been paid to it in the bioethics literature. How health professionals come to terms with the difficulty of understanding what constitutes informed consent—given knowledge about human nature and the complexities of information processing—remains problematic and is the subject of ongoing debate. Although the issue of uncertainty related to informed consent cannot be resolved here, understanding the difficulties involved permits thoughtful and careful decision making on the part of the APN, along with the recognition that collaboration or the marshalling of other resources on the patient/subject's behalf may be warranted.

INFORMED CONSENT AND ITS LIMITS

For current purposes, then, although it is important to note that the difficulties inherent in protecting human research subjects have not been resolved, the results of research endeavors have often greatly improved human quality of life and lifespan. For such reasons, society continues to appreciate the ongoing need for human subject experiments and explorations. For many people, participating in a research study holds the potential of direct benefit, especially for those whose mental or physical condition cannot be relieved by any available treatment. In addition to the potential positive effects of biomedical research, some qualitative research endeavors have been shown to provide therapeutic effects, too. "Qualitative research is a form of social inquiry that focuses on the way people interpret and make sense of their experiences" (Holloway & Wheeler, 2002, p. 1). Qualitative research endeavors, those designed to understand experienced phenomena such as postpartum depression, victimization, grief, sadness, and moral distress, often provide a therapeutic effect (Shamai, 2003).

With this in mind, the goals of healthcare professionals must include helping people decide whether they wish to participate in research endeavors, for what purposes, and under what circumstances. These are examples of what is meant by respect for persons in research settings. Respect for persons in health care or the healthcare research setting means taking responsibility for understanding who the patient is as an individual with particular needs and concerns and what information that person likely needs to meet his or her own goals. This is true whether a choice is being made about accepting treatment or about becoming a subject of research. Respecting persons, then, means facilitating informed decision making and assisting in making authentic choices. An authentic choice is one that is based on an understanding of what is being proposed and the ways in which a decision once made may affect a person, including the impact it is likely to have on personal lifestyle and goals. As noted earlier, it also means recognizing when persons are not capable of informed decision making and assisting proxy decision makers as they strive to fulfill their responsibilities.

REQUIREMENTS OF INFORMED DECISION MAKING

The following are ethical and legal requirements of informed decision making:

- The provision of knowledge and information appropriate to a person's situation and capacities
- An individual's ability to process and comprehend information and show how it is likely to affect him or her
- Freedom from unduly coercive influences (psychological, physical, or environmental)

These requirements represent the criteria of "disclosure . . . comprehension . . . [and] voluntary agreement" spelled out in more detail in *The Belmont Report* (National Institutes of Health, Office of Human Subjects Research,

1979). In *The Belmont Report* and subsequent discussions, it is recognized that obtaining adequately informed consent under the best of conditions and even with the purest of researcher motivations is difficult. Knowledge development in this area is ongoing. Scholars from various disciplines have been concerned with learning more and have undertaken to study what subjects understand as a result of the consent process and whether this matches the intent of the process. In several research studies, this was shown not to be the case (Hutchison, 1998; Kenyon, Dixon-Woods, Jackson, Windridge, & Pitchforth, 2006; Lynöe, Sandlund, Dalqvist, & Jacobsson, 1991); more research is needed to discover which strategies are facilitative of quality informed consent processes.

Table 6-1 lists the basic and essential elements of informed consent that, with much thought and discussion, have been deemed by regulatory bodies to be necessary but perhaps not always sufficient for a quality informed consent process to occur. Certain circumstances require additional elements to be included. For example, some populations are considered vulnerable for a variety of reasons and require special protections.

A crucial point for the APN is that regardless of whether a person is a subject of research or a patient in need of nursing care, the goals of nursing services are unchanged. Nurses acting in a nursing capacity (i.e., relying upon their professional status as registered nurses) continue to be accountable for practicing in accord with their professional code of ethics (ANA, 1994). Anecdotally, on several different occasions over my years of teaching nursing ethics and more recently in my advisory capacity with the clinical research unit nurses, I have been told by nurses who practice in clinical research settings that they are pressured to ignore nursing concerns related to individuals in favor of maintaining the integrity of research protocols. I believe this is a mistaken understanding, both of the nursing role in research settings and researcher responsibilities. Indeed, the Declaration of Helsinki affirms, "[I]n medical research on human subjects, considerations related to the well-being of the human subject should take precedence over the interests of science and society" (WMA, 2008, Section A5). The complex and uncertain nature of most research requires that "the responsibility for the human subject must always rest with a medically qualified person and never rest on the subject of the research, even though the subject has given consent" (WMA, 2008, Section B15).

For those APNs working in research settings, two recent studies will be of interest (DeBruin et al., 2011; Höglund, Helgesson, & Ericksson, 2010).

■ Table 6-1   Essential Aspects of Research Subject Informed Consent

Interpretation of NIH OHSR Elements	APN Applications in Clinical Research Settings and Advisory Role to a Patient or Family
- Acknowledgment that what is being proposed is a research study and that any questions will be answered by the researcher or designee - The purpose of the study - How long the study will take - Which procedures are experimental and which established	Explain the difference between treatment goals and research goals and how this applies in the particular person's case and relates to the person's goals. Help potential participants to explore in what ways participating might or might not serve their purposes. Explore whether they are feeling any pressure to agree. What are their concerns? Discuss with them what sorts of questions they might want to pose to the researcher or person obtaining consent. If the study cannot benefit the potential participant directly, what would be good reasons for participating (help others later)?
- The important details of the study: tests, procedures, extra visits, possible risks, and expected benefits - What alternative treatments are available if the person decides not to participate	Map it out. Help potential participants understand what this would mean in terms of their lives, time frame, and commitment. Do the potential benefits make it worth the effort? What is the likelihood or magnitude of the risks and benefits? Have any treatments or interventions been used before on other populations? What other treatments exist and what has the experience of these been? Explain that they will continue to receive good care whether or not they agree to participate. People are sometimes fearful that if they don't agree, they will be abandoned by their healthcare provider.

(continues)

■ Table 6-1   Essential Aspects of Research Subject Informed Consent
(*continued*)

Interpretation of NIH OHSR Elements	APN Applications in Clinical Research Settings and Advisory Role to a Patient or Family
- Voluntariness of participation is maintained throughout. Possibility of withdrawal at any time without penalty - They may be withdrawn by their provider or the researcher physician if conditions (theirs or adverse events associated with the study) warrant it - What they can expect if withdrawn - How unforeseen expenses or problems will be addressed	Subjects/patients have the right to withdraw at any time—they do not always understand this. The research team will not necessarily remind them. Some persons may need to be empowered to withdraw when the study becomes too burdensome for them. Primary care providers, not involved in the research, may be the best advocates for the patient. Sometimes the researcher or provider may decide that the person should be withdrawn from the study—they may need help understanding the reason for this and finding appropriate alternative care including hospice or palliative care when warranted.
- How confidentiality will be maintained	Help the person think about how his or her confidentiality will be protected. What might the implications be for the person if personal information got into the hands of the insurance company or an employer?
- Contact information for researcher or resource person	Help subjects/patients think through how to get information in an emergency—who to call and who to inform. If hospitalized, the receiving institution needs to know what protocol is in effect related to interventions they are planning.

Source: National Institutes of Health (NIH), Office of Human Subjects Research (OHSR). (2006). Sheet 6—Guidelines for writing informed consent documents. Retrieved from http://ohsr.od.nih.gov /info/sheet6.html

These studies have started to fill in some of the gaps in knowledge about the daily issues that research nurses face in their disparate settings. They draw attention to some of the tensions faced by research nurses that are not generally discussed in the research regulatory community, yet have critical implications for patient/subject safety and well-being.

CHILDREN AND ASSENT

As Munson (2008) notes, "one of the most controversial areas of all medical research has been that involving children as subjects" (p. 14). Children are especially vulnerable to abuse for obvious reasons, but most particularly because they are dependent on adults to meet their everyday needs and to make decisions on their behalf. Research in the biological, social, cognitive, and psychological sciences has revealed that capacity for reasoning and decision making is developmental and varies related to biological factors, the age of a child, the type of environment in which a child is raised, and the types of experiences a child has had or to which he or she has been exposed. Consequently, in the case of children, the ability to meet the criteria for informed consent, which requires decision-making capacity, must be viewed as occurring along a continuum. It requires understanding a child in context, just as it does for adults. Because it is often difficult to determine just how capable a child is of making informed decisions, legal regulations apply. However, legal regulations alone do not make for ethical practices.

Why enroll children in research at all? Munson (2008) answers this question by pointing out that children are not just small adults. There are differences in biology, metabolism, and biochemistry such that it is necessary to tailor treatments and interventions to their specific needs. Additionally, many illnesses are seen only in childhood, either because the illness is so severe that the child dies or, in the case of infectious diseases, most adults are immune to the disease, having experienced the illness as a child. "To gain the kind of knowledge and understanding required for effective medical treatment for children, it is often impossible to limit research solely to adults" (Munson, 2008, p.15). The same is true of research studies conceived in the social sciences and designed to understand more about how children relate to the world. Addressing the mental health of children requires understanding more about positive and negative influences on their health and ability to adapt to changing conditions.

Legal Requirements

The following is a discussion of the legal protections that exist for children in the United States. APNs working in other countries will need to understand the legal protections that exist in their own countries of practice. However, the information given here will be helpful in thinking about what children need regardless of country of practice. The protection of children and information related to informed participation in the United States is laid out in the CFR (U.S. Department of Health and Human Services, 2005, Title 45, Part 46, Subpart D). Before looking at these regulations in more detail, it is helpful to understand the definitions that the Department of Health and Human Services relies on. Additionally, it is important to know that the age at which a person may legitimately make personal decisions related to health care varies from state to state. Rules about the conditions of obtaining emancipated minor status also vary by state. An emancipated minor is a person younger than 18 years of age who is granted the legal right to make his or her own decisions. It is important that APNs understand their state's rules about emancipated minors.

The fact that rules about appropriate age vary from state to state lends logical strength to the idea that no agreement exists about who is a child and thus not capable of decision making and who is an adult and presumed, all things being equal, capable of personal decision making. CFR definitions are as follows:

(a) *Children* are persons who have not attained the legal age for consent… under the applicable law of the jurisdiction…

(b) *Assent* means a child's affirmative agreement to participate in research. Mere failure to object [is not the same as and should not be considered] assent.

(c) *Permission* means the agreement of parent(s) or guardian to the participation of their child or ward in research.

(d) *Parent* means a child's biological or adoptive parent.

(e) *Guardian* [is one who is officially permitted]… under applicable State or local law to consent on behalf of a child… (U.S. Department of Health and Human Services, 2005 Title 45, Part 46, Subpart D, Section 46.402)

For the purposes of discussing assent and its requirements, it is assumed that the child in question is a nonemancipated minor. Generally, children under the age of 6 years are not considered capable of assent. However, recent research has shown that children with a chronic illness may demonstrate an advanced ability to understand how their illness affects them and are able to manage aspects of it (Alderson, Sutcliffe, & Curtis, 2006).

What, then, are the considerations? The guidelines for IRBs are instructive (U.S. Department of Health and Human Services, 2005). IRBs grant approval for studies involving children when it is felt that the study is well designed and likely to produce results and that every effort is being made to safeguard a child's interests. From my experience on three different IRBs over the past several years, I can say that such committees take this charge extremely seriously. Protocols are read very carefully by committee members, the principal investigator (PI) is charged with answering clarification questions, and the protocol is approved only when all are satisfied that a child subject's well-being is a priority.

For research endeavors that have the probability of no greater than a minimal risk to a child, a child may be enrolled with the permission of one parent and the assent of the child. For children to assent, they need to be given information and allowed to process it in developmentally and circumstantially appropriate ways. This necessitates understanding who the child is in terms of his or her capacities and skills. What constitutes minimal risk has not been well defined and is the subject of ongoing debate in the ethics literature. For the purposes of this discussion, it can be thought of as equivalent to those perils that the child would be likely to encounter in the course of daily life. For example, a child with diabetes would be likely to encounter hypodermic needles more often than other children, so research involving injections would not be considered more than minimally risky for that child.

For research that involves the possibility of more than minimal risk, a child may be enrolled if there is the prospect of direct and likely benefit, no treatment exists that is comparable, and the child's current status is such that the potential benefit is substantial in terms of quality of life. In such cases, the assent of the child is necessary, along with the permission of one parent. Where there is greater than minimal risk and no prospect of direct benefit to the child, the assent of the child and the permission of both parents are needed (where both parents are available). Such situations may be when the child has an incurable disease for which generalizable knowledge is needed to develop ways of preventing or ameliorating the disease in the future for other children. In such situations health professionals are nevertheless charged with minimizing harms and maximizing the child's comfort. This may mean that when the burden becomes too great for the child to bear that the child is withdrawn from the study and offered palliative or hospice care.

APNs AND CONDITIONS OF ASSENT

Parents or guardians may seek the professional opinions of APNs about whether to enroll their child in a study. Additionally, pediatric nurse practitioners may be asked to identify children from their patient populations who are potential subjects for a study. Therefore, it is important to keep in mind possible factors that could endanger a child's welfare either from being inappropriately enrolled in a study or not being enrolled in a study that could potentially provide a benefit.

In addition to understanding the nuances of a research project and ensuring that it is scientifically and ethically sound, as discussed elsewhere, APNs have other responsibilities. In the course of informing and supporting parents or guardians interested in a research study and helping them to determine its appropriateness, the APN should be alert to other factors that could harm a child, such as being persuaded to assent when it is obvious that the child does not wish to participate. Possible factors that would provoke further exploration of a given situation or raise concerns include when parents who are financially burdened talk about the financial or in-kind incentives to participate (perhaps there will be free care or medications); they may need help getting resources from other avenues. On rare occasions, parents may be abusive or influenced by the possibility of secondary gains (e.g., extra attention). Children without a parent or caregiver (e.g., wards of the state) should have an advocate appointed who will look after their interests.

The Ethical Principle of Beneficence

The ideal overall purpose of research on human beings is one of beneficence; that is, the results of empirical endeavors are expected to contribute positively to society and its constituents. In the process of making positive contributions, harms to individuals must be minimized. Researchers are responsible for the physical, mental, and social well-being of subjects. They cannot fulfill this responsibility if they are not willing to understand individual subjects within their contexts, beliefs, values, and plans. Unfortunately, as noted and exemplified earlier, a host of factors can interfere with a researcher's interest in the good of an individual subject. A variety of conflicts of interest can weaken a researcher's willingness to adhere to the goal of beneficence. There may also be financial inducements related to the funding source. It is beyond the purposes of this chapter to detail the commercialization of the biomedical research enterprise that has occurred over the past several decades in the United States and elsewhere; however, this development has raised further possibilities for researcher conflicts and is an important consideration for APNs and others who are concerned about protecting subjects from harm.

Human subjects protection regulations stipulate that conflicts of interests be disclosed in the informed consent process in such a way that the potential subjects understand the implications for them. However, the possible effects of conflicts of interests are not always easy to identify or sort out. This is evident in the expanding body of literature on this topic. The implication for advanced practice is that nurses who frequently find themselves involved in the recruitment or informing stages of the research process have responsibilities to understand the issues involved, so that they can assist their patients or subjects in the decision-making process.

THE TWO BRANCHES OF BENEFICENCE

In the Chapter 1 discussion of ethical principles, the principles of nonmaleficence (do no harm) and beneficence (promote the good) were discussed separately. Philosophically, they are related, but there is disagreement about whether nonmaleficence should be subsumed under the umbrella term of *beneficence*. In research ethics discussions, this is the convention. Beneficence, as noted earlier, is closely related in purpose to the principle of respect for persons.

Beneficence is an obligation both of healthcare professionals and those engaging in research endeavors that involve human beings. For the purposes of undertaking research, "Two general rules have been formulated as complementary expressions of beneficent actions in this sense: (1) do not harm and (2) maximize possible benefits and minimize possible harms" (National Institutes of Health, Office of Human Subjects Research, 1979). Although this seems like a relatively straightforward principle, it is very "complex and ambiguous in application" (Smith, 2000, p. 7). The very nature of most research means that there are unforeseeable risks and potential benefits. Estimating the likelihood, quantity, or quality of the benefits and balancing them against the possibility and likelihood of risk are very tricky tasks. Additionally, although the hoped for benefits may be either to an individual subject or to society, the risks are usually to the well-being of a particular subject.

THERAPEUTIC VERSUS NONTHERAPEUTIC RESEARCH

As noted earlier, in the Declaration of Helsinki (WMA, 2012/1964), the distinction between therapeutic and nontherapeutic research was made. Therapeutic research is that which holds out the hope of treatment for a malady or condition experienced by a study subject and takes place as part of patient care. It is sometimes also called clinical research. Nontherapeutic research is that which aims to contribute more generally to the knowledge base for the benefit of others rather than an individual study subject. Subjects of nontherapeutic research may of course benefit in a variety of ways, for example, feeling good about contributions they are making to health improvements in the future. Capron (1998) and others have called into question the importance of the distinction because it implies that research combined with clinical care is therapeutic. Such research nevertheless involves experimental aspects, and the danger is that the physician, when he or she doubles as researcher, may be lulled into "treating the project as inherently more justified" (p. 143) than nonclinical research. Additionally, for the APN's purposes, both beneficence and respect for persons require attention to the experimental nature of clinical research with its inherent risks.

APNs employed in research settings may be exposed to nontherapeutic research protocols. Nontherapeutic trials often but not always involve healthy volunteers. Some have noted that phase 1 drug trials involving seriously ill persons should be considered nontherapeutic because they are not expected to benefit participants, although participants often do not grasp this fact despite the informed consent process. (**Box 6-2** explains what types of subjects participate in phased trials.) Regardless of whether or how this controversy is resolved, the important point to take away is that research has uncertain aspects, as does clinical care. Beneficence requires that harm to individual patient subjects is reduced and that the individual patient/subject good is considered paramount.

Justice

The third important principle in research ethics is that of justice. For healthcare purposes, the two salient questions related to knowledge development for human good are (1) what constitutes an ethically sound study, and (2) "[w]ho ought to receive the benefits of research and bear its burdens?" (National Institutes of Health, Office of Human Subjects Research, 1979). In Chapter 1, it was noted that the favored conception of justice in healthcare situations is that of justice as fairness. That is, justice means trying to ensure that all individuals and groups have the opportunity to benefit from societal provisions. It is recognized that it is more difficult for the disadvantaged and the impoverished to have their needs met.

Box 6-2   Phases of Drug Trials

Research that involves the development and testing of new drugs generally takes place in four phases. Each phase is distinct and involves different groups of subjects. The following is a synthesis of the pertinent literature over time, including materials from the National Institutes of Health (NIH).

Phase 1	Occurs after testing in animals when feasible. Uses a small group of people. The aim is to see both what is a safe dose and what dose is effective for the purpose designed. May use healthy subjects or subjects with a disease process. Is not designed to benefit the subject, although it sometimes provides a placebo effect (Grace, 2006) and in some cases has an effect on a patient's disease process. Often called safety and efficacy trials. Escalating doses of a drug are given to successive patients or patient groups.
Phase 2	Uses larger groups of people, usually those who have the condition targeted, to further test for safety, side effects, and effectiveness.
Phase 3	Uses a large group of subjects who have the condition the drug is designed to treat. Further tests safety and effectiveness, generally over a longer time frame. The number needed for the study is based on statistical estimates of what is needed to validate findings. Subjects are usually monitored by their physicians and the study's principal investigator.
Phase 4	After the Food and Drug Administration's (FDA's) approval of the drug for general use, these studies monitor for adverse findings over a period of time. Sometimes they are also called postmarketing studies.

However, another problem related to vulnerability that was discussed previously is that historically some persons have been studied because they were convenient, unlikely to object, or easily deceived. Thus, there are three main aspects of justice that are important, as discussed in the following subsections.

FAILURE TO STUDY AN IMPORTANT ISSUE AFFECTING A VULNERABLE GROUP

Justice as fairness requires that healthcare professionals and scientists study issues, psychosocial and biological, that especially affect certain groups of vulnerable people or to which these persons are especially susceptible. For example, to avoid studying factors associated with Alzheimer's disease for the reason that in the later stages of the disease people are not capable of informed consent represents an injustice. Likewise, to avoid investigating problems associated with certain immigrant populations because they require translating documents and information also fails to meet justice criteria.

MINIMIZING HARMS AND MAXIMIZING BENEFITS

This is a very difficult task in view of the complexity and uncertainty associated with much medical research—it requires paying scrupulous attention to all aspects of a project from conception through study termination and publication of findings. It involves understanding the particular risks to both individuals and the group based on the type of vulnerability present.

FAIR SELECTION OF SUBJECTS

Subject selection cannot be based on mere expediency. The history of research ethics provides vivid examples of studies that were carried out upon people who were easily deceived or who could not object. One rule of thumb is that research that uses subjects from vulnerable or disadvantaged groups should be aimed at benefiting those people or their cohort group. *The Belmont Report* proposes the following:

> Justice is relevant to the selection of subjects of research at two levels...
> Individual justice in the selection of subjects would require[s]... fairness... Potentially beneficial research [should not be offered] only to some [favored] patients ... [Nor should] only "undesirable" persons [be selected] (National Institutes of Health, Office of Human Subjects Research, 1979).

Social justice requires that distinction be drawn between the nature of subjects who ought to be included in invitations to participate and who should not based on assessment of benefits and burdens that are likely to accrue further burdens in the absence of the likelihood of significant benefit to their class (National Institutes of Health, Office of Human Subjects Research, 1979). *The Belmont Report* states that there should be:

> an order of preference in the selection of classes of subjects (e.g., adults before children) and that some classes of potential subjects (e.g., the institutionalized mentally infirm or prisoners) may be involved as research subjects, if at all, only on certain conditions. (National Institutes of Health, Office of Human Subjects Research, 1979)

Problems Facing Nurses in Research Roles and Settings

APNs may function in one of several roles related to research. As primary care providers, they may be caring for patients who are on a protocol of some sort. They may be asked to select and recruit patients from their population who would be good subjects for a particular research study. As specialists, they may be asked to be consultants for a research study. The identification of unanswered practice questions may spur the conception of a study where APNs serve as investigators or coinvestigators. Many nurse practitioners and CNSs serve as study coordinators and are responsible for oversight of study integrity and subject safety and well-being. Another role is that of an IRB or Research Ethics Committee member. This is an excellent way for nurses to develop a more in-depth knowledge of the ethical and regulatory issues surrounding healthcare research. All of these roles require different skills and expertise. There is always a period of intense learning for any new role undertaken, and the issues associated with each role cannot be detailed here.

In the United States and elsewhere there is an increasing emphasis on (and available funding for) moving bench science discoveries rapidly into practice settings. This movement encourages interdisciplinary collaboration and facilitates knowledge development that is not possible when separate disciplines work in isolation. The motives for translational research endeavors are laudable, but such research is associated with its own peculiar risks related to human safety. This is perhaps especially true of those studies called first-in-human (FIH) trials. FIH trials are those that move promising scientific findings from preclinical tests and/or testing on animals to testing in humans. There are several problems associated with these trials; for example, the animals used may not actually serve as good proxies for human biology related to the biological innovation. Additionally, there may not have been time for thorough peer review of the innovation via publications and presentations. It is important to understand the nature of risks in order to assist patient or subject decision making. Two recent examples of translational research studies that had disastrous consequences are the case of Jesse Gelsinger in the United States and the TGN1412 trial in the United Kingdom.

The Case of Jesse Gelsinger

Jesse Gelsinger had the mild form of a metabolic problem, ornithine transcarbamylase (OTC) deficiency. This is a genetic problem resulting in the inability to break down ammonia. His disease was identified when he was two years old and was managed with drugs and diet. Others with a more severe form die in childhood from the disease. At several stages in his life he suffered relapses and had to be hospitalized in order to manage his care. At age 17 he suffered a relapse and while being treated learned of a research study for gene therapy that was not meant to benefit him but rather others in the future with a more severe form of OTC deficiency. He volunteered because, as he said, he wanted to help these children. As a result of the trial, in 1999 he developed an overwhelming inflammatory reaction that led to multiorgan failure and death. Although his family was initially supportive of the research team, at a review of the study they learned of several issues. There were a multitude of problems both in the informing process and with researcher conflicts of interest including inadequate consent, unreported problems with prior animal studies, Jesse's own liver enzymes were not within normal limits, and the host institution and the PI having major conflicts of interest. The PI reportedly held $13 million of stock in the company supplying the vector (Gelsinger, 2001; Kong, 2005: Parascandola, 2004). In a memorial, Jesse's father documented the whole story from diagnosis to posthumous review noting of the nurse involved, "[T]he nurse who acted as the informed consent witness when my son was first considered for participation… was the clinical coordinator [initially and she] resigned her position… prior to Jesse's actual participation" (Gelsinger, 2001). Mr Gelsinger got in touch with her and found "that she had resigned because her questions… were not being adequately answered and she was very uneasy about further involvement with the research… not want[ing] to make waves, so she just quit" (Gelsinger, 2001). He thought that she should have been more forceful in expressing her reasons because then "someone would have opened their eyes and seen the danger." (Gelsinger, 2001) Mr. Gelsinger also noted that having an independent person to speak up for the subject, his son, might have prevented his death (Gelsinger, 2001).

The TGN1412 Trial

In 2006, TGN1412, a monoclonal antibody, was used on healthy human subjects for the first time. Its intent is to treat diseases such as rheumatoid arthritis. Eight people were enrolled in the study; two received a placebo and the other six received the TGN1412 in doses much smaller than those that had been tried on animals without ill effect. Within hours all six who received the antibody became seriously ill. Many ethical and scientific issues were discovered when this trial was reviewed; the most salient for the purposes of this discussion is the inadequacy of the informed consent process. There was inadequate information about the level of uncertainty, threats to withdraw the approximately $3,500 incentive if the men left the trial early, and the men were not told of the odds of getting the drug versus getting the placebo. Another problematic finding was inadequate time between subject dosing (with adequate time between subject dosing later subjects could have been spared) (Dresser, 2009) (Emanuel & Miller, 2007; Goodyear, 2006; Milton & Horvath, 2009).

General Common Problems

Other problems commonly faced by nurses related to human subjects of research are discussed in the following list. I do not attempt to propose a course of action for all of these because solutions depend upon more detailed data gathering, and what constitutes good action varies depending on the data. Collaboration and consultation are important problem-solving actions. For more troubling issues, enlist the assistance of the principal PI. If you feel that serious breaches of ethics are occurring and the PI seems uninterested in the problem, then it might be helpful to speak to a member or the chair of the IRB or research ethics committee that approved the study.

1. *Patients who do not seem to understand the goals of the research.* For example, a patient thinks a study is to benefit him when in fact he may be selected to the group receiving a placebo or alternative treatment. For a more in-depth discussion of placebos and randomized control trials (RCTs), see Michels and Rothman (2003). Another example is when the patient thinks the drug is designed to cure, when in fact at best it is to prolong life.
2. *Patients who have expressed a desire to withdraw from the study but are being pressured to continue.* First, it must be ascertained why the patient wants to withdraw, and then a way must be found to support that person in his or her wishes.
3. *Patients who seem to be experiencing a lot of suffering and are not aware of alternatives to a protocol such as hospice or palliative care.* A discussion should be initiated that seeks to discover under what conditions

patients would wish to continue, what patients' goals are, and what is most likely to meet these.

4. *Patients who enter a trial with decision-making capacity but later become cognitively unable to agree to continue or request withdrawal.*

5. *Researchers, colleagues, or surrogate decision makers who appear to be acting unethically.* For example, Ms. Jacques, a 75-year-old woman, is about to be discharged after suffering an acute coronary event with subsequent congestive heart failure (CHF). Ms. Vitale, the critical care unit (CCU) nurse practitioner, is completing her discharge summary when Dr. Gould, one of the CCU attending physicians, asks if he can speak to Ms. Jacques about a study he is doing. He tells Ms. Jacques that he thinks she would benefit from being in this study, which will look at the effect of exercise on CHF. Ms. Jacques says that would be a lot of traveling for her and asks if there are any alternatives. Dr. Gould says, "There isn't anything available where you would be so closely monitored and so well cared for." Ms. Vitale knows this is not exactly true because the local hospital near to Ms. Jacques's home has a cardiac rehabilitation program for which she is eligible. Attending that program would require a lot less traveling, and the unit has a good reputation. Thus, Ms. Jacques's best interests would probably be served by this option.

6. *Surrogate decision makers who seem to be making decisions that are not in subjects' best interests.* For example, Timmy, 10 years old, is being kept in the hospital to complete a drug study. He is experiencing uncomfortable but not life-threatening side effects from the study drug, for which there are alternative treatments with fewer side effects. Timmy has been on these alternatives before and experienced fewer problems. Timmy tells you he wants to go home. You overhear Timmy's stepfather say to his wife (Timmy's mother), "But if we kept him in the study one more week, we could get this week's compensation money."

The following are some questions to assist with ethical decision making in research settings or when assisting a patient with decision making:

- How has the research topic been chosen?
- What issues are investigated and what issues are neglected? Why?
- What is the rationale for subject selection and exclusion?
- Whose interests are served by this project?
- Whose interests are ignored by the project?

- How well have safety issues been addressed?
- How honest, complete, and understandable is the consent form?

Summary

This chapter has provided an overview of ethical issues associated with research conducted in healthcare settings. Such research is necessarily based on the premise that it will further some sort of good or benefit to individuals and society related to health. This chapter provides a basis for understanding the nature and complexity of the research endeavor and identifies the APN's responsibilities related to research subjects as firmly rooted in the goals of nursing to promote individual and social good. Nurses working in clinical research settings sometimes find their professional goals seemingly at odds with the apparent goals of a researcher, who seems more interested in preserving the integrity of a study at the expense of an individual participant's needs. The reality is that the goals of both the nurse and the researcher (who may also be a nurse) are really in concert. Both are ethically charged with ensuring that in the process of the research endeavor, the protection of the individual subject's good remains the priority goal.

Discussion Questions

1. Discuss with peers the ways in which your thinking about the APN's responsibility related to human subjects research has or has not changed as a result of reading this chapter.
2. Imagine that you are an APN in a nurse-run inner-city family practice clinic. The clinic practitioners are trying to decide whether to recruit part of their patient population to an obesity control trial (phase III) at the local university hospital, which involves random assignment to receive either a new drug and support plus exercise sessions, or a placebo and support plus exercise sessions. The purpose is to see if the drug is more effective than support and exercise alone in achieving significant weight loss.
    a. What further information about the study would you need before deciding whether you would recruit patients? What are the implications for provider–patient relationships at the clinic?
    b. You decide that this would be a good opportunity for your population. You are the APN who is most knowledgeable about the

problems and promises of research and the associated ethical issues and have been charged with sharing your knowledge with your colleagues. How would you prioritize the issues? Why?

c. Additionally, because many of your teenage patients suffer from obesity, discuss the potential for them to participate. What special considerations are necessary when recruiting children for experimental research studies?

3. What is the process of informed consent in your country of practice? Is it generally adequate? What do you see as the role of nurses in influencing the process?

4. Imagine that you have a type and stage of lung cancer that even with chemotherapy has only a 20% chance of survival after 3 years. A new drug combination (tested in animals and phase 1 and phase 2 trials) has promise for increasing your chances of survival. What would you want to know?

References

Alderson, P., Sutcliffe, K., & Curtis, K. (2006). Children's competence to consent to medical treatment. *Hastings Center Report, 36*(6), 25–36.

Alexander, M. (2001, August). Thirty years later Stanford prison experiment lives on. *Stanford Reporter, 22.* Retrieved March 31, 2008, from http://news-service.stanford.edu/news/2001/-august22/prison2-822.html

American Nurses Association. (1994). *Position statement: The nonnegotiable nature of the ANA code for nurses with interpretive statements.* Washington, DC: Author.

Applebaum, P., Roth, L., & Lidz, C. W. (1982). The therapeutic misconception: Informed consent in psychiatric research. *International Journal of Law and Psychiatry, 5,* 319–329.

Axelsen, D. (2001). Race, gender and medical experimentation: J. Marion Sims' surgery on slave women. In W. Teays & L. Purdy (Eds.), *Bioethics, justice and healthcare* (pp. 224–230). Belmont, CA: Wadsworth/Thompson Learning.

Bandura, A. (1986). *Social foundation of thought and action.* Englewood Cliffs, NJ: Prentice Hall.

Bandura, A. (1999). Moral disengagement in the perpetration of inhumanities. *Personality and Social Psychology Review, 3,* 193–209.

Beecher, H. (1966). Ethics and clinical research. *New England Journal of Medicine, 274,* 1354–1360.

Benedict, S., & Kuhla, J. (1999). Nurses participation in the euthanasia programs of Nazi Germany. *Western Journal of Nursing Research, 21*(2), 246–263.

Capron, A. (1998). Human experimentation. In R. Veatch (Ed.), *Medical ethics* (2nd ed., pp. 135–184). Sudbury, MA: Jones and Bartlett.

Chambliss, D. (1996). *Beyond caring: Hospitals, nurses and the social organization of ethics.* Chicago, IL: University of Chicago Press.

Council for International Organizations of Medical Sciences. (2012). First meeting of the new CIOMS working group on research ethics in Geneva. Retrieved from http://www.cioms .ch/index.php/12-newsflash/221-the-first-meeting-of-the-new-cioms-working-group-on-research-ethics-was-held-4-5-september-2012-in-geneva

DeBruin, D. A., Liaschenko, J., & Fisher, A. (2011). How clinical trials really work: Rethinking research ethics. *Kennedy Institute of Ethics Journal, 21*(2), 121–139.

Dewey, J. (1980). *The quest for certainty.* New York, NY: Putnam Publishing—Perigee Books. (Original work published in 1929.)

Doris, J. M., & The Moral Psychology Research Group. (2010). *The moral psychology handbook.* New York, NY: Oxford University Press.

Dresser, R. (2009). First-in-human trial participants: Not a vulnerable population but vulnerable nonetheless. *Journal of Law, Medicine, and Ethics, 37*(1), 38–50.

Dunn, C., & Chadwick, G. (2001). *Protecting study volunteers in research: A manual for investigative sites.* Boston, MA: Center Watch.

Eagleman, L. (2011). *Incognito: The secret lives of the brain.* New York, NY: Pantheon.

Emanuel, E. J., & Miller, F. G. (2007). Money and distorted ethical judgments about research: Ethical assessment of the TeGenero TGN1412 Trial. *The American Journal of Bioethics, 7*(2), 76–81.

Faden, R. R., Lederer, S. E., & Moreno, J. D. (2003). US medical researchers, the Nuremberg doctors trial and the Nuremberg Code. In E. J. Emanuel et al. (Eds.), *Ethical and regulatory aspects of clinical research* (pp. 7–11). Baltimore, MD: The Johns Hopkins University Press.

Festinger, L. (1957). *A theory of cognitive dissonance.* Stanford, CA: Stanford University Press.

Gelsinger, P. (2001). Jesse's intent. Retrieved from http://www.circare.org/submit/jintent.pdf

Glannon, W. (2006). Phase I oncology trials: Why the therapeutic misconception will not go away. *Journal of Medical Ethics, 32*, 252–255.

Goodyear, M. (2006). Editorial: Learning from the TGN1412 trail. *British Journal of Medicine, 332*, 677–678.

Grace, P. (2006, February). The clinical use of placebos: Is it ethical? Not when it involves deceiving patients. *American Journal of Nursing, 106*(2), 58–61.

Häyry, M., Takala, T., & Herissone-Kelly. (2007). Development, research and vulnerability. In M. Häyry, T. Takala, & P. Herissone-Kelly (Eds.), *Ethics in biomedical research: International perspectives* (pp. 1–6). New York, NY: Value Inquiry Books.

Höglund, A. T., Helgesson, G., & Eriksson, S. (2010). Ethical dilemmas and ethical competence in the daily work of research nurses. *Health Care Analysis, 18*, 239–251.

Holloway, I., & Wheeler, S. (2002). *Qualitative research in nursing* (2nd ed.). Malden, MA: Blackwell.

Hope, T., & McMillan, J. (2004). Challenge studies of human volunteers: Ethical issues. *Journal of Medical Ethics, 30*(1), 110–117.

Hutchison, C. (1998). Phase I trials in cancer patients: Participants' perceptions. *European Journal of Cancer Care, 7*(1), 12–22.

International Council of Nurses. (2011). Nurses and human rights. Retrieved from http://www.icn.ch/images/stories/documents/publications/position_statements/E10_Nurses_Human_Rights.pdf

Jewish Virtual Library. (2008). Bone, muscle, and nerve regeneration and bone transplantation experiments. Retrieved from http://www.jewishvirtuallibrary.org/jsource/Holocaust/bonexp.html

Kahneman, D. (2011). *Thinking fast and slow*. New York, NY: Farrar, Straus & Giroux.

Katz, J. (1992). The consent principle of the Nuremberg Code: Its significance then and now. In G. J. Annas & M. A. Grodin (Eds.), *The Nazi doctors and the Nuremberg Code: Human rights in human experimentation* (pp. 227–239). New York, NY: Oxford University Press.

Kenyon, S., Dixon-Woods, M., Jackson, C., Windridge, K., & Pitchforth, E. (2006). Participating in a trial in a critical situation: A qualitative study in pregnancy. *Quality and Safety in HealthCare, 15*(2), 98–101.

Kimmelman, J. (2007). The therapeutic misconception at 25: Treatment, research, and confusion. *Hastings Centre Report, 6,* 36–42.

Kong, W. M. (2005). Legitimate requests and indecent proposals: Matters of justice in the ethical assessment of phase I trials involving competent patients. *Journal of Medical Ethics, 31,* 205–208.

Lynöe, N., Sandlund, M., Dahlqvist, G., & Jacobsson, L. (1991). Informed consent: Study of quality of information given to participants in a clinical trial. *British Journal of Medicine, 303*(6803), 610–613.

Michels, K., & Rothman, K. (2003). Update on unethical use of placebos in randomised trials. *Bioethics, 17*(2), 188–204.

Milgram, S. (1974). *Obedience to authority*. New York, NY: Harper & Row.

Miller, F., & Wertheimer, A. (2007). Facing up to paternalism in research ethics. *Hastings Center Report, 37*(3), 24–34.

Milton, M. N., & Horvath, C. J. (2009). The EMEA Guideline on First-in-Human Clinical Trials and Its Impact on Pharmaceutical Development. *Toxicologic Pathology, 37,* 363–371.

Mohr, W., & Mahon, M. (1996). Dirty hands: The underside of marketplace healthcare. *Advances in Nursing Science, 19*(1), 28–37.

Munson, R. (2008). *Intervention and reflection: Basic issues in medical ethics* (8th ed.). Belmont, CA: Wadsworth/Thomson Learning.

Nagel, T. (1991). *Equality and partiality*. New York, NY: Oxford University.

National Institutes of Health, Office for Human Research Protections. (2004). Title 45 Code of Federal Regulations, Part 46, 102(d). Retrieved from http://www.hhs.gov/ohrp/humansubjects/

National Institutes of Health, Office of Human Subjects Research. (1979). The Belmont Report: Ethical principles and guidelines for the protection of human subjects of research. Retrieved from http://www.hhs.gov/ohrp/humansubjects/guidance/belmont.html

Parascandola, M. (2004). Five years after the death of Jesse Gelsinger has anything changed? *Research Practitioner, 5*(6), 191–200.

Parascandola, M. (2007). Use of prisoners in research. *Research Practitioner, 8*(1), 12–24.

Ramsey, P. (2001). Judgment on Willowbrook. In W. Teays & L. Purdy (Eds.), *Bioethics, justice and healthcare* (pp. 245–249). Belmont, CA: Wadsworth/Thompson Learning.

Rothman, D. (1991). *Strangers at the bedside*. New York, NY: Harper Collins—Basic Books.

Savitt, T. L. (2001). The use of blacks for medical experimentation and demonstration in the Old South. In W. Teays & L. Purdy (Eds.), *Bioethics, justice and healthcare* (pp. 215-224). Belmont, CA: Wadsworth/Thompson Learning.

Sellman, D. (2005). Towards an understanding of nursing as a response to vulnerability. *Nursing Philosophy, 6*(1), 2-10.

Shamai, M. (2003). Therapeutic effects of qualitative research: Reconstructing the experience of treatment as a by-product of qualitative evaluation. *Social Service Review, 77*(3), 455-467.

Smith, M. B. (2000). Moral foundations. In B. Sales & M. Folkman (Eds.), *Ethics in research with human participants* (pp. 3-10). Washington, DC: American Psychological Association.

Swazey, J., Anderson, M., & Louis, K. (1993). Ethical problems in academic research. *American Scientist.* Retrieved from http://www.americanscientist.org/issues/page2/ethical-problems-in-academic-research

Tavris, C., & Aronson, E. (2007). *Mistakes were made (but not by me): Why we justify foolish beliefs, bad decisions and hurtful acts*. Orlando, FL: Harcourt.

U.S. Department of Health and Human Services. (1949). *Nuremberg Code. Trials of war criminals before the Nuremberg Military Tribunals Under Control Council Law*, No. 10, Vol. 2 (pp. 181-182). Washington, DC: U.S. Government Printing Office. Retrieved from http://www.hhs.gov/ohrp/archive/nurcode.html

U.S. Department of Health and Human Services. (2005). DHHS, 2005 Title 45, Part 46, Subpart D, Section 46.402. Additional protections for children involved as subjects in research. Retrieved from http://www.hhs.gov/ohrp/humansubjects/guidance/45cfr46.html

Verplaetse, J., de Schrijver, J., Vanneste, S., & Braeckman, J. (2009). *The moral brain: Essays on the evolutionary and neuroscientific aspects of morality*. Dordrecht, Netherlands: Springer.

Vollman, J., & Winau, R. (1996). Informed consent in human experimentation before the Nuremberg code. *British Medical Journal, 313*, 1445-1447.

Weiner, B. (1992). *Human motivation: Metaphors, theories and research*. Thousand Oaks, CA: Sage.

Weston, A. (2005). *A practical companion to ethics* (3rd ed.). New York, NY: Oxford University Press.

Wheelwright, P. (1988). *The Presocratics*. New York, NY: Macmillan.

World Medical Association. (2012/1964). About the WMA. Retrieved from http://www.wma.net/en/60about/index.html

World Medical Association Declaration of Helsinki. (1964/2008). Retrieved from http://www.wma.net/en/30publications/10policies/b3/17c.pdf

Zimbardo, P. (2005). Professional profile. Retrieved from http://zimbardo.socialpsychology.org/

SECTION III

ETHICAL ISSUES IN ADVANCED PRACTICE SPECIALTY AREAS

CHAPTER 7

Nursing Ethics and Advanced Practice: Neonatal Issues

Peggy Doyle Settle

Never give out while there is hope; but hope not beyond reason,
for that shows more desire than judgment.
—WILLIAM PENN, *Some Fruits of Solitude*, 1682

Introduction

Good nursing care in the neonatal intensive care unit (NICU) is achieved when nurses are empowered to advocate for infants and their families. As in all areas of nursing, the goals of good nursing care in the NICU include the alleviation of suffering and the protection, promotion, and restoration of health in the care of both the infant and family (American Nurses Association [ANA], 2001). The Council of International Neonatal Nurses (COINN, 2010) asserts that "[K]ey roles for neonatal nurses include advocacy, promotion of a safe environment, research, participation in shaping health policy and in patient and health systems management for infants and their families." Factors influencing good nursing care include a nurse's knowledge and experience, available technology, and an understanding of health policy implications of treatment and supportive environments. Ethical issues and dilemmas arise in the NICU when the goals of good nursing care conflict with the goals of other disciplines and/or family members or when there is uncertainty about what constitute reasonable goals. This chapter reviews ethical issues that are unique to the neonatal setting. Strategies and tools for exploring or resolving these issues are discussed, including the best interest standard, collaborative decision making with healthcare professionals and parents, and understanding medical futility in the newborn period. These issues and many others contribute to the complexity of nursing care in the NICU. Advanced practice neonatal clinical nurse specialists (CNSs), nurse practitioners (NPs), and nurse administrators are in pivotal roles to facilitate discussions with direct care nurses and other health team members when ethical issues arise that jeopardize the delivery of good nursing care. While the author's context of practice is the United States, the ensuing discussion is relevant to those working in NICU settings in other countries. Some important and pertinent differences related to international NICU practice are highlighted. All NICU nurses in advanced practice settings are encouraged to discuss their particular concerns about group ethics in specialty practice associations and/or interdisciplinary ethics meetings and to draw upon the knowledge of those with ethics training and expertise in order to gain clarity about best actions.

The Context of Care

The care of critically ill newborns is an ethical and emotional challenge for all members of a healthcare team. Uncertainty is a constant in NICU settings. Many critically ill and/or premature infants receive available treatment and recover with no or minimal sequelae (Berger, Steurer, Woerner, Meyer-Schiffer, & Adams, 2012; Lantos, Mokalla, & Meadow, 1997; Meadow, Lee, Lin, & Lantos, 2004). However, other NICU infants require prolonged medical treatment, and even with such treatment they still may have only a very small chance of recovery (Catlin, 2005). Although some progress is being made in prognostication (Ambalavanan et al., 2012), it is not always easy to determine which babies can recover and which will have serious ongoing problems that will impinge on their quality of life (QOL). The rapid pace of technological developments adds further uncertainty to the decision-making process. Problems that cannot be treated very well currently may well have an effective intervention down the road. Moreover, literature suggests that medical treatment decisions and outcomes vary based on geographic location and the technical capabilities of institutions (Berger et al., 2012; Vohr et al., 2004). These variations mean that there may be different treatments applied and different outcomes seen for two infants with similar problems merely as a result of country or area of location. Health policies in different countries influence medical treatment decisions, causing further variations in treatment and outcomes among countries (Rebagliato et al., 2000). These variations also pose ethical issues in the delivery of good nursing care. For example, based on sociodemographic factors, one family with a critically ill infant may be offered the option of discontinuing treatment, whereas another family may not be offered the same option (Orfali, 2004; Orfali & Gordon, 2004).

Before describing the ethical issues encountered with critically ill and premature newborns, a review of the technological advancements and healthcare regulations affecting treatment decisions is necessary. This will create a more in-depth understanding of the factors influencing care. In addition, the unique role of the direct care NICU nurse is included to fully describe the context of care.

The Historical Context of Care

The specialty of neonatology was established in the United States in 1966 and in many other countries shortly thereafter. Circa 1970 when the principal author of this text (Grace) was undertaking her basic nurse training in Liverpool, United Kingdom, she recalls being seconded from Walton Hospital to Alder Hey Children's Hospital for a pediatric rotation and being placed on a combined "preemie"/cystic fibrosis unit. The preemie side delivered "intensive care" for premature infants suffering from respiratory distress.

Innovation in neonatal care was followed by the regionalization of neonatal services. This involved the transport of critically ill and premature newborns in specially equipped vehicles to tertiary care centers. Transport from rural or other areas where the sophisticated technology and healthcare professional skills needed to maintain the lives of these infants were not available improved chances of survival. However, this transport also often resulted in the separation of infants from their parents and placed infants directly in the healthcare team's control (Pinch, 2002). Treatment decisions for these newborns were made by the healthcare providers directly involved in their care with little input from the parents (Pinch, 2002).

Technology provided some previously nonexistent opportunities but also led to some problematic practices. As technology became more sophisticated, healthcare providers were able to initiate, sustain, and in some cases prolong the lives of extremely early born infants. In the United States public disclosure of certain ethically questionable medical practices regarding critically ill infants who were liable to have a protracted clinical course led to amendments in federal legislation that aimed to provide additional protection for these infants. Additionally, given the reported variations in NICU patient outcomes, healthcare providers questioned if treatment should always be offered to this patient population simply because it is now available. Providers must consider under what circumstances it is permissible or even obligatory to withhold life-prolonging treatment.

The Technological Context of Care

The ongoing fundamental physiologic needs of the critically ill and premature infant are warmth, respiratory and nutritional support, and prevention and treatment of infection (Pinch, 2002). Landmark technological developments of each decade are listed in **Table 7-1**.

Despite the technological advances of each decade, few standardized treatment protocols were developed and few clinical trials aimed at developing guidelines related to NICU practice were conducted. Healthcare providers initiated treatments for infants with whatever resources were available (Pinch, 2002). The development of biological and technological innovations that can be applied to the care of high-risk infants continues. These developments enable NICU teams to provide life-sustaining treatment to extremely low-birth-weight (ELBW) infants born at 22 to 23 weeks gestation, now

■ Table 7-1   Landmark Technological Innovations

1950s	Mechanical ventilator for newborn
	Phototherapy as a treatment for hyperbilirubinemia
	Ventricular shunt for newborn
1960s	Total parental nutrition
1970s	Regionalization of high-risk care
	Continuous positive air pressure (CPAP)
1980s	Pulse oximetry trials
	Open fetal surgery
	Neonatal surfactant therapy introduced
	Cryosurgery for retinopathy
1990s	Laser surgery for retinopathy
2000s	Nitric oxide

Source: Pinch, W. (2002). *When the bough breaks: Parental perceptions of ethical decision making in the NICU.* Lanham, MD: University Press of America, pp. 8–11.

considered the threshold of viability (Brinchmann & Nortvedt, 2001; Orfali & Gordon, 2004; Pinch, 2002; Sayeed, 2005).

The morbidity and mortality rates related to this "rescue philosophy" (Pinch, 2002, p. 13) of care for ELBW infants are variable. The long-term developmental outcomes related to the application of life-sustaining treatments range from minimal to severe neurodevelopmental complications (Hack et al., 2002; Wilson-Costello, Freidman, Minich, Fanaroff, & Hack, 2005). Few prognostic indicators exist to accurately determine long-term outcomes (Stoll et al., 2010). This poses decision-making dilemmas regarding whether and when to initiate, and under what conditions to continue, ongoing treatment of ELBW infants in view of the potential unpredictable complications resulting from their early birth (Medlock, Ravelli, Tamminga, Moo, & Abu-Hanna, 2011).

Legislation

Understanding the history behind current laws pertaining to the care and treatment of critically ill and premature infants is an important aspect of an advanced practice nurse's (APN's) knowledge base. In the United States, some laws are federally based and some vary from state to state. Laws regulating neonatal practice, of course, also vary from country to country and depend upon underlying cultural ideologies and values. NICU APNs must understand the reasoning behind their country's regulations and the effect of these regulations on practice. Where laws begin to affect "good practice," nurses have obligations to work toward change. This may require interdisciplinary discourse and action.

A review of U.S. regulations permits an appreciation of the complexity of the conflicts surrounding treatment decisions. These regulations also exemplify how public (and professional) misunderstandings and political maneuverings can cause problems for practice. The law honors parents' rights to make medical decisions on behalf of their infant with two exceptions. The first exception is an emergency situation, where life-saving treatment is required and parents are not available to give consent. This exception requires that healthcare providers determine and provide the most appropriate medical treatment. The second exception occurs when the court determines that parents are not acting in the best interest of their child. This exception enables the court to override the parents' medical decisions for their child (Hurst, 2005) in the interests of protecting the child. Legislation

■ Table 7-2   Legislation Related to Newborn Infant Care

Law	Year	Implications
Rehabilitation Act, Section 504	1983	Nontreatment equivalent to civil rights violation. Act not upheld in court
Child Abuse Amendments	1984	Nontreatment considered neglect
Emergency Medical Treatment and Labor Act Section 1867 of the Social Security Act	1997	Healthcare providers must offer emergency services, even when this is potentially futile
Born Alive Infant Protection Act	2001	Ensures that neonates are afforded legal status and protections under the law at birth

related to medical treatment decisions for handicapped or prematurely born infants is provided in **Table 7-2**.

This legislative agenda evolved over three decades in response to increased public reporting of what were seen as troubling end-of-life decision-making practices by physicians and parental refusal of medical treatment for critically ill and handicapped infants (Anspach, 1993). Duff and Campbell (1973) first reported on end-of-life decision-making practices in their Yale, New Haven, NICU. They studied infant deaths over a 2-year period and identified two categories of infant deaths. Causes of death for infants in category 1 resulted from pathologic conditions. Category 2 infant deaths were associated with severe impairments, usually resulting from congenital anomalies. The deaths of these infants resulted from withdrawal or discontinuation of treatment. This disclosure, along with others, prompted wide public and professional debate over treatment decisions for handicapped and extremely early born infants (Anspach, 1993; Singh, Lantos, & Meadow, 2004).

The "Baby Doe Rules" resulted from these widely publicized cases involving the death of handicapped newborns who were denied medical treatment. The primary case, Baby Doe, occurred in 1982. This case involved the parents' refusal to allow physicians to treat medical conditions that were diagnosed at the baby's birth. Baby Doe was diagnosed with Down syndrome, tracheoesophageal atresia, and other problems. Conflict arose between the involved pediatricians regarding the most appropriate course of treatment, and legal action was eventually sought by the birth hospital.

Baby Doe's pediatrician and parents elected not to repair the infant's atresia and to withhold fluids, with the intention of not prolonging the infant's life. This decision was upheld in court and Baby Doe died 6 days later (Munson, 2008). In 1983, a similar situation involving "Baby Jane Doe," an infant with spina bifida, an abnormally small head, and hydrocephaly again brought public attention to the issue of withholding treatment for newborns with disabilities.

Responding to these and other cases, the U.S. Department of Health and Human Services amended regulations of the Rehabilitation Act, Section 504, which included strict guidelines regarding the treatment of sick or handicapped newborns. The Baby Doe Amendments defined child abuse as including the withholding of fluids, food, and medically indicated treatment from disabled infants. This legislation stipulated that failure to provide medical treatment was a violation of an infant's civil rights (Kopelman, 2005). To enforce these regulations, hospitals were required to post notices with hotline numbers for any professional or lay person to report instances of suspected medical neglect. Investigations of reported neglect included medical record review, private investigations, and court orders to force medical treatment that had been refused by parents. The investigations revealed no instances of medical neglect, but the threat of federal investigations prompted many hospital administrators and healthcare providers to alter their practices regarding treatment decisions for these infants. Treatments were often given even where little hope of survival or a reasonable QOL existed.

The first set of Baby Doe Rules was challenged and invalidated in 1986 (Kopelman, 2005). A second set of Baby Doe Rules was enacted in 1984 as amendments to the Child Abuse and Protection and Treatment Act. This legislation forbade the withholding of indicated treatment. Healthcare providers were required to institute care to handicapped or preterm infants regardless of their gestational age or the benefit or futility of treatment. These regulations distinguished between merely prolonging life with measures that are considered futile and care that is beneficial irrespective of the infant's probable handicap (Avery, 1998). The regulations along with definitions of the 1984 Child Abuse Amendments (CAA) are included in **Table 7-3**.

Controversy within the healthcare community regarding the Baby Doe Rules continues. In 2009, a symposium was held to mark the 25th anniversary of the rules. Hosted jointly by Georgia State University's College of Law and Emory University's Center for Ethics, the symposium focused on the contemporary significance of the laws (Scott, 2009). The varied perspectives

■ Table 7-3 U.S.C.A. Title 42, Chapter 67, Sec. 5106a. Grants to States for Child Abuse and Neglect Prevention and Treatment Programs

(B) an assurance that the state has in place procedures for responding to the reporting of medical neglect (including instance of withholding of medically indicated treatment from disabled infants with life-threatening conditions), procedures, or programs, or both (within the State child protective services system) to provide for
(i) coordination and consultation with individuals designated by and within appropriate health-care facilities;
(ii) prompt notification by individuals designated by and within appropriate health-care facilities of cases of suspected medical neglect (including instances of withholding of medically indicated treatment from disabled infants with life-threatening conditions); and
(iii) authority, under State law, for the State child protective services system to pursue any legal remedies including the authority to initiate legal proceedings in a court of competent jurisdiction, as may be necessary to prevent the withholding of medically indicated treatment from disabled infants with life threatening conditions

of speakers highlighted ongoing controversies about these laws. Little has changed except that the numbers of premature infants in need of or able to receive care has increased for a variety of reasons, including technological advances. One question that persists and is not answered by these laws is how low must the odds of survival be, or how severe must the burdens of treatment be, to justify allowing parents to refuse medical treatment for their infant (Scott, 2009, p. 806).

Some professionals believe that the CAA regulations limit the parents' right to decide (Kopelman, 2005; Sayeed, 2005). Many physicians have altered their practices related to end-of-life decision making for the handicapped and critically ill newborn as a result of these rules, which in fact remain untested. Others consider the regulations related to state funding for child abuse prevention grants (Hurst, 2005), stipulating that the language of the regulations contains no sanctions against medical providers for violating the law. The American Academy of Pediatrics (AAP) recommends individualized treatment decisions by clinicians and families using the best interest standard (AAP, 2007; Hurst, 2005). Application of the Baby Doe Rules is perceived as limiting clinician discretion and preventing individualized care (Kopelman, 2005; Sayeed, 2006). The guidelines recommended by the AAP are perceived by some as not consistent with the law (Sayeed, 2006), creating further ambiguity for healthcare providers in the NICU.

The Emergency Medical Treatment and Active Labor Act (EMTLA), Section 1867 of the Social Security Act enacted in 1997, imposed specific obligations on Medicare-participating hospitals to offer emergency services and medical screening for emergency medical conditions to all patients presenting themselves to their hospitals (Romesberg, 2003). This act was intended to prevent the dumping of poor and indigent patients by emergency departments. It allows for no exceptions, futile care or otherwise. The law stipulates that if a patient can be stabilized, then the healthcare providers must act to do so (Hurst, 2005). Legal precedent has been established that enables parents to request the initiation of treatment even in cases where treatment may be incompatible with life (Romesberg, 2003).

The most current legislation affecting the neonate in U.S. society is the Born Alive Infant Protection Act (BIPA) of 2001. This act defines being born alive as displaying signs of life including the following:

> breathing, beating heart, pulsation of the umbilical cord or definite movement of voluntary muscles, regardless of whether the umbilical cord has been cut, and regardless of whether the expulsion or extraction occurs as a result of natural or induced labor, cesarean section or induced abortion. (H.R. 2175 107th Congress 2nd session)

This regulation, initially understood as anti-abortion rhetoric (Sayeed, 2005), raised little concern in the healthcare community. Clinicians responding to the delivery of marginally viable newborns are instructed by the Neonatal Resuscitation Program (NRP) steering committee to retain their current approach to treatment for the care of the marginally viable newborn (AAP, 2007). However, it is evident from recent discussions in the literature that new concerns are being raised about the intent and potential effects of this legislation (Sayeed, 2005, 2006). One major concern is specifically related to the absence of language regarding standards of practice, best interest of the neonate, or the parents' decision-making authority. And although there is no mandate for medical treatment where none is currently indicated, the worry is that a "prudent" lay person attending a birth and seeing what he or she takes to be a viable infant in need of emergency medical care could call for care to be initiated. A further concern is that literal interpretations of the legislation could result in overtreatment of infants born at lower and lower gestations (Sayeed, 2006). Recent research regarding delivery room treatment decisions for marginally viable newborns and end-of-life decisions in the NICU is inconsistent with policy (Singh et al., 2004). Although the law continues to evolve, there are no clear legal answers (Hurst, 2005), especially related to the treatment or protection of those at the margins of viability. Furthermore, the moral responsibilities of healthcare professionals related to the care and treatment for such infants are still unclear. Treatment of very premature neonates continues to vary significantly across NICUs (Stoll et al., 2010).

The Role of Direct Care Neonatal Nurses

Direct care NICU nurses fulfill a unique role in caring for infants and their families. NICU nurses encounter ethical issues daily and are in a position to both understand the implications of a medical condition as well as be familiar with a family's customs, feelings, and attitudes (Catlin, 2007). The number and types of dilemmas that confront those involved with care of critically ill or premature babies are likely to increase as a result of advances in technology and pharmacology, parental involvement in decision making, and varying availability of resources (Spence, 2000).

The National Association of Neonatal Nurses (NANN) recognizes the NICU nurse as a contributor to the ethical decision-making process (Catlin, 2007) through direct care and family education. The COINN evolved to encourage dialogue and support among neonatal nurses across countries and to promote the idea that nurses are instrumental in the delivery of good care to newborns, both premature and term. Yet NICU nurses report they are more likely to be involved in clinical decision making than ethical decision making (Romesberg, 2003). In addition, the theoretical differences between physicians' and nurses' approaches to care (Catlin, 2007), along with the existence of a multicultural society where differing beliefs and values abound, are factors affecting the ability to reach consensus about the best course of action in ethical dilemma situations. Settle (2013) found that NICU nurses are likely to talk with each other or to a physician about a treatment decision disagreement leading to an ethical dilemma. Moreover, NICU nurses in this study were likely to request a team meeting to discuss ethical issues. This finding suggests that APNs in all roles can mentor, counsel, and coach direct care nurses to explore with their peers, as well as their physician colleagues, their experience of dilemmas in daily practice.

The parental role in the NICU has evolved over the past century to family-centered care (FCC) as best practice. FCC is also a COINN value (COINN, 2010). The FCC framework is based on respect, information sharing, collaboration, and confidence building, with collaborative partnerships as the foundation of encounters between nurses and parents (Fegran, Helseth, & Slettebo, 2006; Harrison, 1993). Although implementation of FCC is variable and NICU nurses have different experiences with the approach, both parents and nurses share a common concern—the vulnerable infant. NICU nurses provide a constant presence in the care of infants, and the relationships they develop with families are crucial in determining how parents move from involvement to participation in the care of their infants. Parents are dependent on nurses to help them integrate new knowledge, enabling them to act in their child's best interest. It is essential for NICU nurses to consider the vulnerability parents experience because they are dependent on nurses to care for their child and do not have the clinical expertise to interpret the meaning of changes in their infants' conditions. Parental participation can be achieved by encouraging nurses to create opportunities for participation. Nurses must also be alert and responsive when parents initiate caregiving activities. APN administrators, CNSs, and NPs can enable direct care NICU nurses to reflect on their competence and willingness to involve parents in their infant's care (Fegran et al., 2006).

In summary, the context in which the NICU nurse provides care to critically ill and premature infants is influenced by geographic context, technological capability, and clinicians' interpretations of the laws regulating care. The direct care NICU nurse is in the crucial role of ensuring that parents receive appropriate information concerning the prognosis and treatment options for their infant. This can be achieved by facilitating discussions with all clinicians involved in care along with the family. Hurst (2005) encourages nurses to facilitate the transparent communication processes advocated by many national associations, including the AAP and NANN. However, the workplace has been identified as a barrier to initiating transparent conversations among healthcare providers and parents, which results in ethical conflict (Corley, Minick, Elswick, & Jacobs, 2005). Early indicators of ethical conflict include signs of disagreement, patient suffering, nurse distress, ethics violations, unrealistic expectations, and poor communication

(Pavlish, Brown-Saltzman, Hersh, Shirk, & Nudelman, 2011). The APN is in a central role to identify early indicators of ethical conflict and influence the discussions among nurses and between other members of the healthcare team. Regular multidisciplinary ethics meetings provide the opportunity for disciplines to share perspectives, as well as to hear the perspectives of their colleagues. With a broader view, a more comprehensive plan of care can be developed for the infant and family, as well as the healthcare team. One mechanism to enhance transparent communication and influence the discussions among all clinicians in the NICU is regular multidisciplinary ethics rounds. A monthly ethics meeting that includes residents, medical students, nurses, administrators, respiratory therapists, nutritionists, occupational and physical therapists, as well as a chaplain, can help give voice to the concerns of every member of the healthcare team. Cases for discussion can be identified by any member of the team, and the APN can notify staff of the particular situation to be discussed. The most important conditions of these rounds are confidentiality and the willingness to hold multiple perspectives. As team members share their professional obligations and personal insights, attendees develop a more comprehensive understanding of other disciplines, as well as the parents' perspectives. This cross-disciplinary sharing can lead to improved communication, decreased distress, and less patient suffering. When especially difficult issues arise, it may be important to draw on the resources of a person with ethics or mediation expertise. In the United States, hospitals are required to have recourse to ethics expertise; elsewhere, forming liaisons with academic ethics experts is an important strategy.

The Best Interest Standard

Most, if not all, decisions made in the care of newborns use the best interest standard. It is derived from the ethical principles of beneficence and nonmaleficence (Steinberg, 1998) as discussed in earlier chapters. These principles, along with considerations of the value of life and QOL, serve as a decision framework that enables healthcare providers to determine which interventions will benefit an infant, produce the least amount of harm, and include the cultural traditions of the parents. Before describing the best interest standard decision-making model, it is helpful to review the principles related to the standard to promote a detailed understanding of the decision-making process affecting the care of both healthy and high-risk infants.

Beneficence

Beneficence refers to activities that assist others. Beauchamp and Childress (2009, p. 1997) outline some specific moral rules related to beneficence that include the following:

- Protect and defend the rights of others.
- Prevent harm from occurring to others.
- Remove conditions that will cause harm to others.
- Help persons with disabilities.
- Rescue persons in danger.

Beneficence requires positive actions, may include favoritism, and if not followed, seldom leads to legal challenges. Special relationships, such as the nurse–patient relationship, require specific beneficent actions related to role responsibilities. According to the ANA (2001), "The primary commitment of the nurse is to the health, welfare and safety of the client."

Beneficence also includes the concept of utility. Utility in this context involves the use of analytic techniques applied to health policies that provide information regarding the benefits of a treatment compared to the detriment or costs (Beauchamp & Childress, 2009). Cost-effectiveness analysis (CEA) and cost–benefit analysis (CBA) are the two most commonly used analytic techniques used to evaluate the impact of medical technologies on health and safety. Both tools are used to identify the value of outcomes, one in monetary terms and one in both monetary and nonmonetary terms. QOL cases or cases describing a more complex view of cost than just economics can be assessed with CEA. With CEA costs in terms of such things as pain and symptoms are also factored into the equation. Using a monetary measurement, CBA provides outcomes of both benefit and cost. These analytic techniques are designed to provide information for health policy makers concerning the possible benefits and risks of medical treatments (Beauchamp & Childress, 2009), but they do not always capture "meaning" in relation to family-centered considerations.

Both risk and uncertainty are considered in the analytic techniques of CEA and CBA to determine which medical treatments or policies are beneficial. While both connote a lack of predictability or knowledge of future events, they are different concepts. *Risk* can be defined as the likelihood and extent of negative outcomes. A risk–benefit analysis is the ratio of expected benefits to risks. It involves the probability of an individual experiencing harm and focuses on the acceptability of the harm related to the good that is anticipated (Beauchamp & Childress, 2009).

With insufficient evidence, there is an inability to predict or know an outcome. This results in *uncertainty*. There is always uncertainty in risk assessment. The challenge for the analyst in risk assessment is recognizing that their values and attitudes may influence a prediction, either positive or negative (Beauchamp & Childress, 2009). In the NICU, APNs must be aware that their values and attitudes contribute to their perceptions of the potential benefits and harms of treatments. The APN must communicate the reasons for a specific plan based on this assessment with the direct care nurse and family.

Nonmaleficence

Nonmaleficence, described by Beauchamp and Childress (2009), refers to the obligation not to harm others by intentionally causing pain, disability, mental harm, and death. This principle focuses on a person's actions related to creating situations, participating in acts, and/or not acting that result in tribulations or the risk of tribulations to others. Rules outlined by Beauchamp and Childress (2009) regarding nonmaleficence include; "do not kill . . . cause pain or suffering . . . incapacitate . . . cause offense [or] deprive others of the goods of life" (p. 153). Nonmaleficence also requires a person to try to anticipate potential harms and minimize these.

There are healthcare guidelines that specify requirements of nonmaleficence for treatment and nontreatment decisions. Beauchamp and Childress note that only some of these remain helpful for decision making. Certain distinctions such as between starting and withdrawing life-sustaining treatments (where withdrawing was seen as less morally permissible than not starting) and ordinary versus extraordinary interventions do not withstand critical philosophical analysis (Beauchamp & Childress, 2009).

Beauchamp and Childress (2009) contend that relying on such guidelines may lead to over- and undertreatment. They advocate that healthcare providers consider a detailed assessment of the benefits and burdens of a treatment and determine individual medical treatment plans with the greatest benefits and least burdens to the infant, family, and society. The following descriptions of benefits and burdens related to treatment better capture good decision making:

> If balance of benefits outweighs burdens, the obligation is to treat.
> If no reasonable hope of benefit exists, the obligation is not to treat.

> If a reasonable hope of benefit exists with significant burdensomeness, the treatment is optional. (Beauchamp & Childress, 2001, p. 133)

Other considerations regarding treatment decisions for infants include absolute value and QOL. Historically, societies and all major religions have considered the absolute value of life one of the most important values. The absolute value of life criterion is considered objective, with a biological and medical definition. However, this value is diminishing in importance. Ethicists currently are focusing their attention on the QOL criterion, which may not always benefit infants and small children (Steinberg, 1998). The QOL criterion may be biased and is not applicable to infants or young children who are incapable of verbally stating a personal QOL view. Dangers may exist in prioritizing the QOL definition over the "absolute value"; there is concern about a "slippery slope" in the absence of precise boundaries regarding making life and death decisions (Steinberg, 1998). What is meant by "slippery slope" is that over time, an accepted practice for certain types of cases might cause health professionals to relax their views of the importance of human life in other cases. The worry is that this would permit unjust deaths or inadequate treatment for some patients who may still derive some benefit from treatment. As Beauchamp and Childress (2001) note, "The best interest standard has sometimes been interpreted as highly malleable, thereby permitting values that are irrelevant to the patient's benefits and burdens" (p. 103). They give the example of parents giving permission for the donation of an organ from one child to a brother or sister in need where the rationale given is that it will benefit the donor to know that he or she has helped a sibling. The best interest standard is supposed to protect the interests of individuals who do not have decision-making capacity and for whom beliefs and values are unknown. A surrogate decision maker is appointed or approved to consider the benefits of various treatments and the alternatives to treatments for the infant or individual in question.

Thus, the best interest standard protects a patient's interest by requiring a surrogate decision maker to consider the benefits of various treatments and the alternatives to treatments. "The surrogates consider pain, suffering and restoration, as well as loss of functioning when determining the highest benefit among available options" (Beauchamp & Childress, 2001, p. 102). The best interest decision makers for an infant include the parents, the healthcare team, and if necessary the legal system. The decision-making framework requires the healthcare team to gather relevant medical data and to determine which treatment provides the most benefits with the least amount of pain and suffering.

Information must be shared with family decision makers or others who have been granted decision-making responsibility in a way that takes into account the knowledge and educational level of the ultimate decision maker. Long-term benefits and burdens are important aspects of the consideration. In addition, the healthcare team must establish and maintain therapeutic relationships with parents and include the sociocultural and religious preferences of families in the decision-making process (Steinberg, 1998).

In summary, the best interest standard of decision making for handicapped and critically ill infants is derived from the ethical principles of beneficence and nonmaleficence. The principle of beneficence describes the obligations to protect from harm, prevent harm, and remove conditions that will cause harm to others, although this last obligation applies more to those who have the physical capacity to harm others. The principle of nonmaleficence describes the obligation to refrain from actions that intentionally cause harm and to take into consideration possible harm when making treatment decisions. Decision makers must consider all possible treatments and select those that provide the highest benefit and the least harm. QOL and the absolute value of life measures are to be integrated into treatment decisions as well. Thus, the APN in the NICU is required to act positively by protecting infants and their families from harm, removing the conditions that cause harm, and helping persons with disabilities. This is accomplished by facilitating positive acts by other health team members in the care of infants in the NICU.

CASE STUDY: BEST INTEREST

The transport team at Rolin Hospital was contacted to transport a term infant with possible seizure activity for a workup from a community newborn nursery. While the transport physician obtained necessary and relevant medical data, other members of the team including the nurse and respiratory therapist prepared the transport equipment for departure. The time of the transport call was 6:30 p.m., and the staff for the night shift were just arriving on the unit.

The region was experiencing a severe snowstorm, with blizzard conditions reported in several areas. The oncoming nurses reported treacherous weather conditions and extreme difficulty driving. The nurse assigned to transport that night had witnessed several cars and small trucks that skidded off the roads. Other nurses arriving reported many car accidents. The arriving transport nurse questioned the safety of the transport and strongly suggested that the team delay or refuse the transport because she believed that traveling would endanger the team. The attending physician disagreed with the transport nurse's suggestion and directed the team to proceed with the transport.

The transport physician obtained a current medical history of the infant at the community hospital. The male infant, now 12 hours old, presented at delivery with clear amniotic fluid, a nuchal cord times one (one loop of the umbilical cord wrapped around the neck during delivery), Apgar scores of 6 at 1 minute and 8 at 5 minutes of life. He was taken to the newborn nursery of the delivery hospital, where he was noted as having a typical physical and clinical course. The baby was described by nurses as vigorous and after the initial evaluation, he spent the majority of time in the mother's room. The parents then reported time-limited jerky movements consistent with seizure activity, and this was subsequently observed by community hospital medical and nursing staff as well. Oxygen saturations were noted to be greater than 98% in room air, and the infant remained vigorous after the episode. After the initial episode, no further jerky movements were noted; however, the referring pediatrician requested the infant be transferred to further evaluate the possible seizure activity. No information regarding the parents' concerns was available for discussion with the physician.

The options for the transport team at Rolin Hospital were to risk the transport in treacherous conditions or to refuse the transport. The seeming "ethical dilemma" the team faced was deciding what on balance was in the best interest of this newborn infant and the transport team. The NICU nursing director was contacted by the transport nurse to discuss her concerns and resolve the situation. An ethical dilemma is one where there is no good alternative or way to decide which of two or more actions is preferable. Is this case a true dilemma, or might a preferable action be determined after an exploration of the facts?

Using the Best Interest Standard to Explore the Case

According to the best interest standard, this situation requires the NICU nursing director to facilitate a discussion regarding the transport of this otherwise healthy infant with neurological symptoms during a severe snowstorm. The discussion needs to include the benefits of transport to a NICU with the diagnosis of suspected seizures as well as the burdens of remaining in a hospital that may not be equipped with appropriate technology and personnel. In addition, the discussion requires the consideration of the risks of transport during a severe snowstorm. Possible risks to the infant include potential weather-related accidents and harm related to the slow traveling time if he should become compromised during the journey. Additionally, an accident could damage the transport vehicle and the special equipment in which the infant is housed during transport. This type of damage could cause physiologic instability and possible harm to the infant. The speed with which the infant is returned to the NICU may create a situation where the transport team is unable to optimally provide needed interventions such as intubations for mechanical ventilation.

The NICU nursing director also must consider the benefits and burdens for the transport team. The reported travel conditions indicate that travel is currently dangerous, and the oncoming shift witnessed many travel accidents. This transport would require the team to travel in severe storm conditions twice, increasing the chances of harm to the team. Harm to the team members is in and of itself an ethical consideration. The loss of services to other infants that might accrue is an additional burden to be factored into the decision-making process. To make a decision that considers the best interests of the team and the infant, the NICU nursing director requires more information.

Relevant Facts

The male infant is 12 hours old. He was delivered by spontaneous vaginal delivery with Apgar scores of 6 at 1 minute and 8 at 5 minutes. He had a nuchal cord times one and weighs 8 pounds and 6 ounces. He is noted to be a vigorous infant with good tone and has voided and passed stool. His neurological exam revealed no negative findings, and no further episodes of jerky movements have been observed. His oxygen saturations remain at 98%–100%. The nursing director at Rolin Hospital contacts the NICU physician to further discuss this transport. Specifically, the nursing director is interested in what data regarding the infant are so concerning to the physician that a transport is considered urgent enough to risk traveling in the severe weather.

The nursing director also requests to speak with the ambulance company that provides the transport and obtains an updated weather forecast. By collecting all of the relevant data regarding the ability of the transport team to respond, the healthcare team can make the best decision for the infant and transport team. The nursing director requests a conference call with the NICU physician and transport nurse.

Who Are the Decision Makers?

The healthcare providers in both NICUs along with the parents are the decision makers for this infant. All are in agreement that it is in the infant's best interest, all things being equal, to be transported to the NICU for further evaluation of his neurological symptoms, but not all agree on the urgency of the transport. The severe snowstorm in progress alters the situation and must be factored into the decision making. The NICU transport nurse has rightly questioned the decision regarding the safety of the transport. The NICU physician informs the NICU nursing director that there is no other information concerning the medical history of this infant. The infant continues to room-in with the mother and is breastfeeding uneventfully. The lack of specialty physicians at the community hospital is the reason the NICU physician is adamant that the transport occurs. The nursing director informs the physician that the storm is expected to decrease in severity in about 2 hours. The NICU physician and community hospital physician discuss the coverage that will be needed for at least 2 more hours and reach agreement regarding physician availability in the community hospital and the possibility of a consult from the specialists at Rolin Hospital should there be changes in the infant's status. The transport team is in agreement that the infant will remain at the community hospital until the storm lessens in intensity, and then he will be transported to the NICU at the larger hospital.

After the problem is resolved, the nursing director decides that it is important to put into place a policy that will guide future similar decisions. She plans a meeting for the purpose of policy making related to transport safety. She involves the NICU physicians, members of the transport team, the NICU CNSs and NPs, the shift charge nurses, and a member of the hospital ethics committee who serves as the NICU resource for difficult cases. Although policy making cannot anticipate all problems that can occur, guidelines are helpful in pointing to possible resources and avenues of action. Additionally, discussion of such issues after the fact is educational and permits insights about important considerations in such situations.

Collaborative Decision Making

Collaborative decision making in the NICU means that all pertinent voices are encouraged and heard as an important part of the data necessary for good (beneficent) or least harmful (nonmaleficent) care of an infant that takes into account both long- and short-term implications. The involved physicians, APNs, direct care nurses, and family members or guardians all have important perspectives. The importance of collaboration has not always been, and is not always, understood. A collaborative environment is difficult to institute and maintain even under the best of circumstances when all are willing to participate (Grace, Willis, & Jurchak, 2007). It involves trust and respect for a variety of viewpoints, as well as the treatment of each perspective as equally relevant.

As with other aspects of neonatal care, decision making is in the process of evolving from a process of closed communication that tends to leave out family members and paternalism, where healthcare professionals determine appropriate actions, to one of transparency and collaboration. Although the importance of family involvement is in general now more valued than it has been in the past, it is still not always honored. The following discussion provides an argument for the importance of family involvement and the role that APNs can play in encouraging this.

Until the past decade or so parents assumed a more passive role in the care of their critically ill and/or premature infant. They tended not to be involved in clinical decision-making processes because of barriers in communication and the hierarchical structure of the NICU (Pinch, 2002). The barriers parents faced included a lack of pertinent medical knowledge and an inadequate understanding of information provided to them by professionals, including the short- and long-term implications of treatment. In addition, in some studies aimed at gaining clarity about this problem, parents reported being overwhelmed by technology, terminology, a lack of continuity of relationships, and reluctance to voice concerns (King, 1992; Penticuff, 2005; Pinch & Spielman, 1990). The reluctance to participate in the process or to voice concerns was identified as stemming, in part, from parents' fear of being labeled "difficult" and the consequences that could have for their baby (Hurst, 2001). In addition, the decision-making process for most aspects of an infant's care became part of the medical decision-making agenda as technological advances were made and the ability to save very premature and critically ill infants became possible. The parents' point of view was ignored or neglected. Harrison's (1993) publication of the FCC principles and the AAP endorsement of them created momentum for parents and professionals to achieve a more active partnership regarding the care of high-risk infants. The FCC principles are listed in **Table 7-4**.

Several studies conducted both in the United States and elsewhere have pointed to the desire and need of parents to participate in decision making related to their infant (Brinchmann, Førde, & Nortvedt, 2002; McHaffie,

■ Table 7-4   Family-Centered Care Principles

1. Family-centered neonatal care should be based on open and honest communication between parents and professionals on medical and ethical issues.

2. To work with professionals in making informed treatment choices, parents must have available to them the same facts and interpretation of those facts as the professionals, including medical information presented in meaningful formats, information about uncertainties surrounding treatments, information from parents whose children have been in similar medical situations, and access to the chart and rounds discussions.

3. In medical situations involving very high mortality and morbidity, great suffering, and/or significant medical controversy, fully informed parents should have the right to make decisions regarding aggressive treatment for their infants.

4. Expectant parents should be offered information about adverse pregnancy outcomes and be given the opportunity to state in advance their treatment preferences if their baby is born extremely prematurely and/or critically ill.

5. Parents and professionals must work together to acknowledge and alleviate the pain of infants in intensive care.

6. Parents and professionals should work together to ensure the safety and efficacy of neonatal treatments.

7. Parents and professionals should work together to develop nursery policies and programs that promote parenting skills and encourage maximum involvement of families with their hospitalized infant.

8. Parents and professionals must work together to promote meaningful long-term follow-up for all high-risk NICU survivors.

Source: Harrison, H. (1993). The principles for family-centered neonatal care. *Pediatrics, 92,* 643–650.

Laing, Parker, & McMillan, 2001; Orfali & Gordon, 2004; Wocial, 2000). These studies reported that parents actively sought out the opportunity to participate in all aspects of their newborn's care including ethical discussions related to withholding or withdrawing life support. All parents desired to be involved with the discussions regarding their infant but varied in their desire to participate in the final decision to withdraw or withhold medical support. As one parent in Brinchmann and colleagues' (2002) Norwegian study stated:

> One has to distinguish between information and discussion. Discussing is something different from making a decision. One can listen to arguments for and against. In making a decision one does not necessarily include all the things one has discussed. But anyway, I think it is important to be part of the discussion. (p. 396)

Although many complex decisions are made in the NICU regarding the care of high-risk infants, parents report their involvement tends to be considered superfluous until the question of redirection of care arises (King, 1992; Pinch, 2002). Both the ANA, in the *Code of Ethics for Nurses with Interpretive Statements* (2001), and the International Council of Nurses (2012) describe the nurse's opportunity and responsibility to preserve, protect, and support the rights and interests of families. Informed parental consent is essential in the delivery of good care for infants and their families.

Direct care NICU nurses, through their close contact with parents, are in a pivotal position to ensure that parents receive information about what is known and what is not known regarding outcomes. They are in a position to understand a family's needs for information and what is required for their comprehension of the information. Through the process of transparency, NICU APNs can model for other healthcare professionals and new nurses the delivery of appropriate information to parents. Transparent communication requires APNs to disclose to parents a healthcare team's reasoning process along with the meaning and implications of technical information. Through the process of transparency, parents are prepared for their decision-making role and enabled to provide informed consent when necessary for their infant.

Neonatal APNs can help parents be adequate decision makers for their infants in the NICU by discussing the burdens and benefits of treatments with parents. Penticuff (2005) reported improved parental understanding with use of an educational process aimed at explaining the types of treatment as well as the burdens associated with treatments. Parents reported increased understanding of the goals of treatment as well as the implications of those situations in which infants were not meeting the goals of treatment. These shared understandings of goals of treatment empower parents to participate more fully in the treatment decisions for their infants. Challenges to the view that parents are the ideal decision makers for their infants come from worries that they may not always make decisions that consider all of the following: their infant's QOL, their own QOL, and the value of their child's life within society. However, whenever possible, parents' wishes should be honored if they are medically reasonable and legally appropriate (King, 1992).

Hurst (2001) described "empowering information" (p. 46) as a determining factor that contributes to collaborative decision making in the NICU. Empowering information is easily accessible, pertinent, and understandable. In addition, empowering information includes the descriptions of a unit's philosophy of care and practice along with how care is organized and delivered to foster supported parental independence. This is achieved through the establishment of trust that has evolved from the development of caring relationships. The APN is in a unique position to model transparency with both the medical team and the direct care nurses. In this influential position, the APN can reduce the barriers parents face to participating in the decision-making process for their infants. APNs play an important role in fostering collaborative decision making in the NICU by ensuring regular meetings, especially when goals of treatment between disciplines conflict.

CASE STUDY: COLLABORATIVE DECISION MAKING

Natalie Smith is a former 29-week gestation infant, now corrected to 38 weeks gestation. Natalie is preparing for discharge home after a complicated course including intubation for 2 weeks due to prematurity and sepsis, along with a cardiac lesion that will be repaired when she is 6 months old. Natalie is now in an open crib maintaining her temperature and has not recently had any apneic or bradycardiac episodes. The main challenge for Natalie is to obtain adequate nutrition from her oral feedings. Her cardiac condition causes her to fatigue easily, and occasionally she requires supplemental gavage feedings to ensure that she receives adequate nutrition and hydration.

Natalie's parents have been very involved in her care and have participated in many meetings with the healthcare team to discuss her medical course and health needs. Natalie's healthcare team and parents are concerned that she is still not able to consistently feed by bottle. A meeting is called with the purpose of discussing the options available to ensure that Natalie will receive the necessary nutrients and hydration for her development and eventual discharge home. It is hoped that she can be discharged to her home soon. Present at the meeting are Natalie's mother and father, her primary nurse, as well as the neonatal nurse practitioner (NNP) assigned to her case. In the course of discussion, the NNP reviews Natalie's progress to date and identifies the single barrier to discharge as Natalie's inability to obtain all necessary fluids via a bottle. Natalie's parents are in agreement that Natalie is not able to complete her bottle feedings. The NNP describes possible options to consider, including keeping Natalie in the hospital until she is able to bottle feed or placing a gastrostomy tube in her stomach. She explains that Natalie's parents can be taught how to care for the feeding tube and administer the amount of feeding that Natalie is not able to take orally. Natalie's parents listen to the options and both agree that neither is acceptable to them. They do not want their daughter to have a surgical procedure because of the risks of reintubation. They are also concerned about the possibility of a prolonged ventilator requirement because of negative experiences with this earlier in Natalie's course of development. Their perception of the current problem is that Natalie will be able to achieve full feedings soon after she gets home. They inform the team that they believe that Natalie is not consuming the necessary amounts of her bottle feedings because of inconsistencies in the approach used by the variety of nurses who care for her. The NNP considers the information the parents are sharing and suggests that they review her entire medical course to put their concerns in context. At the conclusion, the parents again state that they are not interested in and will not consent to a gastrostomy tube.

What Are the Relevant Facts?

Natalie is unable to obtain adequate feedings via the bottle to meet her needs. This is a problem involving the principles of beneficence and nonmaleficence for the healthcare team. Professional obligations include promoting the well-being of the infant and avoiding harm. However, there are also responsibilities to the parents to help them find a solution that will meet their needs and concerns. Viewing this as a family problem rather than just a problem of avoiding harm to Natalie permits the envisioning of alternatives that could work to the benefit of all. The parents have concerns about the course of action proposed and do want Natalie home with them as soon as possible, which is understandable after the long hospitalization that she has had and the future hospitalization that she will face. The healthcare team does need more information about the parents and what they are or are not willing to accept, why they seem so adamant, and whether compromise is possible. It is implied from their concerns about the different feeding styles of the nurses that there may be some trust issues. More information is needed about this. Additionally, it is important to know how often Natalie requires extra feedings and how capable the parents are of monitoring her hydration and nutritional needs should she go home. Would they be capable of learning the gavage techniques used by the nurses? Could a homecare agency provide this service?

Who Are the Decision Makers?

Once Natalie is discharged, her parents will be the ones who make decisions for her. Currently, however, decision making is presumably a team effort. The healthcare team members are the ones who evaluate Natalie's nutritional status, place the tube, and supply the tube feedings when necessary. Indeed, if Natalie's parents objected to a necessary tube feeding, their decision would be overridden if it posed a significant risk to Natalie and there were no other options. This is also true in most other countries. Parental actions that occur outside of a healthcare institution and that put the child at risk for harm may be considered abuse or neglect, which in turn may be grounds for removal of a child from the home setting for safety reasons. However, the ideal outcome is a collaborative endeavor where all parties are willing to listen to each other and try to work out a compromise. Knowing who the parents are, what their fears are, and what their needs for support are in both the short and long term would be helpful. Their fears about the gastrostomy tube placement and possible side effects, including the need for long-term endotracheal intubation, may not be warranted. But if they are making this connection, it is not surprising that they object. Their interest is in protecting their daughter from harm.

Collaborative Resolution

Several possibilities for resolution suggest themselves. First, if a long-term gastrostomy tube placement has not been considered while she was hospitalized, the implication is that her nutrition needs were able to be met by other means; thus the parents may be enabled to meet Natalie's needs with more information and perhaps by learning appropriate techniques. The parents may be wrong in thinking that they will be able to meet Natalie's needs with bottle feeding because they will be more consistent than the nurses. They can be taught how to watch for signs of dehydration and strategies for remedy. Helping the parents to understand the patterns of her fatigue, when it occurs, and what precursors exist could help them pace feedings. Further education and acquisition of necessary skills for the parents will reduce the risks for Natalie. This would also be useful information for the parents to have as they take her home.

One option is to have the parents consistently do the feedings themselves and be involved in monitoring her nutritional and hydration status while she is still in the hospital. This way they could see for themselves what is entailed. Nurses have a responsibility to prepare the parents to care adequately for her at home anyway, and this would include the parents learning how to monitor her nutrition and hydration status.

Although such problems might initially be viewed as dilemmas, they are usually not. Other options may well be available, and thus the challenge is to try to envision what these might be. APNs, with their advanced education and expanded knowledge base, know how to access resources. The NNP in this case has a responsibility to work with the family on discovering options. Perhaps Natalie should remain in the unit long enough to train the parents how to monitor her hydration status and safely give gavage feedings as indicated; Natalie can go home and be monitored by the parents with the adjunct assistance of visiting nurses to help monitor her nutrition and hydration and provide supplemental feedings. Natalie can be brought back for insertion of a gastrostomy tube if her nutritional and hydration status is not maintained.

Questions to Consider

1. Under what conditions might the NNP seek to override the parents' decision?
2. Under what conditions might the visiting nurse seek to override the parents' decision once Natalie goes home?
3. Identify other aspects of collaboration not discussed in the case.
4. In your view, what are the limits of collaboration? Give your rationale.

Medical Futility

Futility may be defined as the inability to achieve a stated purpose. Beauchamp and Childress (2009) note that several meanings for the term *medical futility* can be derived from the literature. Two pertinent meanings in the NICU setting are that what is proposed cannot meet the physiologically desired goal or produce the desired benefit (Beauchamp & Childress, 2009). Additionally, the term *futility* has been divided into *quantitative futility*, that is, the likelihood of benefit is extremely small, and *qualitative futility*, where the quality of benefit is likely very meager (Jecker, 1998). The idea of futility has been used over the last several decades as a clinical criterion in unilateral decisions about prolonging life (Romesberg, 2003). Penticuff (1998) described futility in the NICU as a synthesis of medical and humanistic elements. The medical element is the inability to achieve specific physiologic responses. The humanistic element is the inability to achieve elemental QOL goals. As Truog, Frader, and Brett (1998) noted in their cautions about an overreliance upon futility as a reason to limit care, "A clear understanding of futility has proved to be elusive" (p. 323). Determinations of futility can be especially difficult in the NICU because it is not always possible to predict the likely long-term sequelae of a brain injury.

Although Truog and colleagues (1998) argued that only certain "narrowly defined physiologic" criteria can point to a determination of futility, the concept of futility can be helpful in decision making as long as it is understood that there are often no clear delineations that can be made. For example, one QOL goal for ELBW infants would be to eventually establish a reciprocal relationship with parents or guardians. If an infant is neurologically devastated from a severe intracranial hemorrhage and is blind and deaf, he or she may not have the capacity to establish meaningful relationships with its parents. The philosophical arguments for this are complex and intricate and are beyond the scope of this chapter to discuss in detail. They hinge on the idea that children should be able to experience a meaningful life and not be exposed to a life where the burden of living outweighs the benefits. Munson (2008) gives an illustrative example of when the burden of maintaining a life might outweigh the quality of that life. He describes the short life of a child born with Hallopeau-Siemens syndrome. This terrible collagen deficit disease, which is genetic in origin, causes intractable pain and discomfort from continual blistering of the skin and mucous membranes. There is no treatment for the disease and life is usually short and very painful.

The three interacting factors involved in the analysis of futility in the NICU include (1) the impact of treatment on the probability of mortality, morbidity, and QOL; (2) the extent that treatment produces less pain and discomfort and increased comfort and benefit; and (3) the involvement and decision-making prerogative of the infant's parents (Penticuff, 1998). The use of futility as a clinical criterion in the NICU must be determined individually by each infant's response to treatment and other supportive data. In the case of the ELBW infant, decisions to redirect the goals of care, from that of prolonging life with pharmacological and technological interventions to providing comfort measures only, should be based on the infant's response to treatment and the parents' QOL goals for their infant, not solely on the infant's gestational age or birth weight.

Palliative care programs are increasingly available in newborn intensive care units both in the United States and internationally as an option to consider when there is no hope of meeting treatment goals. The transition to palliative care can be staged to include no escalation of treatment, complete review of current medical interventions to determine if any can be discontinued due to the burden to the infant, and increased parent involvement during end-of-life care. Parents can contribute to the plan of care and make informed choices regarding what will and will not be provided to their infant during this time. Neonatal APNs can provide education describing the principals of palliative care and present the position statement from the NANN to all members of the healthcare team (NANN, 2010). With a consistent approach, the healthcare team can support the parents, infant, and each other through a very difficult and emotional time. Chapter 13 provides an expanded discussion of the role of palliative care for infants and children as well as adults.

CASE STUDY: MEDICAL FUTILITY

Mrs. M. experienced an uneventful early pregnancy but ruptured her membranes at what was estimated to be 24 weeks gestation and began to labor. She was admitted to the labor and delivery unit by her obstetrician. A NICU consult was requested. The consulting neonatologist met with Mr. and Mrs. M. while Mrs. M. was in early labor. The neonatologist informed them of the medical course their infant would likely experience and some of the possible complications of such an early delivery. In addition, they were informed that the NICU team would respond to Mrs. M.'s delivery and provide the necessary treatment for her baby.

Mr. and Mrs. M. requested that no medical treatment be administered because they did not believe their prematurely born infant would survive. Mrs. M. had no previous experience with prematurely born infants and did not want her child to suffer because she could not carry her infant to term. The information Mr. and Mrs. M. received from the neonatologist only confirmed that their wishes of no intervention at delivery were reasonable. However, the neonatologist informed Mr. and Mrs. M. that the technology to sustain the infant's life was available and that some infants born this early do survive in the NICU with the highly advanced technological and nursing care provided there. Moreover, Baby Doe and related laws have caused many providers and institutions to be nervous about the legal ramifications of delivery practices when the delivery is very premature. Thus, a neonatologist may be moved by personal or institutional policy to attend those births suspected to be problematic for whatever reason, including prematurity. The neonatologist in this case saw herself as being legally required to attend the birth and to provide care if the baby seemed "like it could live," and she conveyed this message to the family. She went on to note that many babies survive with minimal handicaps if the necessary interventions are initiated. However, she assured the couple that she would communicate the consult findings and request of no intervention to the NICU delivery team.

Mrs. M. delivered a 560-gram female infant. The infant emerged pink and crying, and a heart rate was noted to be greater than 100 beats per minute. Based on the current legislation and the infant's condition at birth, the NICU team provided warmth and cardiopulmonary support in the form of ventilation, oxygen, and fluid though intravenous catheter for this ELBW infant.

Nurse S. admitted Baby M. to the NICU and assumed the role of the baby's primary nurse. She was aware of the neonatology consult and parents' request, as well as the reasons given for instituting treatment. Initially, Baby M. responded to treatment and required minimal interventions. Mr. and Mrs. M. started to become more optimistic. Nurse S. proceeded to establish a therapeutic relationship with Baby M.'s parents. She communicated with them daily and included them in aspects of care they were interested in, such as obtaining their daughter's temperature and changing her diaper, and she discussed the baby's status with them. She talked with them about their lives and expectations, and they told her about their cultural backgrounds and beliefs. Nurse S. was concerned about the family receiving adequate external support because they had no support structure in the area. Unfortunately, on day 7 of life, the baby suffered a severe intracranial hemorrhage that extended well into the brain as identified on ultrasound. Nurse S. requested a family meeting to inform the parents of this finding. During this meeting, the parents requested that the treatment to their daughter be stopped and that comfort measures only be offered.

Questions to Consider

Using the preceding discussion, explore this case in class or with colleagues.

1. What data would support a determination of futility and a redirection toward palliative care?
2. As the NNP on duty, if a determination of futility were made, what would be your responsibilities to the baby? To the parents? To Nurse S.?
3. Suppose the team concludes that it is too early to determine whether the continuation of treatment is futile. How would you approach the family? What would your role be related to Nurse S.?
4. Given the ambiguous status of the laws governing the treatment of babies who are born at the borderline of viability (500 grams or 22 weeks approximately) and the arguments that these laws can limit healthcare professionals' ability to serve the babies' best interests, what if any are an APN's responsibilities to be politically active in challenging these laws?
5. What strategies can be used by APNs to inform the public?

Summary

Advanced nursing practice in neonatal settings can be both very rewarding and very difficult. It is rewarding when an infant begins to thrive and is eventually discharged with minimal injury. It is difficult when an APN is faced with ambiguity and uncertainty about an infant's short- and long-term prognoses or when an infant is suspected to be experiencing ongoing suffering. Not only are these infants extremely vulnerable physically, but their parents also are faced with emotional turmoil and crisis during a time that for many others is full of anticipation and joy. For this reason, ethical NICU practice is concerned with the needs of the family unit. Paradoxically, in the United States at least, although the healthcare system is beginning to take seriously parental interests in children's well-being and to understand the importance of involving the parents in the decision-making process, concerns about the law may trump ethical concerns about the good of an individual baby and its family unit.

Much more could be said about ethical issues associated with NICUs. Questions have been raised about the antecedents of the current increase in premature births and whether more money should be diverted to this area of concern than is currently. There is concern about the issue of nurses being able to maintain their sense of personal integrity and about issues of moral distress and burnout. These problems were not discussed in great detail in this chapter but were discussed earlier in the book and will be further elucidated later related to other specialties. When nurses experience prolonged distress in their workplace, they may leave their jobs or become more resistant to noticing ethical issues. Either case is liable to contribute to the problem of providing good care for these infants and appropriate support for their families.

Discussion Questions

In the collaboration case presented earlier in this chapter, the parents would not consent to a gastrostomy tube for their baby. Although there were options available to redress the issue in that case, alternative scenarios might be more difficult to resolve. Suppose the mother does not speak English. She and her husband are living in the United States for a year related to his lecturing appointment. Their baby has been in the NICU for several weeks. Usually, the husband serves as the translator. However, he has to go back to Turkey (they are of Kurdish origin) and the mother is currently the sole decision maker. The baby is almost ready for discharge, but in this case a gastrostomy tube is necessary if the baby is to go home. The mother is unable to understand the request for consent to the procedure, which the nurse thought the husband had explained to her. The only available interpreter who speaks her language is Turkish (there have been conflicts for several decades between the Kurdish and Turkish peoples). When the interpreter arrives and the mother discovers his origin, she is horrified (this is reported by the interpreter) and will not talk to him.

1. What are the important issues here?
2. How would you take into account cultural beliefs and values in your discharge planning?

3. What avenues of action are available?
4. If you are not familiar with a culture's beliefs and values, how could you go about gathering information about these?
5. What is the role of empathy or self-reflection in such cases?

References

Ambalavanan, S., Carlo, W. A., Tyson, J. E., Langer, J. C., Walsh, M. C., Parikh, N. A., . . . Higgins, R. D. (2012). Outcome trajectories in extremely pre-term infants. *Pediatrics, 130*(e115–124).

American Academy of Pediatrics. (2007). Non-initiation or withdrawal of intensive care for high-risk newborns. *Committee on Fetus and Newborn Pediatrics 2007, 119,* 401–403.

American Nurses Association. (2001). *Code of ethics for nurses with interpretive statements.* Washington, DC: Author.

Anspach, R. (1993). *Deciding who lives: Fateful choices in the intensive care nursery.* Berkeley, CA: University of California Press.

Avery, G. B. (1998). Futility considerations in the neonatal intensive care unit. *Seminars in Perinatology, 22*(3), 216–222.

Beauchamp, T., & Childress, J. (2001). *Principles of biomedical ethics* (5th ed.). New York, NY: Oxford University Press.

Beauchamp, T., & Childress, J. (2009). *Principles of biomedical ethics* (6th ed.). New York, NY: Oxford University Press.

Berger, T. M., Steurer, M. A., Woerner, A., Meyer-Schiffer, P., & Adams, M. (2012). Trends and centre-to-centre variability in survival rates of very preterm infants (< 32 weeks) over a 10-year period in Switzerland. *Archives of Disease in Childhood, Fetal and Neonatal Edition, 97*(5), F323–F328.

Born Alive Infant Protection Act. (2001). Retrieved from http://www.nrlc.org/Federal/Born_Alive_Infants/BAIPLaw0405.html

Brinchmann, B. S., Førde, R., & Nortvedt, P. (2002). What matters to the parents? A qualitative study of parents' experiences with life-and-death decisions concerning their premature infants. *Nursing Ethics, 9*(4), 386–404.

Brinchmann, B. S., & Nortvedt, P. (2001). Ethical decision making in neonatal units—the normative significance of vitality. *Medicine, Healthcare & Philosophy, 4,* 193–200.

Catlin, A. (2005). Thinking outside the box: Prenatal care and the call for a prenatal advance directive. *Journal of Perinatal & Neonatal Nursing, 19*(2), 169–176.

Catlin, A. (2007). Commentary on NANN position statement 3015: NICU nurse involvement in ethical decisions (treatment of critically ill newborns). Ethical issues in newborn care. *Advances in Neonatal Care, 7*(5), 269.

Corley, M. C., Minick, P., Elswick, R. K., & Jacobs, M. (2005). Nurse moral distress and ethical work environment. *Nursing Ethics, 12*(4), 381–390.

Council of International Neonatal Nurses. (2010). Scope of neonatal nursing document. Retrieved from http://www.coinnurses.org/1_documents/resources/p_statement/Scope_Neonatal_Nurs_Doc.pdf

Duff, R., & Campbell, A. (1973, November 12). Shall this child die? *Newsweek*, 70.

Fegran, L., Helseth, S., & Slettebo, A. (2006). Nurses as moral practitioners encountering parents in neonatal intensive care units. *Nursing Ethics, 13*(1), 52–64.

Grace, P. J., Willis, G. G., & Jurchak, M. (2007). Good patient care: Egalitarian inter-professional collaboration as a moral imperative. *American Society of Bioethics and Humanities Exchange, 10*(1), 8–9.

Hack, M., Flannery, D., Schluter, M., Cartar, L., Borowski, E., & Klein, N. (2002). Outcomes in young adulthood for very-low-birth-weight infants. *New England Journal of Medicine, 346*(3), 149–157.

Harrison, H. (1993). The principles for family-centered neonatal care. *Pediatrics, 92*, 643–650.

Hurst, I. (2001). Vigilant watching over: Mothers' actions to safeguard their premature babies in the newborn intensive care nursery. *Journal of Perinatal & Neonatal Nursing, 15*(3), 39–57.

Hurst, I. (2005). First rule: Choose your battles wisely. *Pediatrics, 116*, 288.

International Council of Nurses. (2012). *Code of ethics for nurses*. Geneva, Switzerland: Author. Retrieved from http://www.icn.ch/about-icn/code-of-ethics-for-nurses

Jecker, N. (1998). *Futility*. University of Washington, School of Medicine Ethics Website. Retrieved from http://depts.washington.edu/bioethx/topics/futil.html

King, N. (1992). Transparency in neonatal intensive care. *Hastings Center Report, 22*(3), 18–25.

Kopelman, L. (2005). Are the 21-year-old Baby Doe Rules misunderstood or mistaken? *Pediatrics, 115*, 797–802.

Lantos, J. D., Mokalla, M., & Meadow, W. (1997). Resource allocation in neonatal and medical ICUs. Epidemiology and rationing at the extremes of life. *American Journal of Respiratory and Critical Care Medicine, 156*, 185–189.

McHaffie, H. E., Laing, I. A., Parker, M., & McMillan, J. (2001). Deciding for imperiled newborns: Medical authority or parental autonomy. *Journal of Medical Ethics, 27*, 104–109.

Meadow, W., Lee, G., Lin, K., & Lantos, J. (2004). Changes in mortality for extremely low birth weight infants in the 1990s: Implications for treatment decisions and resource use. *Pediatrics, 113*(5), 1223–1229.

Medlock, S., Ravelli, C. J., Tamminga, P., Mol, B. W. M., & Abu-Hanna, A. (2011). Prediction of mortality in very premature infants: A systematic review of prediction models. *PLoS ONE, 6*(9), 1–9.

Munson, R. (2008). *Intervention and reflection: Basic issues in medical ethics* (8th ed.). Belmont, CA: Wadsworth/Thomson Learning.

National Association of Neonatal Nurses. (2010). Palliative care for newborns and infants position statement. *Advances in Neonatal Care, 10*(6), 287–293.

Orfali, K. (2004). Parental role in medical decision-making: Fact or fiction? A comparative study of ethical dilemmas in French and American neonatal intensive care units. *Social Science & Medicine, 58*, 2009–2022.

Orfali, K., & Gordon, E. J. (2004). Autonomy gone awry: A cross-cultural study of parents' experiences in neonatal intensive care units. *Theoretical Medicine, 25,* 329–365.

Pavlish, C., Brown-Saltzman, M. A., Hersh, M., Shirk, M., & Nudelman, B. A. (2011). Early indicators and risk factors for ethical issues in clinical practice. *Journal of Nursing Scholarship, 43*(1), 13–21.

Penn, W. (1682). Some fruits of solitude in reflections and maxims. In the *Modern History Source Book.* Retrieved from http://www.fordham.edu/Halsall/mod/1682penn-solitude .asp

Penticuff, J. H. (1998). Defining futility in neonatal intensive care. *Nursing Clinics of North America, 33*(2), 339–352.

Penticuff, J. H. (2005). Effectiveness of an intervention to improve parent-professional collaboration in neonatal intensive care. *Journal of Perinatal & Neonatal Nursing, 19*(2), 169–176.

Pinch, W. (2002). *When the bough breaks: Parental perceptions of ethical decision making in the NICU.* Lanham, MD: University Press of America.

Pinch, W., & Spielman, M. L. (1990). The parent's perspective: Ethical decision-making in neonatal intensive care. *Journal of Advanced Nursing, 15,* 712–719.

Rebagliato, M., Cuttini, M., Broggin, L., Berbik, I., de Vonderweid, U., Hansen, G., . . . Saracci, R. (2000). Neonatal end-of-life decision-making. Physicians' attitudes and relationship with self-reported practices in 10 European countries. *Journal of the American Medical Association, 284,* 2451–2459.

Romesberg, T. L. (2003). Futile care and the neonate. *Advances in Neonatal Care, 3*(5), 213–219.

Sayeed, S. A. (2005). Baby Doe redux? The Department of Health and Human Services and the Born-Alive Infants Protection Act of 2002: A cautionary not on normative neonatal practice. *Pediatrics, 116*(4), 577–585.

Sayeed, S. A. (2006). The marginally viable newborn: Legal challenges, conceptual inadequacies, and reasonableness. *Journal of Law and Medical Ethics, 34*(3), 600–610.

Scott, C. (2009). Baby Doe at twenty five. *Georgia State Law Review, 25*(4), 801–833. Retrieved from http://digitalarchive.gsu.edu/cgi/viewcontent.cgi?article=2391&context=gsulr

Settle, P. D. (2013). Nurse activism in the newborn intensive care unit: Actions in response to an ethical dilemma. *Nursing Ethics* (in press).

Singh, J., Lantos, J., & Meadow, W. (2004). End-of-life after birth: Death and dying in a neonatal intensive care unit. *Pediatrics, 114,* 1620–1626.

Spence, K. (2000). The best interest principle as a standard for decision making in the care of neonates. *Journal of Advanced Nursing, 31*(6), 1286–1292.

Steinberg, A. (1998). Decision-making and the role of surrogacy in withdrawal or withholding of therapy in neonates. *Clinics in Perinatology, 25*(3), 779–790.

Stoll, B. J., Hansen, N. I., Bell, E. F., Shankaran, S., Laptook, A. R., Walsh, M. C., . . . Higgins, R. D. (2010). Neonatal outcomes of extremely preterm infants from the NICHD neonatal research network. *Pediatrics, 126*(3), 443–456.

Truog, R., Frader, J., & Brett, A. (1998). The problem with futility. In J. Monagle & D. Thomasma (Eds.), *Health care ethics: Critical issues for the 21st century* (pp. 323–329). Gaithersburg, MD: Aspen. Reprinted from *New England Journal of Medicine, 326*(23), 1560–1565.

Vohr, B., Wright, L., Dusick, A., Perritt, R., Poole, W., Delaney-Black, V., . . . Mayes, L. C. (2004). Center differences and outcomes of extremely low birth weight infants. *Pediatrics, 113*, 781–789.

Wilson-Costello, D., Freidman, H., Minich, N., Fanaroff, A., & Hack, M. (2005). Improved survival rates with increased neurodevelopmental disability for extremely low birth weight infants in the 1990s. *Pediatrics, 115*, 997–1003.

Wocial, L. D. (2000). Life support decisions involving imperiled infants. *Journal of Perinatal & Neonatal Nursing, 14*(2), 73–86.

CHAPTER 8

Nursing Ethics and Advanced Practice: Children and Adolescents

Nan Gaylord
(with assistance from Laura A. Hart)

So many people feel so overwhelmed and disempowered by the stresses of modern life that they convince themselves they can't make a difference. So they don't even try. They bury their talents in the ground and let their spirits wither on the vine of life.

I hope they will bestir themselves at least to say every day as an anonymous old man did, "I don't have the answers, life is not easy, but my heart is in the right place."

—MARIAN WRIGHT EDELMAN, *Guide My Feet: Prayers and Meditations for Our Children*, 2000

I've learned that people will forget what you said, people will forget what you did, but people will never forget how you made them feel.
—MAYA ANGELOU, Interview with Oprah Winfrey, December 2000

Introduction

The health care of a child requires the child's parents' involvement for success. Children are integrally dependent on their parents for their physical care, emotional support, transportation, and nutrition; parents are ultimately responsible for their children and their children's well-being. Therefore, ethical concerns of children involve their parents. Caretakers for children are most often their parents; however, it is acknowledged that there are other persons who care for children besides parents. This chapter uses the term *parents* to encompass all of those persons who may assume the primary responsibility for children, whether those are grandparents, aunts, foster parents, or other appointed guardians. Assurance of who does have legal custody, and thus is legally permitted to give consent for interventions or other actions on behalf of a child in the absence of a parent, should be ascertained where healthcare-related interventions are needed. This chapter focuses on the primary care of infants and children, whereas Chapter 13 discusses ethical issues associated with end-of-life decision making and palliative care issues related to infants and children. Although this author's context of practice is the United States, references to international pediatric advance practice roles and settings are made as well. The ethical issues involving children's care tend to apply across settings, but legal regulations are bound to differ among countries of practice as they do across U.S. state boundaries. Thus, it is important for nurses to understand the legal boundaries of their practice settings; these boundaries factor into decision making but do not necessarily determine what the ethical action is in a given situation. Parents have a vested interest in, and generally the legal capacity to consent for, the care provided to their children. Parents generally care about their children and are ultimately responsible for addressing their health needs. For the most part, this means parents make healthcare decisions that are in their children's best interest. Therefore, overriding the parents' request for, or denial of, care for their children should not be undertaken lightly; the consequences of those decisions are ones with which parents must live. But it should also be recognized that parents may not have the appropriate clinical information to make a good decision. They may not have fully grasped the implications of a given course of action for their child's life.

The rights-based autonomous person ethical stance in health care for adults is not appropriate in the care of children because a one-to-one relationship with a healthcare provider is not possible when caring for children. Additionally, inclusion of as many support persons as necessary into a child's care, upon request of a child or parent, is advantageous for children who require significant adaptation in the home or community. It has been noted that to nurture a healthy, happy child in today's world may take a village. "And we have learned that to raise a happy, healthy and hopeful child, it takes a family, it takes teachers, it takes clergy, it takes business people, it takes community leaders, it takes those who protect our health and safety, it takes all of us" (Clinton, 1996). Therefore, inclusion of family members and family supporters is a component of the health care of children, and those invited persons are not excluded from information or care as they may be in the autonomous patient model of care.

Related to the care of children, the principle of autonomy centers around informed consent, and the question to be answered is, "Is the healthcare decision made knowing all the risks and benefits?" Therefore, the major ethical concerns evidenced in the care of children are parental consent or refusal, adolescent consent or refusal, and child assent or refusal. *Assent* is the term used in the United States to denote understanding and affirmation of a child to a proposed course of treatment or to be involved in a research trial. The outcomes of healthcare decisions in the ethical care of children should be to promote the parents' ability to care for their child, the child's ability to care for him- or herself, and collaboration between the healthcare provider/system and the family.

Although Gilligan's (1982) ethical feminist perspective has received criticism in the rights-based healthcare arena (as discussed in Chapters 1 and 3), an ethic of care is applicable to the care of children. This perspective emphasizes the importance of understanding relationships among people and associated responsibilities. Persons do not make decisions in isolation from considerations of context and the effects of these decisions on others. Good communication in this ethical stance is valued because it is the foundation of stable, caring relationships. This relationship focus gives rise to the moral orientation of care. The pediatric provider, including the advanced practice nurse (APN), practicing with this ethical focus, strives to be the kind of person who fosters relationships by presenting a caring attitude when others, such as pediatric patients and their families, are encountered. This interest and concern are manifested through "attentiveness to the other's particular needs and unique life circumstances and through the expression of compassion when faced with great need or vulnerability on the part of the other" (Keller, 1996). Communication about health information within the context of relationships and responsibilities is important, and adversarial encounters diminish the capacities of such relationships (child to provider, parent to provider, child to parent) to promote healing and growth. It is essential that the pediatric healthcare provider values, maintains, and promotes those relationships that a child is physically and emotionally dependent upon, as well as other relationships by which a child's sense of self and security is nurtured.

Frequently Encountered Concerns

In this chapter cases are used to explore important issues. Several case studies follow. They demonstrate frequently encountered ethical concerns in the care of children and adolescents. These cases arose within the U.S. healthcare system, but the ethical analysis is pertinent to similar situations encountered in pediatric advanced practice settings elsewhere.

CASE STUDY 1: IMMUNIZATIONS

Sarah is seen by her healthcare provider for her 12-month well-child visit. The nurse practitioner notes that the child's development is on track. The physical examination reveals no concerns and the child has no signs of contagious illnesses. Several immunizations are recommended at this health screening visit. However, when the nurse practitioner initiates the conversation about immunizations, Sarah's mother quickly responds, "I do not want her to have these shots." Upon questioning Sarah's mother about her rationale for not immunizing Sarah against vaccine-preventable childhood illnesses, her mother states that she has been told by friends and family that vaccines pose serious health risks and that she is not willing to expose Sarah to them.

Questions to Consider

1. When can parents refuse immunizations?
2. How can the ethics of care model (that emphasizes relationships rather than 'autonomy' as an important consideration in decision making) assist in the resolution of these issues?
3. When does the greater good for the population outweigh parental (individual) rights?
4. In what cases do interventions for the child override parental rights/consent?

Case Discussion

The risks of the diseases that are prevented by the recommended immunizations are higher than the risks of receiving the vaccines. For instance, if the measles, mumps, and rubella (MMR) vaccine is refused and the child contracts measles, the possible sequelae of the disease include the following:

> Measles virus causes rash, cough, runny nose, eye irritation, and fever. It can lead to ear infection, pneumonia, seizures (jerking and staring), brain damage, and death. The risk of MMR vaccine causing serious harm, or death, is extremely small. Getting MMR vaccine is much safer than getting measles, mumps, or rubella. (Centers for Disease Control and Prevention [CDC], 2012)

In the United states, all healthcare providers who administer immunizations through the Vaccines for Children Program are required to provide parents with the vaccine information sheet (VIS) relative to the vaccine received. **Table 8-1** lists the information provided by the CDC in the MMR VIS.

When a parent reads the VIS, with all the potential problems listed, concern is frequently generated, yet parents still for the most part provide consent for administration of the vaccines. In two research studies, however, parental consent was influenced strongly by both trust in the provider and

■ **Table 8-1   Effects of the MMR Vaccine**

The information provided by the CDC in the MMR VIS notes that some persons may experience the following:

Mild Problems

- Fever (up to 1 person out of 6)
- Mild rash (about 1 person out of 20)
- Swelling of glands in the cheeks or neck (about 1 person out of 75)
- If these problems occur, it is usually within 6–14 days after the shot. They occur less often after the second dose.

Moderate Problems

- Seizure (jerking or staring) caused by fever (about 1 out of 3,000 doses)
- Temporary pain and stiffness in the joints, mostly in teenage or adult women (up to 1 out of 4)
- Temporary low platelet count, which can cause a bleeding disorder (about 1 out of 30,000 doses)

Severe Problems (Very Rare)

- Serious allergic reaction (less than 1 out of a million doses)
- Several other severe problems have been known to occur after a child gets MMR vaccine. But this happens so rarely, experts cannot be sure whether they are caused by the vaccine or not. These include:
  - Deafness
  - Long-term seizures, coma, or lowered consciousness
  - Permanent brain damage

Source: Centers for Disease Control and Prevention, 2012.

the quality of the communication, rather than an adequate understanding of the information provided (Benin, Wisler-Scher, Colson, Shapiro, & Holmboe, 2006; Wu et al., 2008). Furthermore, this research suggested that many mothers, both those who consent and those who do not, may have very little knowledge about vaccination and indeed may not have enough information to realistically qualify as being informed. Evidence shows that healthcare providers have a strong positive influence on a parent's decision about whether to vaccinate (Omer, Salmon, Orenstein, deHart, & Halsey, 2009). Therefore it is important that healthcare providers spend adequate time discussing vaccine safety concerns and benefits with parents in order to improve immunization rates.

Parents refuse immunizations for multiple reasons, including religious beliefs, cultural values, and safety concerns. There have been clinical monographs and studies (Diekema & Committee on Bioethics, 2005; Healy & Pickering, 2011; Wu et al., 2008) describing parents' rationales for vaccine refusal, and most propose that additional health information and education are needed for parents to make fully informed choices regarding vaccines.

The European Centre for Disease Prevention and Control (ECDC, 2012) also has as a core aim of improving immunization rates across Europe in light of recent outbreaks of measles and other infectious diseases for which there are vaccinations. The strength of immunization programs varies across countries. "Communication and vaccine delivery strategies need to address all these (associated) challenges. Programmes need to tailor their approaches to reach both vaccination sceptics and socially disadvantaged groups. Scientific evidence on the benefits and safety of vaccines should be made easy available to enable both policy makers and the public to make informed and rational decisions" (ECDC, 2012). Healthcare providers who spend more time and effort discussing vaccine safety concerns and vaccine benefits with parents are likely to improve immunization rates in countries where immunizations are easily accessible and considered an important public health measure. Most parents and grandparents of today are not familiar with vaccine-preventable diseases and the morbidity and mortality associated with those diseases, so their focus may be more on the possible side effects of the vaccines for their own child. In some European and other countries, vaccines are either not readily available to the poor or are unaffordable. This puts a burden on healthcare providers to argue for the importance to all of making vaccination easily accessible and affordable, as well as adequately informing parents and guardians about the benefits in relation to the risks of not vaccinating.

Refusing Immunizations

In the United States, once fully informed of the pros and cons of vaccines, parents still have the right to refuse immunizations for their child. Indeed there are certain high-risk children who should not receive vaccines, but, for those who are eligible, vaccines are highly recommended. What is the concern if parents refuse the vaccinations that are recommended for their child? The unimmunized child is unlikely to acquire the vaccine-preventable disease in a community where the immunization rates are high. In fact, it may be in the individual child's best interest not to receive the vaccine and expose the child to vaccine-associated risks. Yet that child is benefiting from the actions of other children's parents who consented for their children to receive the vaccine and exposed them to vaccine-associated risks. When the incidence of the disease is low because of a high community immunization rate, an occasional parental refusal is not problematic. The problem becomes more serious when more parents refuse vaccines, as is beginning to happen. Then the vaccine-preventable disease increases in incidence and even some of those children who are vaccinated will contract the disease because no vaccine is 100% effective.

Although immunizations are required upon school entry in all 50 U.S. states, and in many other developed countries, all states and most countries allow medical exemptions. Most states and some countries also offer exemptions on the basis of religious beliefs opposing vaccination, and a few states allow exemptions for personal, nonreligious reasons (Paul & Donn, 2011). During the 2009–2010 school year, up to 5.8% of kindergarteners in the United States received nonmedical exemptions from state vaccination requirements (CDC, 2011). According to Omer and associates (2009), the mean exemption rate in states allowing nonmedical exemptions continues to rise, and children living in areas with high levels of exemptions are at a significantly higher risk of contracting vaccine-preventable diseases than children in areas with higher rates of compliance. Unimmunized children in these areas are 35 times more likely to contract measles and 5.9 times more likely to contract pertussis than children who receive recommended immunizations (Fernbach, 2011). Between January 2008 and April 2008, there were 5 measles outbreaks with a total of 64 reported cases in the Unites States. All but one of the persons who contracted measles were unvaccinated; 67% of the school-aged children affected had obtained a nonmedical exemption and 13 cases occurred in children too young to be vaccinated (Omer et al., 2009), which highlights the risks unvaccinated children pose to other members of the community.

This is the status in the United States currently. For APNs working in other countries, it is important to understand the rules of their country related to immunizations and to be ready and willing to provide information, education, and where necessary, to advocate for easy access. Following are some of the common arguments and misunderstandings related to vaccinations.

The U.S. Supreme Court has ruled on several occasions that individual states may require vaccination and that "the very concept of ordered liberty precludes allowing every person to make his own standards on matters of conduct in which the society as a whole has important interests" (Malone & Hinman, 2003). In other words, restrictions on personal liberty are sometimes permissible when the possibility of serious or widespread harm exists within a society. No U.S. state currently mandates, nor has the nation been willing to mandate, immunizations for children yet. In the United States, however, vaccines are available for all children via the national Vaccines for Children Program. Access to vaccines is facilitated via local health departments and private healthcare offices. The United States has attempted to protect children from vaccine-associated risks by reporting reactions to the Vaccine Adverse Event Reporting System (VAERS). This national program is a postmarketing safety surveillance program. That is, it keeps track of vaccines that have received Food and Drug Administration (FDA) approval to be widely distributed. If the VAERS discovers that a vaccine seems to be causing unanticipated or serious problems, the FDA and the CDC will investigate further. Compensation to persons injured by vaccines is available through the National Vaccine Injury Compensation Program. For adverse reactions to vaccines, there is reimbursement for healthcare expenses, payment for projected healthcare expenses, and compensation for pain and suffering. Vaccines are not without side effects and some do have serious adverse effects. Therefore, health professionals cannot reassure families that there is no risk. However, they can discuss the risks versus benefits of immunizations. APNs can try to determine what the needs and capacities of a child's decision maker are related to comprehending information and exchange information with them accordingly.

Refusing Families Who Refuse Vaccinations

Controversy exists within the U.S. medical community about whether a provider should refuse to continue providing care for families who choose not to immunize their children. Those in favor of disengaging these families from care argue that when unvaccinated children present to the clinic and spend time in the waiting room and other common areas, they are putting children who cannot be immunized, due to age or medical status, at risk for the diseases that they may potentially be carrying. Furthermore, if families who do not vaccinate are disengaged from the practice, the providers can relatively confidently assure parents that the children who receive care at the clinic have been vaccinated to the fullest extent possible. If these families are not disengaged, however, physicians argue that it is necessary to disclose to all families that there may be, at any point, a child inside the clinic who could potentially be harboring a devastating but vaccine-preventable illness (Block, 2012). Ethically this stance is not defensible as stated as there is no guarantee that the child will not be exposed outside of a clinic.

The American Academy of Pediatrics (AAP) does not endorse the dismissal of nonvaccinating families on the grounds that an ongoing, trusting relationship with a provider is more likely to yield a positive outcome than fostering distrust by discharging a family (Diekema & Committee on Bioethics, 2005). In a recent survey of pediatricians, it was reported that an average of 32% of parents who initially refuse a vaccine will change their mind after educational efforts by the pediatrician (Paul & Donn, 2011). This and other evidence indicate that providers can have an overall positive effect on parents' decision to immunize (Fernbach, 2011). If a provider is quick to dismiss a family when they do not see eye to eye on vaccinations, he or she has forfeited future opportunities for educating the family about the risks of vaccine-preventable diseases and the benefits of immunizations. For this reason, the AAP recommends that discharging patients should be done only as a last resort (Diekema & Committee on Bioethics, 2005).

The Ethics of Care Model

At this point, the decision about whether or not to vaccinate a child is made by parents, hopefully after they are adequately informed. The transfer of this information by healthcare providers, specifically APNs, requires knowledge and time (Healy & Pickering, 2011). It has been demonstrated that the time to explain the targeted diseases, the rationale for the development of vaccines, the potential sequelae of disease processes, vaccine-associated risks, and the anticipated side effects of vaccines affects the decision of parents. It may be, too, that a parent does not consent to vaccines at an initial visit, but the relationship of the APN or other provider with the child and parent is ongoing and the discussion can continue at the next visit.

As a child develops an understanding of health issues, pressure is frequently put on the parent by the child, and a child may request a vaccine in the presence of his or her parent. However, if it is the case that a parent consents and the child refuses, then it becomes important to explain to the child in age and developmentally appropriate language why a vaccine is important. The use of an ethic of care means that a provider enlists a child's cooperation and involvement through open and honest communication about possible discomforts and how these will be relieved. However, if a child fails to assent, this does not trump his or her parents' consent and request for vaccine administration, although patience and explanation by the provider are essential to the maintenance of the relationships involved. The AAP's Committee on Bioethics (1995) stresses the importance of trying to gain a child's assent and encourages involving children in discussions about their health care to "foster trust and a better physician [provider]-patient relationship, and perhaps improve long-term health outcomes." However, they do also recognize that there may be occasions when a provider does not try to elicit a child's assent if the treatment is necessary and will be given regardless. In such cases, it is the healthcare provider's responsibility to lessen the child's fear and apprehension and minimize the child's distress. The process of gaining a child's assent should include at minimum all of the following elements:

1. Helping the patient achieve a developmentally appropriate awareness of the nature of his or her condition.
2. Telling the patient what he or she can expect with tests and treatment(s).
3. Making a clinical assessment of the patient's understanding of the situation and the factors influencing how he or she is responding (including whether there is inappropriate pressure to accept testing or therapy).
4. Soliciting an expression of the patient's willingness to accept the proposed care. Regarding this final point, we note that no one should solicit a patient's views without intending to weigh them seriously. In situations in which the patient will have to receive medical care despite his or her objection, the patient should be told that fact and should not be deceived. (AAP's Committee on Bioethics, 1995, p. 316)

Although assent is important, it is also important not to view consent simply as a one-time event involving a test of a child's understanding or ignorance. The consent process can nurture and enlarge children's understanding, trust, and confidence in caring for themselves, and this is especially true in children with chronic illnesses. Over time, as children learn about their diseases and in the process of maturing, they begin to acquire more and more responsibility for their care. Through a child's personal growth and in the process of parental–child, healthcare provider–child interactions, the responsibility for managing an illness may be transferred from parent to child over time. In a U.K. study by Alderson, Sutcliffe, and Curtis (2006) involving children's understanding of their diabetic condition, children and parents repeatedly showed "an awareness of their own responsibilities and capabilities that suggests they would regard parents' overruling of children's responsible health care decisions as a violation of parental responsibility and loving family intimacy" (p. 33).

In the case of vaccination refusal for a minor child by his or her parent, when an unimmunized person reaches the age of consent (18 years of age in most states and countries), he or she will of course be free to seek immunizations independently. In some states and some health departments, immunizations may be provided to adolescents as young as 14 without parental consent. The AAP's Committee on Bioethics (1995) introduced another concept, parental permission, into the consent discussion, stating that children of these ages may actually provide consent for their own treatment. By law, parents are informed of their child's decision; however, parental consent is not required. Discussion around the age of consent for immunizations is now complicated by the human papillomavirus (HPV) vaccine because an adolescent may seek care for sexual health at the age of 14 without parental consent, and this vaccine was developed to prevent cervical cancer. The question of whether this vaccine falls into the sexual healthcare category or the traditional immunization schedule that requires parental consent is presently being debated (Luciani, Prieto-Lara, & Vicari, 2011).

Overriding Parental Consent for the Greater Good of the Community

With the passage of time and because vaccine-preventable diseases are no longer common and thus familiar to the public, it is anticipated that the numbers of persons refusing vaccines will continue to increase. When outbreaks of these diseases do occur (as they almost inevitably will), persons who are not vaccinated will seek the vaccine, but not before many more will acquire the disease. At some point, health professionals may need to reevaluate more lenient school exemption policies or introduce mandatory immunizations for school entrance, as was the intent of mandatory immunization laws when originally instituted. Parents today have a choice, and providers should continue to ensure that this decision is well informed and that the long-term as well as short-term risks and benefits are understood. This is important both to protect children from future problems and also others for whom acquiring these infectious diseases could be deadly, such as those with compromised immune systems.

In the United States, child education is mandatory. A child is required to attend school (or receive home schooling) until he or she is 16 years of age, whether parents agree that education is important or not. This requirement is for the community's good as well as the individual's, but permission or consent is not required by the individual or his or her parents. Thus, a precedent exists for ensuring a good by limiting the liberty to dissent. In health care, one example of when parental consent for treatment is not required is when a child has tuberculosis. Treatment for tuberculosis is mandated for the common good whether the parents agree or not because treatment is required to prevent the disease's spread to others. Thus, the risk of likely and serious harm to others is a valid limit on the freedom to act according to one's own will. Generally, superseding the parental right to consent or to refuse health care is reserved for cases when the best interests of a child are at risk. For the most part, parents are left alone to nurture their children in accordance with their own values and beliefs.

Overriding Parental Rights/Consent in the Best Interest of the Child

In the United States and many other developed countries, when a child's life is threatened by his or her parents' refusal to consent to a needed treatment, parental neglect exists. When the parent is making an obviously poor choice that will affect a child's well-being, or the parent's beliefs are endangering a child's physical health, healthcare providers, child protection professionals, and ultimately the courts will step in and override the parents' rights to make decisions for or sometimes even to care for the child. Sometimes it is ethically ambiguous whether, and to what extent, a treatment will meet its goals. An example is an experimental chemotherapy regimen. In such cases, a team process of ethical decision making may be required, as discussed further in Chapter 13. Most frequently, poor parental decision making occurs in the community setting and as a consequence of child abuse or neglect. However, in the healthcare setting, if parents are refusing lifesaving interventions that are well supported by evidence, healthcare providers can request that the courts give them permission to intervene with those measures necessary for the safety, well-being, or benefit of a child. The reason for this is that a child is considered to have the right to live long enough to be able to decide for him- or herself what beliefs are acceptable. The following is a case that exemplifies this particular problem—a parental belief system that may put a child at risk of death or serious impairment.

CASE STUDY 2: PARENTAL REFUSAL OF BLOOD FOR A CHILD

A 7-year-old male presented with his parents to the outpatient surgery unit for a tonsillectomy. After preoperative arrangements were complete, the patient was taken to surgery. A tonsillectomy was performed without difficulty, but a substantial amount of blood was lost during the procedure. After the patient was taken to the postanesthesia recovery room, a complete blood count was drawn from a blood sample and revealed normal results, with the exception of a hemoglobin (8.2 gm/dL) and hematocrit (30.4%), which had decreased in comparison to the baseline results of a hemoglobin (12 gm/dL) and hematocrit (40%). After the results were evaluated, the surgeon ordered 1 unit of packed red blood cells to be given. However, when the surgeon, Dr. J., went to discuss the blood transfusion with the parents, they became very upset and told Dr. J. that a blood transfusion would not be possible because of their religious beliefs. The surgeon explained the risks for the patient in not receiving the blood transfusion, including the possibility of hypovolemic shock resulting from inadequate circulating blood volume. Inadequate circulation decreases tissue perfusion and can result in organ failure and death. The parents continued to insist that their son not receive the blood transfusion, despite the surgeon's medical advice (see Chapter 12 for further discussion of the beliefs of Jehovah's Witnesses and the anesthesia provider). The parents were informed that, unfortunately, a court hearing would be necessary to overrule their authority and permit this intervention, which was seen as necessary for their son's safety. However, they continued to insist that their son not receive a blood transfusion.

During the emergency court hearing, the presiding judge ruled in favor of giving the patient a blood transfusion. The judge stated that although he respected the religious beliefs of the parents, the life of the child had to be considered more important. Thus, the child received the blood transfusion. However, at a difficult time the family was exposed to further distress. This may have been unavoidable, but often such problems can be anticipated. Some interpretations of the Jehovah's Witness belief system imply that treatment forced against a person's will is not considered a sin and thus no disciplinary measures such as expulsion will occur. According to a recent BBC Radio 4 program (2009) exploring the status of Jehovah's Witness beliefs, "children who are transfused against their parents' wishes are not rejected or stigmatised in any way by the church." Understanding these nuances of the religion can lessen a parent's anxiety about their child's status within the religion.

Case Discussion

In primary care settings, healthcare providers usually are familiar with a family's beliefs and values. These are good places to have discussions with families about what their beliefs and values mean in the context of highly technological healthcare settings and how they can best communicate these to providers should they ever need to be hospitalized. In this case, surgery was elective and scheduled ahead of time. Thus, problems could have been anticipated and alternatives or options explored. Cases such as these can be prevented or at least anticipated if parents express their beliefs prior to the intervention, especially if the intervention is nonemergent. Communication between the surgeon, the preoperative nurse, the parents, and the child could have elucidated the religious beliefs of the family. Autologous or family-member-directed blood donation may be permissible, depending on the belief system. In such cases, blood could be garnered ahead of time and stored for use if needed (storage is time sensitive). Anticipation of problems can lessen the possibility of conflict between a family and healthcare professionals. Additionally, a decision to override parents' wishes should be made only after careful consideration and with reasonable certainty that a child really is at risk. In this case, other surgeons might have been willing to observe the patient for evidence of circulatory compromise rather than treat him immediately, although a court order might still have been obtained for precautionary purposes (in the event of an emergency or deterioration). The child could be admitted for observation and monitoring of the hematocrit/hemoglobin levels for the next

24 hours because these levels are reported as borderline indications for transfusion after acute blood loss (Chao, 2011), although not enough information is provided in this clinical scenario to determine if that was the case. There are, however, probably no surgeons willing to chance losing a child from excessive bleeding from a tonsillectomy, and they would err on the side of providing the lifesaving measure by overriding the parents' refusal to consent.

Other examples of court intervention for lifesaving healthcare interventions include effective treatments for cancer that parents are refusing, minor interventions in the intensive care nursery for infants who will live with minimal impact from their prematurity, and parents who are incompetent to make decisions for themselves or their children for whatever reason. In the United States, APNs who suspect child abuse are obligated to report the abuse to the appropriate authorities, and parents lose their rights as parents if the children are judged to be in danger and/or neglected and there is no possibility of reeducation or remediation that would keep the family together while securing the child. These children are removed from the home and placed in foster care or with another family member until an appropriate intervention is decided. Various reporting measures exist, depending upon the country of practice. APNs who interact with children should make themselves aware of such resources and regulations. As a reminder, ethical obligations may be at odds on occasion with legal regulations in some cases.

For parents to lose their ability to consent for healthcare decisions or to have the court mandate care of a particular child requires that the intervention is life saving and that the child will die without it. Until that point, parents can decide what care is and is not appropriate for their own child. Again, for the most part parents are left to nurture their children in accordance with their own values and beliefs.

CASE STUDY 3: THE REQUEST FOR BIRTH CONTROL

Julie, a 15-year-old high school freshman, comes into the healthcare setting and requests a pregnancy test and birth control. She is also complaining of a sore throat and cough. You have not seen Julie before and know nothing about her, her family, and her current situation. No one has accompanied her to the visit. What should your response be to Julie's request?

Questions to Consider

1. Based on Julie's age, what services is the APN able to provide?
2. What services may not be provided?
3. What other consent/assent issues arise when caring for adolescents?
4. How can the ethics of care model assist in the resolution of these issues?

Discussion

Confidential assessment, pregnancy testing, and provision of a birth control method for adolescents seeking contraception, as in the given case, are permitted in every state and in many developed countries. For all women, including adolescents in the United States, reproductive health services are accessible and confidential based on the Title X of the Public Health Service Act, which was signed into effect in 1970 by President Nixon. In 1977, family planning services, including the availability of contraception, were extended to minors under the age of 16 as a result of the Supreme Court's decision in *Carey v. Population Services International* (Planned Parenthood, 2008). Clinics supported by Title X funds have been able to serve adolescents requesting these services since 1977 without parental consent or permission. In some states, age eligibility has been expanded to include persons as young as 13 years of age. In other countries, provision of services depends on the funding arrangements of the healthcare system and who is considered capable of consenting to treatment. For example, in the United Kingdom, a law was established to guide determinations of competence for personal decision making as a result of the case of *Gillick v. West Norfolk and Wisbech Area Health Authority* in 1985. Regarding contraception and abortion, "The House of Lords ruled that such advice and treatment can lawfully be given to girls under the age of 16 without the consent or knowledge of their parents provided that they have *'sufficient understanding and intelligence'*"; Hayhoe, 2008, pp. 764–770. Australian laws also permit confidentiality for those under 16 who are deemed mature enough by physicians. However, the fact that the laws of many countries lean on the side of adolescent decision making does not relieve providers of the responsibility to help adolescents receive the support they need.

Services the APNs Can Provide

In the United States, currently only 26 states have laws that allow the provision of contraceptive services to adolescents without parental consent (down from 36 in 2008), even though it has been approved at the national level. All 50 states permit the treatment of sexually transmitted infections (STIs) in adolescents without parental consent of notification (Guttmacher Institute, 2012a). New parental notification laws (PNLs) have recently been initiated by lawmakers at the urging of conservative parents and interest groups. These parents were concerned about not knowing when their children sought these services and believed it to be a parent's right to know. Additionally, the proposed PNLs were intended to help adolescents by increasing their social and emotional support in sexual decision making. Research shows, however, that adolescents are more likely to seek care, return for follow-up care, and disclose sensitive information when a healthcare professional can ensure confidentiality (Duncan, Vandeleur, Derks, & Sawyer, 2011).

Because current guidelines for adolescent health care stress the importance of confidentiality, professional organizations have not been supportive of PNLs. The Association of Women's Health, Obstetric and Neonatal Nurses (AWHONN) "supports the implementation of legislation and public health initiatives that would ensure that young people have access to affordable, adequate and confidential health care services," and "the expansion of state laws that protect adolescent confidentiality in the health care setting" (AWHONN, 2009, p. 128). The American Congress of Obstetricians and Gynecologists reinforces this by stating, "The potential health risks to adolescents if they are unable to obtain reproductive health services are so compelling that legal barriers and deference to parental involvement should not stand in the way of needed health care for patients who request confidentiality" (2011, p. v).

Services That Cannot Be Provided

If Julie is pregnant and is considering an elective termination of the pregnancy, 37 states require parental involvement (Planned Parenthood, 2007), 21 states require parental consent, and 11 states require parental notification (Guttmacher Institute, 2012b). In addition, Julie cannot consent to the evaluation and treatment of her complaints of sore throat and cough. Full legal consent for healthcare interventions, other medical procedures, and pharmacologic therapeutics is given to all persons at 18 years of age, so evaluation and treatment, if indicated, would require parental consent. For those APNs in settings outside the United States, it is important to understand the legal status of their own country. In the United States, exceptions exist in the case of a class of persons who are deemed "emancipated minors." In the United States, differences in state regulations can make it very difficult for providers who work across states or who change their state of practice. See **Box 8-1** for the AAP's Committee on Bioethics description of the settings in which minors have the authority to make health decisions.

In those health centers where a majority of the patients are adolescents, parental consent may be acquired in the form of "blanket" consent, meaning that the available services are listed and the parent acknowledges with a signature that the child may receive the listed services. This arrangement acknowledges the adolescent's ability to make healthcare decisions and to be responsible for doing so. It also permits the adolescent's confidentiality to be maintained over a wide range of services that are normally available only with parental consent as required by law.

Other Consent/Assent Issues

Another consent issue to be explored in Julie's case is that of sexual activity—Is her sexual activity voluntary? Most of the time, adolescent sexual activity

---

Box 8-1   Minors' Healthcare Decision-making Authority

Laws designate two settings in which minors have sole authority to make healthcare decisions. First, certain minors are deemed "emancipated" and treated as adults for all purposes.

Definitions of the emancipated minor include those who are:

1. self-supporting and/or not living at home;
2. married;
3. pregnant or a parent;
4. in the military; or
5. declared to be emancipated by a court.

Second, many states give decision-making authority (without the need for parental involvement) to some minors who are otherwise unemancipated but who have decision-making capacity ("mature minors") or who are seeking treatment for certain medical conditions, such as sexually transmitted diseases, pregnancy, and drug or alcohol abuse.

is voluntary—not planned, but voluntary. It is important, however, to ask how old the boy/man is that she is having sexual relations with to assess voluntariness. Significant age differences change the power differential, and voluntariness can be questioned even when the adolescent says the sex is consensual. When the male is 5 years older than a minor, statutory rape should be considered and reported to the police and the sexual assault crisis center if concerns are raised (or as the law of the state requires). When a minor female is reporting sexual activity as voluntary but the activity involves another family member and is an incestuous relationship, a report should be made to the child protection agency. Any nonconsenting sexual activity is reported to the police and sexual assault crisis team as rape and appropriate support given to the adolescent.

Overriding Parental Rights

Parental rights to make healthcare decisions for adolescents can be overridden as they can for younger children. For example, anorexia nervosa is a condition that sometimes involves family complicity or influence. As such, it may require family therapy to address the complex issues inevitably involved. This requires clinical judgment on the part of the APN to evaluate and communicate concerns appropriately and allow early interventions. A child may need to be admitted to the hospital for treatment and observation whether the parent agrees with the APN or not. Or the family may need to be referred for counseling to a professional who has expertise in the evaluation and treatment of eating disorders.

CASE STUDY 4: THE ADOLESCENT AT RISK

An adolescent girl 13 years of age presented to a private primary care health center in an affluent neighborhood for a well-child check. At the initial well-child visit, however, the APN, a pediatric nurse practitioner (PNP), became concerned because the health history and physical exam, as well as her interactions with the girl, and answers given to questions about her diet and activities, all indicated the possibility of anorexia nervosa. Additionally, the girl's father and mother had recently divorced and her father had moved overseas for his job. The PNP discussed her worries with her physician colleague who, while acknowledging that the family was under stress, discounted her concerns about an eating disorder, saying, "It's 'genetic' in that family; all the women in the family are thin—look at her mother."

The physician had for several years served as the primary provider for the father (before he moved overseas), the mother, and the daughter but had wanted the nurse, an experienced PNP, to assume the ongoing care of the adolescent because "she is difficult." The PNP was puzzled by the explanation of the girl's weight as genetic and was worried that her colleague was missing the boat. The issue of conflicts among professionals is discussed in more detail in Chapter 5 along with strategies to resolve collaboration problems. The PNP will have to address this problem with her colleague eventually. However, for current purposes the conflict is about doing the right thing for the girl, and this means raising a sensitive issue with her and her mother.

Despite the sensitive nature of issues such as weight and mental health, a responsibility exists to address them with patients and, in the case of adolescents, with the adolescent and the family. A tactful, empathetic, and nonjudgmental approach is required. The approach should be tailored to knowledge of the persons in question and introduced in ways that are most likely to permit a therapeutic course of action. When the problem involves an adolescent, the situation is complicated by having to address entrenched parental attitudes and possibly the parent's facilitation of the adolescent's behavior. In this case, the PNP discussed some of her concerns with the mother and daughter, although she did not label her concerns as anorexia nervosa. She did, however, discuss the stresses of adolescence, introduced some information about ways adolescents try to cope with the anxieties related to their development, and suggested that the daughter might benefit from both nutritional and psychological counseling.

Despite the PNP's carefully considered discussion, the mother became very indignant. "We don't want her getting too fat; she'll become unpopular. I know, I have seen what happens when you can't control your weight. You're just fine, aren't you?" At this point, the daughter nodded but did not say anything. The PNP was worried but did not think she had enough evidence to pursue the issue further at that point, and the adolescent did not seem to be in any imminent danger. The PNP was able to get the two to agree to a follow-up visit in 1 month.

Two weeks later the mother and daughter returned. The adolescent was now suffering from respiratory symptoms and fatigue. She was diagnosed with mononucleosis. At 5 foot 4 inches and 98 pounds, her weight at the first visit had been a little worrying, but though thin, she had not seemed emaciated. Now her weight had dropped to 93 pounds, and she looked pale and listless. The PNP's concerns about anorexia were strengthened by this second visit and her current evaluation. She discussed with the mother and daughter the nature of and possible contributors to mononucleosis, effective treatment options, exercise limits, and a nutrition plan before raising the issue of the daughter's weight again and her seeming unhappiness. This time the daughter did not disagree about being unhappy and the mother seemed worried. The PNP's approach, based on a developing understanding of both the mother and daughter and their relationship, was empathetic and when the PNP was alone with the mother she acknowledged the fact that it must be very difficult for her to be raising her daughter alone. They reached agreement that the daughter needed help, which permitted further options to be explored.

This represents the best-case scenario, where an understanding of professional responsibility to address difficult issues, along with clinical judgment and compassion, facilitated a parent to act in the best interests of her child. It will not always be the case that a parent or child will agree to accept the help that is needed. At the end of the chapter, a discussion question related to the problem of reluctance to receive appropriate help is raised for further exploration. When APNs encounter difficult problems that seem beyond their capacity to address, it is important that they seek the counsel of an expert colleague rather than avoid dealing with the problem. In this case, consultation with and possible referral to a colleague who has expertise in the diagnosis and treatment of eating disorders would be helpful.

Case Discussion

Eating disorders have the highest mortality rate (4%) of any mental illness, and it is estimated that only 1 in 10 people suffering from an eating disorder receive any treatment (National Association of Anorexia Nervosa and Associated Disorders, 2012). Early intervention is thought to improve cure rates, so the time to intervene with families assertively, despite their reticence to discuss the situation, is at the diagnosis, or possible diagnosis, because the psychological aspects and family component of this disease process also require intervention. In addition to healthcare services, outpatient management of anorexia nervosa should include individual counseling, family counseling, and nutrition counseling. The ethical ramifications of anorexia revolve around many patients' refusal to acknowledge the diagnosis and needed treatment.

CASE STUDY 5: ENACTING AN ETHIC OF CARE

A 16-year-old female patient accompanied by her grandmother presented with a chief complaint of nausea and vomiting. A urine sample was collected to rule out a urinary tract infection based on the vagueness of some of her complaints. After leaving the room, the APN decided to run a pregnancy test on the collected urine as well. The grandmother and patient were told that the purpose of the urine was to ensure no infection; there was no mention of the pregnancy test, nor were questions about sexual activity asked of the patient. It was determined the patient had acute gastroenteritis and was treated appropriately.

Several weeks later, the grandmother called very upset because a pregnancy test was done on her granddaughter without either of them knowing about it. She complained that no one discussed this test with her at the time of the visit and that her granddaughter was not asked about having sex. She also pointed out that she was sure her granddaughter was not sexually active and said that she was not paying for the test. The purpose of the test was explained to her, as well as the reasons for performing it. She was told that the test was part of the routine workup for menstruating females presenting with nausea and vomiting. The grandmother was still upset.

This situation could have been handled differently by being honest with the patient about the test ordered and the rationale for the order. Asking for a sexual history in front of parents/grandparents opens the door for them to talk with their adolescent about it when they arrive home. Even if parents/grandparents/legal guardians have the right to refuse the test, it is important that the concern about pregnancy as a cause of the presenting symptoms be mentioned, and if the female patient is pregnant, the chart should reflect the discussion and refusal of the test. Adolescents may not always tell the truth in front of their parents, and therefore, if possible, evaluation of adolescents without parents at some point during the visit is preferable. If that opportunity is not possible or refused by one or the other, then the provider cannot avoid sensitive topics. According to the ethics of care model, the trust relationship between provider and patient/parent was damaged in the clinical case given. The damage could have been avoided with an open, frank discussion of possible concerns.

Another similar concern is when an adolescent is seen alone and the parents receive the healthcare bill outlining exactly what services were provided. Payment for services may need to be addressed with the adolescent prior to being seen. In states where it is legal for the adolescent to seek sexual health care without parental consent, sending the bill or insurance statement to the house may be problematic. Adolescents may need counsel on the financing of healthcare services, and referral to health department/free clinics may be appropriate for the adolescent population if it is requested that parents not know about services received.

When confronting healthcare concerns with adolescents, the adolescent's web of relationships must be considered. Requirements for parental notification do not encourage supportive family relationships but demand information about an adolescent when the adolescent might not be ready to share it. There are adolescents who would never enlist parental participation in their care, and some parents are more helpful than others in difficult situations. If an adolescent is encouraged to talk about who will help with the presenting problem, most will name a supportive adult, but it is not always their parent. Frequently, an APN is enlisted to talk with a designated adult in the presence of the adolescent about the problem at hand. Whether that adult is the parent or not, it is helpful that assistance has been enlisted willingly by the child, and the other adult can facilitate parental involvement if it is deemed appropriate or important. The APN's understanding of the issue can actually be distorted if the only perspective available is that of the adolescent in question. The adolescent may have misinterpreted parental concerns or attitudes as interfering, judgmental, or punitive. In the ethics of care model, the maintenance and encouragement of significant supportive relationships available to the adolescent are important. Such relationships permit uncovering the nuances of a situation and allow a concerned provider to work in concert with an adolescent and his or her support system toward a satisfactory outcome for difficult problems.

An adolescent, however, needs to know under what circumstances parental consent is required and what information will be given to parents regarding the treatment needed. Consent for treatment may be required, but confidentiality regarding an adolescent's healthcare visit can be maintained with the adolescent as long as the adolescent is not in danger of harming him or herself or others. In its policy position statement on confidentiality in adolescent health care, the AWHONN states that providers "should establish environments within the limits of the law in which adolescents' rights to confidential health care are protected," in order to "increase adolescents' comfort about disclosing sensitive healthcare information; to provide more effective care; and to bolster patient satisfaction" (2009).

As patients progress through their teen years, the responsibility for consenting to health care gradually becomes more the adolescent's than the parents', even when parents are present and are the official consenters. The adolescent, in the absence of cognitive problems, will be legally responsible for personal healthcare decision making at 18 years of age, if not earlier. However, being responsible and informed does not happen when the birthday candles are blown out. Development of the necessary maturity for making sound decisions is gradual. It is facilitated by the existence of supportive others and with opportunities to practice decision making in safe environments. Unfortunately, not all adolescents will have the benefit of ideal circumstances. APNs are ideally situated to understand this and to provide the needed resources and assistance.

Summary

APNs and all healthcare providers who are caring for children serve as advocates for children. Children vary in their developmental stages and levels of maturity, and they cannot legally represent themselves, except in specific circumstances, so often their voices are heard only when others express needs on their behalf. The provision of health care for children in any setting requires attention to (1) the web of relationships in a child's life, (2) the parents' interests, and (3) the child's needs. Consideration of the parents' and child's understanding of healthcare decisions is important in both parental informed consent and the child's consent at times and assent at others.

Inherent in the communication style between APNs, other healthcare providers, the child, and the family is the ethical term *respect for persons*. Communication with both parents and children is important, and it may guide interaction patterns in healthcare encounters throughout life. APNs should analyze their communication styles. Some styles demonstrate more caring attitudes than others. One study (Hansson, Kihlbom, Tuverno, Olsen, & Rodriguez, 2007) looked at nonverbal communication of physicians. The more positive styles (general politeness, actively showing efforts to set the stage for a respectful encounter, and showing sensitivity by responding to parents' needs in a respectful manner) were associated with a respect for integrity when parents were interviewed after healthcare encounters with their children. The study had only 21 subjects, but it is significant in that it acknowledges that nonverbal communication is important in the healthcare encounter. Additionally, the study also recognizes that time and communication skills are required of the healthcare provider for informed decision making by parents.

Excellent communication skills with children and families are important because in ethical concerns, problems, and dilemmas with children there is frequently no good answer and the best answer is often not good. The answer may not be decided immediately, and it may require days, months, or years of conversation for everyone to reach consensus. The plan of care is agreed upon by all involved parties—it is not that one side wins or loses. APNs and other health providers cannot make children or parents act/behave/perform as prescribed or as they would, and achieving consensus on the plan of action may take effort by all involved.

There are other clinical cases with ethical components that have not been discussed in this chapter. Examples include children as organ donors, parental/family presence during procedures and resuscitation, complementary therapies, withdrawal of support in the pediatric intensive care unit/neonatal intensive care unit, end-of-life care for children, substance abuse screening in schools, growth hormone administration, increasing use of psychostimulants in children, and technology-dependent children in the home and community and the moral obligation of parents to care for them. This latter issue is increasingly important in relationship to the resources available or unavailable to these children and their families. The case studies chosen and discussed set an ethical framework for discourse and evaluation of other moral concerns in the care of children.

The final ethical principle guiding the care of children is that of justice. It is the moral responsibility of APNs to ensure that their most vulnerable population, a nation's most treasured resource, has access to care. Access ensures the health of a nation's children so that they may develop their full potential as a nation's future leaders and workforce. The American Nurses Association's *Code of Ethics for Nurses* Plank 3 (2001) states that "the nurse promotes, advocates for and strives to protect the health, safety and rights of patients." The International Council of Nurses' (2012) *Code of Ethics for Nurses* similarly states "In providing care, the nurse promotes an environment in which the human rights, values, customs and spiritual beliefs of the individual, family and community are respected." Health care for children includes access to (1) well-child care to detect and intervene in healthcare concerns early and receive vaccines to prevent disease, (2) timely intervention into acute illnesses to prevent long-term sequelae of illnesses, and (3) coordinated care and interventions for children with special healthcare needs.

> *Better the occasional faults of a government that lives in a spirit of charity than the constant omissions of a government frozen in the ice of its own indifference.*
> —FRANKLIN D. ROOSEVELT

Discussion Questions

1. Case Study 4—*The Adolescent at Risk*—had the potential for a positive resolution because of the considered actions of the PNP and the receptiveness of the family. However, the mother may well have continued to deny the need for assistance based on her own problems and issues. With colleagues or classmates, discuss what would be required if the mother and/or daughter continued to deny that a problem existed.
2. How have your own attitudes toward stigmatized issues such as psychiatric illness and eating disorders changed over time, if at all? What rationale can you give for your beliefs?
3. What does it mean to say parents are responsible for their children's health behaviors? What does it mean to say adolescents are responsible for their health behaviors?
4. There is an ongoing debate about the relationship of autism to vaccines. The debate persists despite the fact that there is little to no supporting evidence of a relationship between the two. What is the APN's responsibility related to understanding the status of knowledge related to such controversial issues? How do you address healthcare-related questions that patients raise and that have not yet been satisfactorily answered in the literature?

Acknowledgments

The author is grateful for the contributions of Juliet Gladson, RN, MSN; Lori Heston, RN, MSN; Andrea Heaton, RN, MSN; and Miriam Allman, RN, MSN. Many of their suggestions, cases, and examples remain from the first edition of this chapter.

Laura A. Hart provided research assistance, suggestions for case studies, and other revisions for this second edition.

References

Alderson, P., Sutcliffe, K., & Curtis, K. (2006). Children's competence to consent to medical treatment. *Hastings Center Report, 36*, 25–34.

American Academy of Pediatrics, Committee on Bioethics. (1995). Informed consent, parental permission, and assent in pediatric practice. *Pediatrics, 95*(2), 314–317. Retrieved from http://www.cirp.org/library/ethics/AAP/

American Congress of Obstetricians and Gynecologists. (2011). *Guidelines for adolescent health care* (2nd ed.). Washington, DC: Author.

American Nurses Association. (2001). *Code of ethics for nurses with interpretative statements.* Retrieved from http://www.nursingworld.org/codeofethics

Angelou, M. (2000, December). Oprah talks to Maya Angelou. O, *The Oprah Magazine.* Retrieved from http://www.oprah.com/omagazine/Oprah-Interviews-Maya-Angelou/1

Association of Women's Health, Obstetric and Neonatal Nurses. (2009). Position statement: Confidentiality in adolescent health care. *An official position statement of the Association of Women's Health, Obstetric and Neonatal Nurses.* Retrieved from http://www.google.com/url?sa=t&rct=j&q=awhonn%20position%20statement%20on%20adolescent%20confidentiality&source=web&cd=1&ved=0CCwQFjAA&url=http%3A%2F%2Fwww.awhonn.org%2Fawhonn%2Fbinary.content.do%3Fname%3DResources%2FDocuments%2Fpdf%2F5H1e_PS_ConfidentialityInAdolescent.pdf&ei=bsa9Uc_2Fo_s0gXZmoGgDA&usg=AFQjCNG56ow5A6GN98IU5193j5ElU6F44A&bvm=bv.47883778,d.d2k

BBC Radio 4. (2009). Ethics and religion. Jehovah's Witness ethics. Retrieved from http://www.bbc.co.uk/religion/religions/witnesses/witnessethics/ethics_1.shtml

Benin, A. L., Wisler-Scher, D. J., Colson, E., Shapiro, E. D., & Holmboe, E. S. (2006). Qualitative analysis of mothers' decision-making about vaccines for infants: The importance of trust. *Pediatrics, 117*, 1532–1541.

Block, S. L. (2012). Families that refuse to vaccinate their infants. *Pediatric Annals, 41*(4), 142–144.

Centers for Disease Control and Prevention. (2011). Vaccination coverage among children in kindergarten. United States, 2009-10 school year. *Morbidity and Mortality Weekly Report, 60*(21), 700–704.

Centers for Disease Control and Prevention. (2012). Vaccination information statement for MMR vaccine. Retrieved from http://www.cdc.gov/vaccines/pubs/vis/downloads/vis-mmr.pdf

Chao, J. (2011). Transfuse or not to transfuse: For post-op anemia. *American Journal of Clinical Medicine, 8*(1), 11–14.

Clinton, H. R. (1996, August 27). Speech given at the Democratic National Convention in Chicago, IL. Retrieved January 20, 2008, from http://www.pbs.org/newshour/convention96/floor_speeches/hillary_clinton.html

Diekema, D. S., & Committee on Bioethics. (2005). Responding to parental refusals of immunization of children. *Pediatrics, 115*, 1428–1431.

Duncan, R. E., Vandeleur, M., Derks, A., & Sawyer, S. (2011). Confidentiality with adolescents in the medical setting: What do parents think? *Journal of Adolescent Health, 49*, 428–430.

Edelman, M. W. (2000). *Guide my feet: Prayers and meditations for our children.* New York, NY: Harper Collins Perennial.

European Centre for Disease Prevention and Control. (2012). Health policy topic spotlight – Immunizations. Retrieved from http://ecdc.europa.eu/en/healthtopics/spotlight/Spotlight_immunisation/Pages/Situation_in_EU.aspx

Fernbach, A. (2011). Parental rights and decision making regarding vaccinations: Ethical dilemmas for the primary care provider. *Journal of the American Academy of Nurse Practitioners, 23*, 336–345.

Gilligan, C. (1982). *In a different voice*. Cambridge, MA: Harvard University Press.

Guttmacher Institute. (2012a, August 1). State policies in brief: An overview of minors' consent law. Retrieved from http://www.guttmacher.org/statecenter/spibs/spib_OMCL.pdf

Guttmacher Institute. (2012b, August 1). State policies in brief: Parental involvement in minors' abortions. Retrieved from http://www.guttmacher.org/statecenter/spibs/spib_PIMA.pdf

Hansson, M. G., Kihlbom, U., Tuvemo, T., Olsen, L. A., & Rodriguez, A. (2007). Ethics takes time, but not that long. *BMC Medical Ethics, 8*, 1472.

Hayhoe, B. (2008). Decision-making in children and young people: Gillick competent? *InnovAiT, 1*(11), 764–770. DOI:10,1093/innovait/inn091

Healy, C. M., & Pickering, L. K. (2011). How to communicate with vaccine-hesitant parents. *Pediatrics, 127*, S127–S133.

International Council of Nurses. (2012). *Code of ethics for nurses*. Geneva, Switzerland: Author. Retrieved from http://www.icn.ch/about-icn/code-of-ethics-for-nurses/

Keller, J. (1996). Care ethics as a health care ethic. *Contexts: A Forum for Medical Humanities*, 4. Retrieved January 19, 2008 from http://www.uhmc.sunysb.edu/prevmed/mns/imcs/contexts/care/carejean.html

Luciani, S., Prieto-Lara, E., & Vicari, A. (2011). Providing vaccines against Human Papillomavirus to adolescent girls in the Americas: Battling cervical cancer, improving overall health. *Health Affairs, 30*(6), 1089–1095.

Malone, K. M., & Hinman, A. R. (2003). Vaccination mandates: The public health imperative and individual rights. In R. A. Goodman et al. (Eds.), *Law in public health practice* (pp. 262–284). New York, NY: Oxford University Press.

National Association of Anorexia Nervosa and Associated Disorders. (2012). Eating disorder statistics. Retrieved from http://www.anad.org/get-information/about-eating-disorders/eating-disorders-statistics/

Omer, S. B., Salmon, D. A., Orenstein, W. A., deHart, P., & Halsey, N. (2009). Vaccine refusal, mandatory immunization, and the risks of vaccine-preventable diseases. *New England Journal of Medicine, 360*, 1981–1988.

Paul, S., & Donn, S. (2011). Legal right to refuse: What to do when parents are hesitant to have their child immunized. *AAP News, 32*(2), 16.

Planned Parenthood. (2007). Fact sheet: Laws requiring mandatory parental involvement for minors' abortion. Retrieved from http://www.plannedparenthood.org

Planned Parenthood. (2008). Fact sheet: America's family planning program: Title X. Retrieved from http://www.plannedparenthood.org/files/PPFA/Title_X.pdf

Wu, A. C., Wilsler-Sher, D. J., Griswold, K., Colson, E., Shapiro, E. D., Holmboe, E. S., & Benin, A. L. (2008). Postpartum mothers' attitudes, knowledge, and trust regarding vaccination. *Maternal & Child Health Journal, 12*, 766–773.

CHAPTER 9

Nursing Ethics and Advanced Practice: Women's Health

Katharine T. Smith and Pamela J. Grace

No woman can call herself free who does not own and control her body.
— MARGARET SANGER

Introduction

The advanced nursing practice specialty of women's health concentrates on addressing health issues that are of particular concern to women. However, many of the issues that arise in women's health clinical settings are also encountered in other areas of advanced practice; thus, this chapter provides insight, approaches to care, and strategies facilitative of health that have broad applications. Additionally, many countries do not have the luxury of an advanced practice nurse (APN) role in women's health. The needs of women are addressed variously in the primary care setting, reproductive health clinics, and so on. Moreover, movements to change health policy and political obstructions to women's health often require collaborative efforts informed by women's situations and those with in-depth understanding of the effects of environmental conditions on women. Thus, this chapter contains information and strategies pertinent to providing healthcare services to women across the lifespan and in a variety of settings.

In the United States, Canada, and elsewhere, other APNs such as adult health and family nurse practitioners (NPs) are educated to be knowledgeable about women's health, have many of the same professional skill sets as women's health nurse practitioners (WHNPs), and have overlapping scopes of practice. What, then, differentiates women's health advanced practice nursing from other specialty practice? It is the concentrated focus on the experiences associated with being female and the ways in which this cultural identity affects a patient's health and well-being that is permitted by the APN's scope of practice. In this sense, women's health APNs can also serve as resources and consultants for other specialties. The discussions in the chapter can be helpful to a wide variety of APNs, point-of-care nurses, and allied health providers, who in the course of their daily practice may be confronted with issues arising from the concerns of women. Although some progress has been made in improving the condition of women worldwide, women's issues continue to be underaddressed (Global Alliance for Women's Health, 2007).

Through studies in nursing, women's health nursing, ethics, and clinical practice, the first author (Smith) has encountered problems stemming from two societal influences on women as a group. Because of their ties to the cultural identity of women and their implications for many of the ethically difficult cases encountered by WHNPs, understanding the bases of these influences is important, not only for women's health practitioners, but also for practitioners in all advanced practice settings who care for women. The first influence is that of historically and culturally established gender-based power imbalances that are pervasive throughout many societies. When people feel powerless, they may not be able to discern what their own needs and wishes are and consequently may not be able to articulate these to others. There are degrees of powerlessness; however, many issues encountered both in women's health and primary care settings prove especially difficult to resolve because their roots are deeply embedded in the culture of a given society and a societal view of women as not quite equal to men. For example, a defense lawyer's response to the recent case of the assault, rape, and murder of a woman in New Delhi, India was that "she deserved it, respectable women are not raped" (Caulfield, 2013).

Issues faced by APNs include patients experiencing intimate partner violence (IPV), those who have been sexually assaulted, those who have reproductive control issues, or those who live in poverty and have children for whom they are the sole support. The second influence often affecting ethical issues in women's health, regardless of setting, is rooted in societal expectations to fulfill certain roles based on gendered identities. Women's health issues are inherently tied to women's expected roles as mothers, professionals, caregivers, wives, and friends. Many ethical issues in women's health arise from the complicated factors involved in women negotiating their identity through a balance among these roles. In addition, WHNPs may also find themselves caring for more than simply their female patients.

As reproductive health specialists, WHNPs often care for male patients suffering from reproductive problems and transgender patients who may identify as either male or female. Also, good care of women often means working for change and this necessarily involves the whole of society. Influencing misogynist attitudes is an important aspect. Because of this diverse patient population, it is also important to consider not just how an identity as a woman may affect a patient's health, but the overall effects of gendered identities more generally.

As discussed in Chapter 1, feminist ethics approaches are aimed at exposing the power imbalances and underlying assumptions present in a case, based on gender, race, class, or other factors. Additionally, philosophical understandings of nursing and its purposes in concert with a feminist ethic of care direct APNs to engage with their patients in a process that permits a holistic understanding of the patient as a unique individual inseparable from his or her context. The human rights stance described in Chapter 6 depends on women being considered of equal moral worth to men. This stance clashes with cultural beliefs about a woman's value in many countries. Using these perspectives to explore women's health concerns yields a fuller account of the issues. If practice is interested in caring not just for female patients, but for patients who are affected by their cultural gendered identity, then APNs must work to understand the complex ways in which this identity has influenced each patient's life, experiences, and healthcare needs. Traditional principles of healthcare ethics are helpful for further clarifying specific issues and in moral decision making within this feminist care perspective but will not be the primary approach taken here. This chapter analyzes ethical issues in women's health in a way that is based on the value of an ethic of care, first attempting to understand the complexities of a client's unique experience, and then applying both feminist and traditional ethical principles to develop possible courses of ethical action.

The following is a discussion of salient issues often seen in the women's health advanced practice setting. Each issue is highlighted using a case study scenario likely to be seen in clinical practice. The discussion will begin by discussing the issues involved in gaining trust from clients who may have backgrounds that are very different from their practitioners. The chapter continues with cases concerning violence against women, coercion, assisted reproductive technologies, maternal–fetal conflicts, genetic testing, and providing care for transgender clients.

Gaining Trust: Setting the Groundwork for an Ethically Sound Practice in Women's Health

Trust is one of the most, if not the most, important aspect of a successful relationship between a WHNP and his or her client. In the exam and consultation rooms, clinicians are speaking with clients about the most intimate parts of their lives—sexuality, reproductive choices, and personal relationships. Without building trust and mutual respect, WHNPs cannot even begin to elicit the information needed from their patients to develop, in concert with them, appropriate plans of care. Often, WHNPs serve communities that are much different from their own. From women in rural communities or urban communities to incarcerated women, racially and ethnically diverse populations, to LGBTQ women and transgender individuals, WHNPs will more likely than not be faced with trying to gain trust from clients whose backgrounds are drastically different from their own. Therefore gaining the trust of clients, demonstrating that, as a clinician, the WHNP is aware that his or her situated experience may be different from a client's and that the WHNP is willing and interested in learning about the client's experiences in a nonjudgmental way, will lay the groundwork for being able to work through ethically difficult situations. WHNPs taking a feminist perspective on ethically difficult cases must work to understand the unique experiences of their clients situated in the cultural context in which they live.

There are many different ways to gain such trust and each clinician will develop his or her own style in this process. The following are a few suggestions for the beginning clinician who may be working with a new community different from his or her own. When the WHNP encounters a patient who has a background that he or she is unfamiliar with, it is necessary to remember that the patient knows more about her past and cultural experiences than does the WHNP. The WHNP should be honest about his or her knowledge level and act as the learner. At the same time, patients do not want to be tokenized or responsible for educating their providers. For this reason, it is also important to do as much research as possible ahead of time to be familiar with common practices, health disparities, and belief systems. The most important strategy is the one a clinician would use with any patient, regardless of how similar the patient's background is to his or hers. Each client should be approached as a unique individual whose experience and background is integral to her health and well-being. The WHNP should enter the exam room with a nonjudgmental, open mind and seek to learn from the patient what the important influences are on the patient's life and place in the community. Approaching each patient in such a manner will lay the groundwork for a feminist approach, not just to clinical care, but also to aid in working through ethically difficult situations. Only by understanding patients as unique individuals who are situated within particular cultural contexts can clinicians begin to develop clinically and ethically sound plans of care.

Frequently Encountered Concerns

The following is a discussion of concerns frequently encountered by WHNPs. Each concern is introduced with a case study drawn from clinical practice and concludes with practice guidelines for working through similar ethically challenging cases. Each case is evaluated based on the ethical decision-making guidelines set forth in Table 2-6. The considerations from the guidelines are italicized, as not all guiding considerations are relevant to all cases.

Violence Against Women

CASE STUDY 1: INTIMATE PARTNER VIOLENCE

Joan Blundell is a 28-year-old very anxious female patient who comes into a primary care clinic. She is accompanied by a male who is very solicitous and is "hovering" around her. Her reason for the clinic visit is abdominal pain. Velda Danboroni holds dual certifications as both a family nurse practitioner (FNP) and a WHNP. When perceived "difficult" patients present to the clinic, they are often assigned to her because her colleagues believe that she handles them well. Velda explains to Joan's companion, Bill, that she needs to evaluate her patient privately. Bill refuses, saying "We have nothing to hide from each other," and "We do everything together... she wants me with her." He is somewhat dogmatic and bordering on belligerent. "She has a pain in her stomach and you had better fix it," he shouts.

Background on Intimate Partner or Domestic Violence and Trafficking

This case exemplifies some typical difficulties that healthcare professionals face in assisting patients whom they suspect may be suffering from IPV or who are victims of human trafficking. IPV, also known as domestic abuse, is prevalent in all countries and across all socioeconomic strata. Many cases of IPV may actually be uncovered in interactions with mothers and their children in pediatric settings (Quist, 2008).

Intimate Partner Abuse

Although both men and women can be the victims of IPV, because this chapter is about women's health primarily, the discussion focuses on women's experience of IPV. Estimates are that IPV affects as many as 20% of all women at some point in their lives. The ripple effects of IPV are widespread and include children, families, and ultimately society (Warshaw, 1998). The Centers for Disease Control and Prevention (CDC, 2010) defines IPV as "physical, sexual, or psychological harm by a current or former partner or spouse. This type of violence can occur among heterosexual or same-sex couples and does not require sexual intimacy." The United Nations Population Fund (UNPF, 2005) asserts that domestic violence is the biggest threat to women's health worldwide. In certain countries where women are not considered equal to men, violence against women is almost certainly even more prevalent but paradoxically more difficult to document. This is because the victims may not have even the ostensible freedom to report the abuse or receive support for it (UNPF, 2005). However, the situation is not much better in those societies where women are officially accorded equality with men. When women do seek help for health issues associated with domestic violence, their experience of the healthcare encounter is overwhelmingly negative (Tower, Rowe, & Wallis, 2011). "There is a tendency to hold women accountable for their situation" (Patterson, 2009, p. 122), despite a growing body of knowledge related to antecedents and patterns of violence. Domestic violence is a chronic malady that saps the self-esteem of women, can endanger them physically, and even puts some at risk of death.

Warshaw (1998) proposed several reasons why healthcare professionals may react negatively to situations of IPV or neglect to screen for it. Among the reasons are their inadequate educational preparation related to the problem and uncertainty about how to raise the question and address it; unexamined social and cultural beliefs that can influence their reaction; the fact that listening to stories of abuse is psychologically disturbing and may lead to distancing or denial of the problem; the fact that professional socialization can have a numbing emotional effect that prevents engagement with the patient;

the inadequacy of local and community resources for IPV patients; and so on. Warshaw's discussion of this issue may seem dated in light of more recent efforts in primary care settings and emergency rooms in Australia, Canada, Europe, the United States, and elsewhere to institute routine screening for IPV. However, the insights remain cogent. The U.S. Preventive Services Task Force (USPSTF, 2013), an independent panel of experts that advises the U.S. Department of Health and Human Services, found insufficient evidence that screening alone is sufficient to reduce harms to women. This finding is in part due to lack of comprehensive studies but may also be related to ongoing provider uncertainty about how to identify and address the problem. What is certain is that inadequate identification of those at risk means that an opportunity to provide a "good" for such patients is lost. A basic under-standing of the causes, patterns, types, responses, possible strategies, and community resources is necessary to address such problems appropriately. Although each woman's experience of IPV is unique, several patterns have been described in the literature. Dutton, Kaltman, Goodman, Weinfurt, and Vankos (2005), informed by prior research, surveyed 406 women who had suffered from IPV. They outlined three patterns:

> Pattern 1: ...moderate levels of physical violence, psychological abuse, and stalking but very little sexual violence
>
> Pattern 2: ... high levels of physical violence, psychological abuse, and stalking but low levels of sexual abuse
>
> Pattern 3: ... high levels of physical violence, psychological abuse, and stalking (p. 489)

Their sample was comprised of more than 80% African American women. The researchers found that African American women were significantly more likely to experience Pattern 1 than other groups. Additionally, in the sample's willing-ness to continue the relationship was 25% with Pattern 1, 16% with Pattern 2, and 5% with Pattern 3. Length of relationship correlated with escalating violence—a movement from Pattern 1 to Patterns 2 and 3. Understanding pat-terns is helpful in identifying those who are being victimized and their risk, but responding appropriately requires further development of skills. However, even if providers are well prepared, their efforts depend for their effectiveness upon good community resources such as shelters and ongoing support. Thus, a fur-ther professional responsibility exists to collaborate with others in the interests of influencing health policies supportive of women's and family health.

Human Trafficking

Human trafficking is a related contemporary problem about which primary care and women's health providers (among others) need awareness. Although human trafficking is not isolated to women, women and children make up the majority of those trafficked. It is estimated that around 800,000 persons annually worldwide are trafficked (Sabella, 2011). Beginning in 2000, and as a result of the growing recognition that human trafficking continued to be a problem in many countries, several sets of regulations were instituted. These include the United Nations Office on Drugs and Crime's (UNODC, 2003) *Protocol to Prevent, Suppress and Punish Trafficking in Persons* and the United States' (2000) anti-trafficking law, the Trafficking Victims Protection Act of 2000, which, like equivalent laws in other countries, is modeled on the U.N.'s protocol. The U.S. law has been reauthorized several times, in 2003, 2005, and 2008. It is now called The Trafficking Victims Protection Reauthorization Act of 2008 (H.R. 7311). Human trafficking is defined by the UNODC (2003) as:

> the recruitment, transportation, transfer, harbouring or receipt of persons... [using] threat or... force or other forms of coercion [including] abduction... fraud... deception... abuse of power or [a susceptible person's] vulnerability or of the giving or receiving of payments or benefits to achieve the consent of a person having control over another person, for the purpose of exploitation. Exploitation... include[s]... the prostitution of others... sexual exploitation, forced labour... slavery or [similar] practices...

These acts have resulted in an increase in research funding for this problem and increased diligence on the part of law enforcement. Additionally, the laws of many countries have instituted special protections and resources for such persons once identified. For example, in the United States, persons may be granted a special visa allowing them residency and those especially at risk may be put into a witness protection program. But it is questionable to what extent nurses are prepared to identify and assist this population. Sabella (2011), in her article entitled *The Role of the Nurse in Combating Human Trafficking*, provides an accessible account of the background, laws, and official assistance that can be given to victims of trafficking. Nurses in other countries need to be informed about the rules and resources for such persons in their counties. All of the following are needed for APNs to respond appropriately to patients or to educate others how to do so: (1) self-reflection about their own experiences and biases related to IPV/human trafficking; (2) knowledge of patterns, signs, and symptoms; (3) ability to engage with a patient who may be untrusting or who has been isolated by her abuser; and (4) knowledge of helpful strategies and community resources. Following a discussion of the case given earlier, some strategies for assisting both women experiencing IPV or who are the victims of trafficking are provided.

Case Discussion

This is a woman's health chapter and thus the case given is that of a woman who may be at risk from abuse, but men can also suffer from IPV and have been trafficked for labor and other purposes. Similar considerations are warranted in the case of a man who seems to be obstructed in speaking for himself. Jumping to immediate conclusions about a situation can be as damaging as not further investigating a provider's suspicions. In either case, a provider can fail to identify the *underlying issue* or may worsen the situation by antagonizing the perpetrator, which in turn can escalate the violence and risks for the patient. Worse, the perpetrator may become suspicious and remove the patient from the clinic or institution.

In the case given, Velda needs to evaluate Joan in the absence of her companion. She needs *more information* before she can determine what is going on and formulate a plan of action. A main principle at stake is Joan's *autonomy*. Joan has the right to make her own choices. However, research on patterns of IPV consistently points to the problem that the accompanying emotional abuse is isolating and undermines a woman's ability to see herself as having choices. In earlier chapters, this was discussed as a problem of moral agency. Moral agency is the ability to be able to make choices that are first in a person's best interests and second in the interests of those around them. This is hierarchical. The development of self-agency necessarily precedes the capacity for moral action toward others. However, self-agency is often what is lacking in situations of IPV. The person is unable to act in her own interests because her self-agency has not been developed or has been dampened or annihilated by the abuser. If Joan does lack the ability to act in her own best interest, that must be factored into her plan of care. The development of trust in the APN and planning for change may take time. For various reasons, including perceived or actual lack of resources, persons who are being abused are rarely able to expediently separate themselves from their abuser. In the

United States, certain states have laws that mandate healthcare provider reporting of suspected IPV or abuse. The mandated reporting by healthcare professionals of suspected abuse in adults remains a controversial topic. The preponderance of ethical arguments and evidence supports the idea that mandated reporting, in many cases, does more harm than good and thus is not ethically warranted (Association of Women's Health, Obstetric, and Neonatal Nurses, 2007; Schumacher, 2011). APNs, in a mandatory reporting state, nevertheless need to use clinical judgment about the well-being of their patients and risks to themselves in determining whether to act in accord with the law. The intent of such laws is to protect persons; when it is unlikely that they will do so in a particular situation, APNs must weigh the options as they must in any such situation. Consulting with others where time allows may be important in determining appropriate actions.

How might Velda approach the issue of separating Joan from her companion in order to gain more information? Various strategies have been used by providers in such situations. What will work depends on the characteristics of the partner and the situation. In this case, Velda remained calm and presented an unsuspicious demeanor. She negotiated with Bill for a period of 15 minutes in which she would be alone with Joan to do the physical exam—which she noted was the routine of the clinic—after that time he could be in the room with Joan (if Joan gave permission) as they discussed treatment. Velda was pretty sure that Joan would allow Bill in the room after that time because of her decision-making deference to him. When alone, Joan nervously, and in response to questioning, tells Velda that she had an abortion 3 weeks ago (Bill does not know) and now has lower abdominal pain, which makes her think she has contracted an infection from her partner. She is afraid of Bill. He has hit her before and once tried to strangle her. She has attempted to leave him several times, but she has few resources and says that "He is always very sorry afterward ... he has had an awful life himself." Velda has several decision points here. She probably cannot attend to all of Joan's needs in 15 minutes, so she must devise a plan that prioritizes the most urgent issues. She knows from the fact of Joan's secret abortion that there are times when Joan is away from Bill. This means there may be other opportunities for Joan to visit the clinic without Bill. First she must assess Joan's risk from Bill. Is it immediate and life threatening? If so, then law enforcement's assistance may be needed. Then she must validate Joan's concerns. She does not deserve the abuse, it is not her fault, and there are resources and options available for her. Velda must assure her that she is not alone in experiencing abuse, that many other people have suffered from similar violence and have managed with assistance to remake their lives. Joan is not responsible for her partner's prior misery. Velda can remind her that abuse can escalate and provide her with both the clinic's phone number and community resources in the event she chooses to go home with Bill. She can provide her with written information about how to develop a safety plan. Then Velda must evaluate Joan's physical signs and symptoms before devising a workable treatment plan that will address any sexually transmitted infection, post-abortion complications, and so on. An acute infection may require hospitalization. It is Joan's prerogative to determine what information may be shared with Bill, but she may require help in determining the extent and nature of the information to be shared and the way in which it should be discussed with Bill. This will require some ingenuity on the part of Velda, and the assistance of colleagues may be needed to formulate a workable plan.

Coercion, Contraception, and Sterilization

CASE STUDY 2: COURT-MANDATED CONTRACEPTION

Twenty-two-year-old Maria presents to a clinic for a consultation and insertion of an intra-uterine device (IUD). IUDs are long-term reversible contraceptive technologies that provide extremely effective birth control for either 5 or 10 years, depending on the type used. Benefits of IUDs include offering effective contraception with no effort required from the user as well as containing little to no hormone, thus providing a safe option for women who cannot use hormonal methods. At the same time, some women suffer from uterine cramping and irregular menstrual bleeding as a result of an IUD. Infrequent but serious risks include uterine perforation and infection. A provider must also consider that an IUD is 100% provider dependent. That is, a patient must return to her clinician to have it removed. If she is unhappy with the side effects, she cannot stop IUD use without accessing further health care.

When discussing the risks and benefits of an IUD, the clinician asks Maria why she is interested in the method. Maria explains that she is seeking an IUD because it is a condition of her parole. She was recently convicted of a crime and due to her history of frequent pregnancies and child neglect she has been court ordered to obtain long-term contraception. She states that she does not particularly care about obtaining an IUD, but she is doing so to fulfill her legal obligations and to become eligible for parole.

Questions to Consider

1. Is it possible for the clinician to ensure patient autonomy in this situation?
2. Does the societal good of inhibiting Maria's ability to have future pregnancies outweigh the importance of her autonomy?
3. If the IUD must be inserted, how can the clinician work to ensure that good is done for Maria and avoid the most harm?

Case Discussion

The main problem is focused on the principle of autonomy. Maria may very much want to use an IUD for long-term contraception, but up front, there is no way to know for sure what her intentions and desires are because she is explaining her choice for an IUD in terms of the court order. Also involved are questions of paternalism. Healthcare providers are always involved in making paternalistic choices for their patients. The goals of clinical practice mandate that providers have expert knowledge that they can use to make decisions that will optimize the good for their patients. In Maria's case, the WHNP may feel that an IUD is the best course of action for Maria's future. The WHNP may also believe that reducing Maria's pregnancies will produce a societal good by reducing the number of children who will need to be cared for by social services. Yet, the goal of WHNPs, especially those taking an ethics of care perspective, is to work closely with patients to understand their unique situations and develop plans of action in concert with them. In this case, the legal system is paternalistically choosing for the patient that the greatest good for her and for society, more broadly, is to require long-term birth control.

Mandating long-term, provider-dependent contraception for Maria is based on certain *underlying assumptions*. These include that a history of frequent pregnancies and child neglect will predict the same future behavior, that the most important way to solve this problem is through preventing Maria from having more pregnancies, and that children born to women like Maria will ultimately become a burden on society. Finally multiple *power imbalances* exist in this case. Most obviously, Maria has little to no power in this decision, as the court has decided for her that long-term contraception be a part of her sentence. Additionally, the WHNP has more power than Maria, for it will be she who will ultimately decide if the IUD is inserted at this visit. This particular power imbalance needs to be taken into account during conversations with Maria. In order to develop an ethically sound plan of care, Maria must not feel that her healthcare provider is coercing her further. Additionally, the WHNP is not completely autonomous in this situation either. She may choose not to insert the IUD, but she may face legal or professional repercussions for not following through with the procedure. This final power imbalance makes it particularly difficult to act on a plan of care if the WHNP's decision is to deny treatment. If she does not work within a supportive professional environment, she may be risking her professional position and or career.

Before an ethically and clinically sound decision can be made, the clinician needs to attempt to fill some of the *information gaps* that currently exist. One of these is the cultural and historical context of coerced contraception and sterilization. Understanding this context will aid the WHNP in considering the *cultural perspectives* that are in play, which undoubtedly affect the choices of the legal system, the patient, and the clinician. The history of compulsory contraception and sterilization in the United States is deeply embedded in the eugenics movement. This movement began in the United States during the Progressive Era, roughly 1890–1920. The historical actors who we now think of as progressives were significantly varied in intention and philosophies, but most worked toward developing a society and government that was better able to comprehensively care for the most indigent and poor of its members (Gendzel, 2011). Many progressive efforts were rooted in the philosophy of eugenics. In the most basic sense, eugenics programs sought to maximize the spread of "desirable traits" among offspring and decrease the inheritance of "undesirable traits." These efforts were significantly based on biased views, which privileged the lifestyles of white middle class families and strived to assimilate working class families into these cultural systems (Jacobs, 2009). These policies by and large affected the lives of marginalized populations, often in brutal ways (Raine, 2012). Eugenics was a pervasive principle that affected healthcare providers, scientists, and social reformers alike. In the beginning, it was part of the social framework of American culture. As time progressed, and policies directly seen as eugenic dissipated, sterilization, contraception, and family policies nevertheless continued in various states that were clearly based on the underlying philosophies of eugenics (Lombardo, 2011).

For years, many legal policies and clinical decision-making processes were based on this principle. Compulsory or legally mandated sterilization or contraception has a long history. Situated within the historical context of the early eugenics movement, mandated sterilization laws culminated with the 1924 Supreme Court decision in *Buck v. Bell*. This famous ruling allowed for mandated sterilization for developmentally delayed and socially outcast individuals. Quoting the ruling, the court concluded, "three generations of imbeciles are enough" (quoted in Raine, 2012). *Buck v. Bell* set the scene for years of state-regulated laws aimed at controlling the fertility of developmentally delayed, socially nonconforming, and marginalized populations. Native peoples, racial minorities, and women living in poverty have historically been victims of such policies (Jacobs, 2009). As political and cultural awareness has evolved, these practices have decreased in number and severity, yet there still exist disparities among coercive sterilization and contraception practices. Even without direct legal mandates, the long-term impact of the eugenics movement on societal beliefs about contraception for minority women may still be affecting some clinicians' attitudes when counseling women about contraceptive methods. In a recent study exploring the experiences of postpartum urban minority women with the contraception counseling they received while in the hospital, one-third of these women reported feeling coerced and racially discriminated against during their counseling (Yee & Simon, 2011). Aside from coercion that comes directly from healthcare providers or the state, many women may feel pressure from family members or community beliefs to make certain reproductive decisions.

In addition to understanding the cultural context in which this case takes place, the WHNP needs to elicit more information from Maria about her situation and her desires. In order to determine whether Maria may autonomously agree with the court order or not and how the WHNP can work to support Maria's empowerment within the situation, she must have a conversation with her that gets to the center of these questions. Examples of questions that could guide this discussion include: What are your feelings about getting an IUD and how do you feel about the court ordering you to get one? How do you foresee the next 5 to 10 years of your life? What are your hopes and desires concerning future family planning? What support systems do you have in your community, and how do you see them affecting your choice?

Finally, the WHNP must decide on an ethically and clinically sound *course of action*. In a situation as complicated as this one, ideally the WHNP will have the opportunity to collaborate with both peer colleagues and clinic management. That way she will have the clinical support of colleagues and the professional support of her management to ensure that she will not face professional repercussions. After having a thorough conversation with Maria, the WHNP learns that Maria may have a personal desire for the IUD to be placed, separate from the court's mandate. She explains that without the court order she would not have considered the long-term method, but afterward she thought about it differently. Thinking that she has no choice in the matter, she has considered the benefits of having an effective long-term method. She expresses apathy about her future family planning choices, expressing neither a desire to become pregnant in the next 5 years nor to fully protect herself against pregnancy. From Maria's story, the WHNP concludes that she has very little to no support system at home. She lives with a friend and she is currently unemployed. She is not in contact with any of her family members.

With this information in hand, the WHNP must now decide whether she will insert the IUD or not. Maria has clearly consented to the insertion, but the WHNP knows that the consent is questionable due to its basis on legal coercion. However, she also knows that because of the legal ramifications for Maria, Maria will seek the insertion elsewhere even if the WHNP does not insert it at this visit. Additionally, knowing the complex history of coercive legal methods of enforcing contraception and sterilization on vulnerable women, she wants to be extra careful to ensure Maria's autonomy and benefit from this experience. After consultation with her colleagues, the WHNP decides that she will move forward with IUD insertion. Before beginning the procedure, she works to ensure as much autonomy as possible for Maria by thoroughly reviewing the risks and benefits of the IUD. She also counsels Maria regarding other long- and short-term contraception options, in case she wants to choose a different one. Explaining that ethically she cannot insert the IUD unless Maria fully consents to the procedure, she asks Maria again whether she consents and asks her to explain her reasoning process. This time, Maria explains that she is interested in the benefits of the method and expresses a desire for the IUD that goes beyond the fact that it is court ordered. The WHNP takes this last conversation as the most influential part of her decision-making process. Maria was able to articulate reasons why she was autonomously (as much as possible) choosing the method. Maria was clearly informed of the risks, benefits, and alternatives to the option and still articulated a desire to receive it. Thus, the WHNP continued with the visit and inserted the IUD.

Assisted Reproductive Technologies

CASE STUDY 3: DESPERATE TO CONCEIVE: INFORMED CONSENT

Karen Walling is a 37-year-old woman who presents to the OB/GYN clinic where Janetta Price is one of the two WHNPs seeing new patients. Her initial reason for the visit is an annual physical including pelvic exam. The WHNPs are prepared to and do provide primary care for patients with uncomplicated medical histories. While discussing her history, Karen confides that she has been living with her boyfriend, Gareth, who is 27 years old, for the past 4 years and they have been hoping to have children. However, they stopped using contraceptives 3 years ago and still have not conceived. Karen has never been pregnant. She used contraceptives in previous relationships. Gareth's sperm count is normal. Karen is seeking information about the possibility of in vitro fertilization (IVF). She tells Janetta that she has heard that people often have twins as a result of fertility treatment and as far as she is concerned that would be a good result, as her boyfriend is from a large family and loves children.

Questions to Consider

1. What are the salient pieces of information in the case that will help Janetta explore possible options with Karen? What other questions would be important to explore with Karen?
2. How does an APN's understanding of existing evidence and ethical controversies surrounding artificial reproductive technologies provide a basis for this discussion?
3. Should everyone have the opportunity to receive IVF or other assisted reproductive technologies? What societal benefits and burdens are there?

Background of Assisted Reproductive Technologies

Dr. William Pancoast is reported to have first used artificial insemination by donor (AID) to impregnate the wife of an infertile couple using the sperm of a medical student. Interestingly, he did not at the time tell them that the sperm was not the husband's (Lynn, 2001). In 1978 in the north of England, Louise Brown became the first baby to be born as a result of IVF. The media dubbed her a "test-tube baby." In-vitro is Latin for "within or in glass." IVF is a form of assisted reproductive technology (ART). In the United States, ARTs have been used since 1981 (CDC, 2013a). There are several types of ARTs (see **Table 9-1**). The development and use of ARTs, although offering great possibilities for some infertile persons or couples, have also caused

■ Table 9-1   Types of ARTs

Term	Process	Preparation
Artificial insemination (AI)	Insertion of sperm into the vagina	With or without prior ovarian stimulation as below
Intrauterine insemination (IUI)	Insertion of sperm into the uterus via cannula	Concentrated sperm from partner or donor sperm
In vitro fertilization (IVF)	Ova fertilized outside of the uterus One or more embryo(s) introduced into the uterus using a cervical catheter (approximately 4 days post fertilization)	Follows a process of ovarian stimulation (8–12 daily injections) and uterus preparation Monitoring of maturation via vaginal utrasound Ova extracted via transvaginal ultrasound aspiration
Zygote intrafallopian transfer (ZIFT)	Ova fertilized outside the body and then placed into fallopian tube (approximately 4 days post fertilization)	Using the same preparation process as above
Gamete intrafallopian transfer (GIFT)	Ova and sperm introduced into the fallopian tube (rarely done)	Using the same preparation process as above
Intracytoplasmic sperm injection (ICSI)	Sperm injected into ova Fertilized egg placed into uterus	Sperm retrieved via masturbation or biopsy
Frozen embryo transfer	Thawed embryo introduced into uterus	Estrogen and progesterone used to prepare uterus

great difficulties for others. The ability to control reproduction has given rise to many thorny ethical issues for human beings. Some claim that the most problematic is the actual or potential ability to determine which embryo with which characteristics will have a chance at being born and vice versa.

Aligned with this are contemporary debates about the permissibility of abortion. ARTs are sometimes used to "screen out" embryos that have genetically undesirable traits, usually those associated with disease or physical anomalies. Such embryos are then destroyed. Additionally, some clinics transfer to the uterus several embryos at a time to enhance the chance of pregnancy (and the clinic's success rate). If several of the embryos implant, a decision may have to be made about selective reduction. There are several processes of selective reduction, some of which are minimally invasive. However, the physical risks include miscarriage of the remaining fetuses. There are also associated risks of psychological distress, as discussed later. However, carrying multiple fetuses to term is also risky for both the mother's health and that of the fetuses.

Certain religions, such as the Roman Catholic Church, are opposed to the use of ARTs altogether, and not just for reasons of potential for abortion. Some in the disability community are worried about the eugenics effect, as discussed earlier, of screening out undesirable conditions and traits. Among their worries is that differences will cease to be tolerated. Feminists are divided as to whether assisted reproductive options increase women's liberty and empower them or are more oppressive because women may feel pressured to use them. Nevertheless, ARTs have become almost a routine solution to infertility and other causes of childlessness such as lack or loss of a partner, in spite of the fact that many of the associated ethical difficulties have not been resolved. ARTs are partly responsible for the rise in prematurity and disability in newborns, as discussed in Chapter 7.

Infertility is defined by the American Society for Reproductive Medicine (ASRM) as "the failure to achieve a successful pregnancy after 12 months or more of timed, unprotected intercourse or donor insemination" (ASRM, 2012). Infertility is estimated to affect up to 12% of the world's populations (World Health Organization [WHO], 2009). The CDC estimates that 10% of women in the United States have fertility issues (CDC, 2013b). The United States, United Kingdom, and Australia, countries at the forefront of the development of ARTs, were keen to develop guidelines about the use of these innovations. More recently the WHO, in concert with the International Committee for Monitoring Assisted Reproductive Technology, has worked to standardize guidelines across countries, but practices remain variable. However, there is now a tentatively accepted glossary that it is hoped will help to "standardize and harmonize international data collection, and ... assist in monitoring the availability, efficacy, and safety of assisted reproductive technology (ART) being practiced worldwide" (WHO, 2009). Regardless of regulation and hoped-for practice standardization, the impact of these technologies on the lives of contemporary people is complex. Thus the task of assisting women (and their partners where these exist) is also complex. It depends on knowing what the controversies are and discerning the particular meaning of these controversies for a particular woman within the context of her life.

Many WHNPs and other primary care providers, while not actually employed in fertility work, may be asked for advice in this area and should be prepared to assist a woman and her partner (if she has one) in their decision making. ARTs are not readily available in many poorer countries for fairly obvious reasons (they are expensive and people are too busy struggling to survive). However, there are increasing reports that women from poorer countries have been solicited both for ova donation and for surrogacy purposes (Crozier & Martin, 2012). Additionally, ARTs may be used for the purposes of detecting genetic anomalies in an embryo and the selection for implantation of an embryo that does not carry a worrisome gene (although the embryo may carry other problematic genetic material that is not detected). This process is called preimplantation genetic diagnosis (PGD or PIGD). (PGD, along with its ethical controversies, is discussed in Case Study 5 later in the chapter.) Ethical problems associated with ARTs and that have implications for society as well as the individuals involved include the issue of gender and trait selection, expense, increased incidence of prematurity and associated physical defects, conflicts of interest for clinics who must show success rates, and adequate informed consent. Certain other aspects of the use of ARTs also remain controversial. Among the philosophically controversial aspects are the following:

- Religious and philosophical considerations about the moral status of embryos. Are they to be considered human beings or not? What are the implications of being considered a human being?
- What underlies the drive for a genetically related offspring? Is it a natural or a socially constructed drive, or are there elements of both? Depending on the perspective, what does this mean for women and society?

- When ARTs are used in conjunction with donors and/or surrogacy, who should be considered the parent(s)? Who assumes responsibility for a child who is considered "defective" in some way? What are the legal ramifications of multiple possible parents?
- Who should have access to ARTs and who should pay? Should menopausal and post-menopausal women have access?
- What are the risks to a woman's health when using ARTs?
- How can WHNPs assist in decision making?
- What are clinic success rates? Do they depend on multiple embryo implantation?

It is beyond the capacity of this chapter to discuss each of these philosophical challenges in detail, but those involved in ART work should be familiar with the arguments that are particularly pertinent to their settings.

The benefits of ARTS are fairly obvious. They allow people who would not previously have had the capacity to reproduce for a variety of reasons to experience parenthood. In many cases, they permit birth of a child who is genetically related to at least one partner. Some common forms of ARTs permit embryonic diagnosis of various genetic disorders and the option not to implant such embryos.

The *drawbacks* associated with ARTs are of three types: physical, psychological, and sociological. The possible physical dangers for women may stem from the drugs used to stimulate the ovaries, the strain of childbirth on the body (exacerbated in the case of increased age), comorbid conditions, and multiple births. The long-term effects of ovarian stimulation have also been noted. A woman using ARTs may be affected psychologically in any of a number of ways. She may have felt family or social pressures to accept IVF because it is an available option. She may be pressured by her partner, stressed by the procedure and its rigorous and intrusive regimen, emotionally labile from the drugs used, have to make a decision about the number of embryos to implant, feel inadequate with failed cycles, and so on. Sociologically, she may be affected by the costs associated with IVF and subsequent pregnancies (especially with increased incidence of multiple births and associated issues of prematurity). Finally, success rates decline with increasing age. In the United States, the CDC approximates success rates for IVF based on mandatory clinic reporting. Success rates are denoted as the percentage of live births for 2010 and rounded: 38% of women < 35 years of age; 34% of women 35–37 years of age; 28% of women 38–40 years of age;

22% of women 41–42 years of age; 17% of women 43–44 years of age; and 13% of women > 44 years of age (CDC, 2011).

Case Discussion

Janetta realizes from Karen's request that there are several *issues* to address. Her focus is on how to provide a *"good"* (*beneficence*) for Karen in terms of understanding the motivation for and strength of her desire for a pregnancy, the support she has, what she knows about the process of IVF—what it involves in terms of time and commitment. She has *more information* to gather and it may be that she will eventually need to talk with both Gareth and Karen. First, she needs to explore with Karen the timing of this request, what has led up to it, what she knows, and what her misperceptions are. Providing the necessary information, tailored to Karen's needs in a low-pressure environment where the provider does not have the same stake in the decision that an IVF clinic might, is crucial. Frith, Jacoby, and Gabbay (2011) from their research interviewing clinic professionals note the boundaries that are drawn in settings (such as IVF clinics) where there is social and ethical controversy about the practice but the everyday work has to be done. In such settings clinicians must "normalize" the practice for themselves. Because many IVF clinics (70%–80%) in the United States, the United Kingdom, and other countries are privately owned and their ratings are based on success rates, they are perhaps more susceptible to conflicts of interest than a primary care or OB/GYN clinic that does not offer such specialized services.

Giving Karen time to think, providing appropriate reading material, and helping her familiarize herself with the process and what it entails are essential. Janetta needs to be available to answer more questions and to help Karen explore acceptable alternatives, such as adoption. In this way she can empower Karen to make a more informed decision that is in line with her life and context. What is her relationship with Gareth like? Does the age difference between them factor into this request? Is he putting subtle or not so subtle pressure on her? It is obvious that Karen does not understand some of the implications of her request from her statements. She thinks it would be good to have twins, but does she understand the dangers associated with multiple births discussed earlier? While Janetta may eventually refer her to a clinic or help her select an appropriate clinic that specializes in ARTs, before she does so she has a responsibility to inform Karen about the process and pros and cons and to prepare her to ask the right questions of the clinic as well as to evaluate the clinic. The more information Karen has the better Janetta's ability to support her autonomous choice in concert with Gareth. An important point to keep in mind is that evidence suggests "[M]any couples embarking on an *in vitro* fertilization (IVF) programme are optimistic with unrealistically high expectations" (Peddie, van Teijlingen, & Bhattacharya, 2005).

The Woman and Her Fetus: A Maternal–Fetal Conflict?

CASE STUDY 4: PRENATAL TESTING

A WHNP is working in an OB/GYN private practice located in a remote rural area. There is an ultrasound machine and trained technician at the office. However, many of the other luxuries that are easily available in more populated areas, such as genetic counselors, level-two ultrasounds, and termination procedures, are not readily available to her patients. Patients are required to travel several hours to access these services. Keisha presents to the clinic for an initial obstetrical visit. This is her first pregnancy. She is 10 weeks pregnant and has no known hereditary risk factors such as cystic fibrosis. She tells the WHNP that her sister, who lives in an affluent urban area, recently had a prenatal screening test that showed she had a very low risk of carrying a fetus affected with Down syndrome or a neural tube defect. The patient wants to know if this is an appropriate test for her. Knowing that the appropriate follow-up resources may not be available and understanding the complex subtleties involved in offering technologically advanced treatment options to women and that the early detection of a possible birth defect can help parents address many of the issues in preparation of their child's birth, the WHNP is conflicted about how to counsel Keisha about her options.

Questions to Consider

1. What if Keisha learns that her fetus is at risk for a birth defect but is financially unable to access the appropriate follow-up care? How will this affect her pregnancy?

2. How will the WHPN ensure Keisha's autonomy while at the same time preventing possible emotional harm to her that may come from knowledge that she cannot act on?
3. What is the risk posed to the current and future health of the fetus if testing is not done, and what is the WHNP's responsibility to the fetus?

Case Discussion

There are two *main problems* present within Keisha's case. The first relates to the principle of autonomy, asking what should the WHNP do if she decides prenatal testing is not in the best interest of Keisha yet Keisha wants to pursue it all the same. Second, the WHNP is faced with the possible conflicting interests of her pregnant patient and the fetus. As a prenatal clinician, she must treat not one patient, but two. This double loyalty often contributes to ethically complicated cases in which an intervention that benefits one may pose a threat to the other. In Keisha's case these issues are less obvious than in other possible cases; yet all the same, there exists a hint of what is often termed, "maternal–fetal conflict." Prenatal testing may benefit the fetus by allowing Keisha to properly prepare to care for a special needs child, yet it may be best for Keisha to not have the testing done.

Questions of autonomy are closely tied to the wealth of possible prenatal tests available to pregnant women. As discussed in Chapter 2, the principle of autonomy is complex and easily affected by influencing factors. One of the complicating factors is an *underlying assumption* held by many in the medical field that increased options inherently increase a patient's autonomy. In the field of women's health, autonomy is all too frequently looked upon simply as a quest for personal choice, which facilitates ignoring the subtle and sometimes coercive influences of the context in which decisions are made. Within this view, a woman is deemed autonomous in her reproductive life if she is granted the ultimate power to give the final consent to treatment. Feminist critiques of the principle of autonomy demonstrate that this understanding may not be comprehensive enough for all instances (Meyers, 2001; Sherwin, 1992). Susan Sherwin (1992) has suggested that autonomy is not something that can be determined on an isolated case basis but rather must be considered in light of the individual's unique and complex life situation. Other scholars have argued that there are forces present within the promise of new technological advances that bear great influence on a patient's choice to pursue treatment, creating constraints on individual autonomy (Sandelowski, 1991). The effect of such influences must be considered if providers are to work to ensure patient autonomy within the field of women's health.

Many scholars debate the benefits of prenatal testing and its effects on informed consent and patient autonomy. Although it is often suggested that new technologies work to increase patient autonomy by offering more choices to women and their partners, many argue that the act of offering an increased number of treatment options may present coercive influences itself. Davies (2001) refers to what she terms the "ambiguity of choice" in regard to decision-making processes about prenatal testing. She contends that although these screening opportunities are offered to increase choices for women, the choice may be more of an illusion than originally understood. She explains that the more choices that are offered to a patient, the more necessary it is for the patient to explain and defend her decision, thereby making it difficult to say no to an offered procedure. In addition, other scholars suggest that women will accept prenatal screening options and other technologically advanced treatment options because they perceive an imperative to "do whatever they can" (Lippman, 2001). These subtle coercive influences that may be present in the offering of screening options make it difficult for an NP to determine whether a patient has agreed to undergo treatment out of her own autonomous decision, out of a pressure to conform to the values of the medical institution, or as a result of coercion (Lippman, 2001).

To address issues of patient autonomy in decision-making processes, NPs have typically attempted to provide treatment options in a "nondirective" way so as not to persuade patients toward one decision or another. However, the previous discussion highlights the ways in which simply providing screening options in a nondirective manner may not preclude the presence of all coercive influences. Instead, it is imperative that the NP know the patient, engage in an exploration with the patient about her ultimate goals for her treatment, and then use this knowledge to aid her in developing a plan of action that will support the patient's identified priorities.

As noted, when debating appropriate courses of action for complicated cases involving pregnant women, many ethicists refer to such a dilemma as a "maternal–fetal conflict." Many practitioners may have *underlying assumptions* that such cases are truly a conflict between mother and fetus. Such assumptions and language can be constrictive because they depict a situation in which the unique aspects of dependence and interconnectedness inherent in the pregnant state are ignored and a view of the fetus and mother as two distinct individuals in direct conflict with each other is adopted. This creates an "adversarial dichotomy" in which the autonomy of one individual cannot be honored without risking the welfare of the other; it proposes mother versus fetus. Examples of cases that fit into this category include pregnant women who continue to use drugs or alcohol throughout pregnancy, women who choose to terminate their pregnancies, and women who face major health risks as consequences of their pregnancies. Approaching such dilemmas from the maternal–fetal conflict perspective can be limiting because it diverts attention away from the details and context of the case, precludes providers from deciding upon a course of action that honors the needs of both stakeholders, and makes it seem as if a provider must choose between patients. Viewing this situation through a feminist ethic of care lens would allow for an evaluation of the details of the experiences within the case so that the practitioner would be better prepared to develop a course of action that benefits both mother and fetus (Marcellus, 2004).

An in-depth discussion with Keisha may allow the WHNP to gain information that will fill some of the *information gaps* present in the case and allow her to mitigate the possible conflicts between what is good for Keisha and what is good for her fetus. Hopefully by learning the complexities of Keisha's life situation she will find that what is best for Keisha is also best for her fetus. Upon further discussion, the WHNP learns that Keisha is not partnered and will therefore be a single parent. She does not have the economic resources to access care outside of the area. Therefore, a simple screening test will only provide Keisha with an estimate of risk on which she will not be able to follow up in order to know more definitively about the health of her fetus. The WHNP also learns that Keisha has decided that pregnancy termination is not an option for her. She expresses that even if it were known that the fetus had a severe birth defect, she would not pursue termination. Therefore the access to termination procedures is not a concern for the WHNP and Keisha. Additionally, the WHNP learns that Keisha has an interest in knowing if her fetus has a relatively high or low risk for health problems. As a single parent, Keisha wishes to have this information in order to begin to access the support she will need to care for her child if the estimated risk of defect is high.

In Keisha's case, as with other similar cases, when the WHNP has gained this knowledge about her patient, she will be able to discuss a plan of action in a way that is suited to the patient's individual needs. For instance, if her patient clearly expresses a desire to utilize all possible treatment options, it is appropriate to offer education about these options, the ways the treatment protocol may look down the line, and what she can expect in the future. For other patients, the WHNP may sense hesitancy to refuse treatment options. In these cases, it may be necessary for the practitioner to not simply provide education regarding the possible options, but also to discuss common feelings about deciding to accept or refuse treatment. In some situations, practitioners may need to give permission to patients to discontinue or refuse treatment and reassure them that it is okay to make such a decision. This process will be different for each patient, clinical situation, and practitioner and will depend heavily on the relationship formed between provider and patient.

In Keisha's individual case, the WHNP decides to counsel Keisha about the screening procedures that are available to her, being clear that the results will only be an estimate and that due to her economic situation they will not be able to determine more definitively what the exact risks are. She counsels Keisha about the details of risk assessment and the possibilities of increased anxieties that may come with knowing about a possible risk and not being able to receive follow-up care. Finally, knowing that as a single parent it is important to Keisha to have as much information as possible to prepare for her new role, the WHNP works to support Keisha's decision to proceed with the first-line prenatal screening tests that are available to her.

Genetic Testing Specific to Women's Health

This section discusses the roles and responsibilities related to discussing genetic issues with patients. Advances in genetic knowledge and science have implications for all healthcare providers. All APNs have responsibilities to understand the basics, but those working in specialty areas need to understand the specific implications of available technology for the health and well-being of their particular populations. Patients trust APNs to help them with their decision making and to find and access resources. APN education in the United States and many other countries includes content on genetics. This knowledge, together with an ethic of care (the intentional focus on an individual and her needs with the object of facilitating her well-being) and the nursing focus on the whole person, helps APNs to discern what individual patients need to make their own decisions related to genetic testing. Women's health, family, and pediatric APNs may be the first ones to identify potential genetic issues based on history taking and/or completing a family tree with a patient. A family tree allows patterns of disease to emerge. Some nurses will be confident enough in their genetic knowledge to provide preliminary counseling. Others will need to refer patients to an appropriate genetic counselor. Genetic counselors are specially trained in one or more of several areas of genetic decision making, for example, reproductive issues, cancer risk, pediatric, and general.

See **Box 9-1** for an overview of the pathophysiology of genetic changes, types and purposes of genetic tests, and strategies for assisting with patient decision making. Two areas of concern for WHNPs are that of whether the family history of a woman or couple point to the possibility of a genetic issue for offspring or for existing family members. Genetic testing that has implications for family members is discussed in the next case study. Genetic testing to screen for the existence of potentially serious genetic mutations is done via preimplantation testing of an embryo usually at around the 8-cell stage. In both cases a thorough exploration of the information, goals of testing, and implications for those involved is needed, and APNs are in ideal positions to provide assistance, resources, and support.

Preimplantation Genetic Diagnosis

There are an increasing number of genetic testing facilities that advertise their tests directly to the public. The availability of genetic tests advertised through direct-to-consumer-marketing means that more and more couples become aware that they may have a problem gene that could be passed on to their offspring. In turn, requests for information about PGD and its possibilities are increasing. In addition to screening for increasing numbers of genetic diseases, PGD allows the identification of which embryos are less likely to implant and can in some cases detect which embryos are likely to develop adult genetically linked diseases. However, while PGD is increasing in sophistication and ability to detect problematic genetic mutations (changes from normal DNA), the associated ethical implications both for individual human beings and societies remain somewhat primitive. One stark question associated with the eugenics problem (or the quest for a perfect race) is the implications for existing human beings of science

Box 9-1   Genetic Testing: Supporting Patient Decision Making

Types and Purposes of Genetic Tests

- A genetic test may be used to confirm *carrier* status. Carrier status means that a person carries a recessive gene, which is likely to pose problems if that person mates with another person who is also a carrier. When this happens, there is a 1:4 chance that each offspring will have the disease, a 1:2 chance that the offspring will be carriers themselves and a 1:4 chance that the offspring will be neither carriers nor subject to the disease.
    - Carrier status simply means that a person has a recessive gene on one of the chromosomes. Multiple genes lie along each chromosome.
    - We have 23 pairs of chromosomes in each body cell nucleus.
    - 22 pairs are somatic (body), the 23rd pair is the sex chromosome (XX = female; XY = male).
    - The genes at corresponding sites on each of the chromosome pair "code" for the same protein. However, one gene is usually dominant, meaning it will be active. Thus the recessive trait will not be expressed unless present in corresponding genes on both chromosomes in the pair. That is, the person inherited two recessive genes: one on the maternally donated chromosome and one on the paternally donated chromosome.

- A genetic test can be used to screen for the presence of a known problem gene.
    - This can be carried out in the process of in vitro fertilization (IVF)—it permits the selection of an embryo that does not have the gene.
    - Newborn screening allows the identification of those at increased risk for genetic disease and in some cases permits disease-preventive actions (e.g., phenylketonuria, which requires dietary modifications).

- A genetic test can be used to *predict* the likelihood of developing a disease.
  - In children—for early-onset diseases such as familial adenomatous polyposis, which if positive, require diligent screening for disease with the goal of early intervention
  - In adults with a family history of genetic disease—if early detection is possible and effective
  - In adults—for life-planning purposes (long process of informed consent required)
  - In adults—if preventive strategies are available
- A genetic test may be diagnostic; it can confirm a suspected diagnosis
  - Useful when it will alter treatment
  - Allows other etiology to be pursued if negative

Important Questions

Perhaps the most important role of nurses in advising is to ensure that the following questions are asked and answered before proceeding. This may mean that the nurse prepares by seeking further information about what is known and what is not known or that the nurse refers the person for formal genetic counseling (see Resources at the end of this box).

- What are the goals of the testing?
  - Use the testing types and purposes above as a guide.
- Does the person understand the goals?
  - Discover what the person thinks that testing will do for him or her.
- What is the meaning of a positive or negative result?
  - What is the probability that a positive result means disease will follow?
  - Can the person live with the knowledge of a positive result in the absence of a cure or treatment?
  - How will the person feel about a negative result if others in the family have tested positive (possibility of survivor's guilt)?

□ A negative result means only that a particular mutation was not found. Many diseases such as cystic fibrosis have numerous mutations, but tests are done only for the most common.

■ What will be done, given positive or negative results?

□ What are the anticipated courses of action?

□ Will this require more frequent screening for disease development?

□ Will a negative result have implications for health insurance?

□ A colleague told of someone who had been treated for breast cancer and had a family history, but when her genetic test was negative for the BRCA gene, the insurance company refused to pay for ongoing surveillance with MRI.

□ What if nothing can be done?

■ Who, besides the person, might be affected by the results?

□ This means understanding the impact the information will likely have on others in the person's family; they may need help in determining when to disclose or when not to disclose to others.

■ What is known about the effects of testing on people's quality of life (QOL)?

□ Research has indicated that some people become depressed when a result is positive, and they cannot enjoy life. Others are relieved at having an explanation of symptoms. The implications are that we should help people to think about these possibilities.

■ Is there a possibility of discrimination in health insurance, life insurance, or job?

□ As of 2008 the Genetic Information Nondiscrimination Act (GINA) was signed into law. Its goal is to the protect against employment and insurance loss as a result of genetic information. The health insurance provisions became effective May 21, 2009; the employment provisions became effective November 21, 2009 (http://www.genome.gov/10002328).

☐ GINA does not protect against loss of life insurance, disability insurance, or long-term care insurance. Military personnel are also not protected by GINA. The Act does not mandate coverage for any particular test or treatment. GINA's employment provisions generally do not apply to employers with fewer than 15 employees (http://www.genome.gov/Pages/PolicyEthics/GeneticDiscrimination/GINAinfoDoc.pdf). Although GINA provides certain protections, the program is far from perfect.

Special Considerations for Children

The general recommendation is that predictive genetic testing not be carried out on children, except in a case in which the gene to be identified signals the probability of an early-onset and serious disease and in which early identification permits effective treatment.

For most genetic testing involving later-onset maladies, children should be allowed to wait until they are of an age when they can decide for themselves. It is important to remember that once a person has received knowledge of positive status, this knowledge is permanent.

Resources

American Nurses Association: http://www.nursingworld.org

ANA's Executive Summary: http://www.nursingworld.org/about/summary/sum99/genetics/htm

The National Society of Genetic Counselors: http://www.genome.gov/

Genetic Information Nondiscrimination Act: http://www.genome.gov/10002328

Government information on genetic testing: http://www.cancer.gov/cancertopics/understandingcancer/genetesting/

Source: Vallent, H. & Grace, P.J. (2011). Ethical Dimensions of Nursing and Healthcare. In J.L. Creasia & E. E. Frieberg (Eds). *Bridge to Professional Practice.* (5th Ed). Elsevier.

successfully eradicating genetic anomalies. Will scientists stop looking for cures? Will the next move be to screen for certain "undesirable traits"?

Decision making around genetic issues and PGD is especially difficult for couples. Studies have supported the idea that a fairly long process of decision making involving several phases is needed for couples to achieve equilibrium. Hershberger and colleagues (2012) found that couples go through "four phases (Identify, Contemplate, Resolve, Engage) of a complex, dynamic, and iterative decision-making process where multiple, sequential decisions are made" (p. 1536). In the first phase, couples are coming to grips with their at-risk status. In the second phase, couples explore their options and think about what they want to do. For almost half of the couples this phase takes around 3 years before moving into the "resolve" stage, where the couples decide on PGD, decline PGD, or oscillate. In the final "engaged" phase, couples carry out their decision. Surprisingly, the authors found that many couples did not access healthcare providers to help them with their decision making. The authors also noted that among those couples who accepted PGD were those with significant genetic implications such as Huntington's Chorea.

For APNs who may be asked for assistance in the identification and contemplation phases, the goal is to help with the information sorting and formulation of goals related to PGD in light of the couples' beliefs and values. Referral to genetic counselors and the provision of support are other strategies. It is not clear whether support groups are available, but this would be a pro-active strategy for an APN whose practice consists of several couples who are contemplating PGD.

CASE 5: FAMILY HISTORY OF BREAST CANCER: SHOULD I GET TESTED?

Paula Harrison is 48 years old with two sons (22 and 27 years old) and a daughter (25 years old). She has a family history of breast cancer. Her mother Eva died at 35 years of age when Paula was just 13. Paula took care of Eva in the last 2 years of her life. Eva had a mastectomy and chemotherapy for metastatic disease, but she succumbed rapidly to the disease after suffering various complications. Eva died within 2 years of diagnosis. Paula recently reunited with her cousin, June, whom she had not seen since they were children. June and her family had been living in New Zealand for the past 40 years. During their conversation, Paula learned that her aunt (June's mother) had also died from breast cancer, at age 50. Paula visits a suburban primary care clinic for the first time. She has moved from another state and a woman at her church recommended this nurse-led clinic. As the clinic's WHNP, Melissa, is gathering her history, Paula asks if she should be tested for the breast cancer gene in light of her family history.

Case Discussion

The main issue here is how to help Paula make a decision that is in her best interest and that of her family members. As usual, more *information* is needed about her experience of caring for her mother at such a young age, the meaning of that, and of the possibility that she may be more at risk for breast cancer than others. What are her family relationships, beliefs and values, supports, understanding of the role of genetics, genetic testing, and their purposes? Once more *information* is gathered about her and her needs, the WHNP can begin to explore the implications of testing for her. Certainly from the information the WHNP has been given there is some reason to suspect a genetic link. Have other members of her family, male or female, had breast or related cancers such as ovarian or pancreatic cancer?

Mutations in the BRCA1 and BRAC2 gene, although relatively rare (approximately 5% of those with breast cancer), put a person at a much higher (5:1) lifetime risk of breast cancer than the general population. Approximately 12% of women without the mutation will develop breast cancer over a lifetime. Of those with the mutation, approximately 60% will develop breast or ovarian cancer. These genes are responsible for tumor suppression and certain mutations in the BRCA1 or BRCA2 genes that fail to protect against tumor growth. There is some question about whether BRCA genes are dominant (only requiring one mutated gene of a pair) or recessive (both genes in a pair). The genes are passed in a dominant pattern but may actually be recessive, only causing problems when the partner gene becomes damaged (Northwest Association for Biomedical Research, 2011). If a person has the gene, there is a 50% chance that it has passed to each of his or her children. Men can also get breast, pancreatic, and prostate cancer. With this in mind, Melissa needs to either refer Paula to an appropriate genetic counselor or explore with Paula the implications of testing or not testing and refer her for counseling once they have addressed the questions they can answer.

Questions to Consider

The following are some questions for the WHNP to keep in mind during the discussion.

1. What are the goals of the testing? In Paula's case, a negative test means that she has not passed the gene on to her children. However, a negative test does not mean that one of the children will not develop cancer; they simply do not have the high risk from cancer imposed by the existence of the gene. However, if she is positive, this has implications for her children and their children. Does Paula understand these goals?
2. What meaning would a positive or negative result hold for her? Once one knows a test result, it cannot be "unknown."
3. Given a positive or negative result, what are the next courses of action? Will Paula need help to discuss the problem with her children? Her cousin June and June's children? Should she discuss the testing with them prior to undertaking it so she can discover what their concerns are? To date, there are no satisfactory resolutions given a positive result. Some patients have opted for bilateral mastectomies and oophrectomy.
4. What is known about the effects of testing on people's quality of life? Some people prefer not to know. Some people experience guilt, especially if it has been passed on to the children.

Given the rapid development of genetic knowledge—including genetic manipulations with the intent of cure—there is some hope that in the future the damaging effects of such genes can be mitigated. Meanwhile APNs are in the ideal situation to support people in their decision-making processes.

Providing Transgender Health Services: Is Informed Consent Enough?

CASE STUDY 6: THE REQUEST FOR TRANS HEALTH SERVICES

A WHNP has been working for 5 years in a reproductive health clinic. This clinic provides comprehensive services, including well-woman care, cervical cancer screenings, sexual transmitted infections testing and counseling, reproductive men's health care, and pregnancy testing, counseling, and termination. In an attempt to be accepting and affirming of a diverse patient population, the clinic advertises that it provides care for many different groups of people including lesbian, gay, and transgender individuals. However, the clinicians are not empowered with practice protocols or specific training in providing health care for transgender people. The clinic regularly sees female-to-male transgender men for healthcare screenings such as annual physicals and pap smears, but they do not provide contra-hormonal therapy, a staple of trans care.

One of the clinicians who regularly works in the clinic has been approached by multiple transgender individuals, both male-to-female and female-to-male, who are seeking hormone therapy. It has become known to the clinician that the local provider who has been serving the trans community has recently retired. These patients have expressed a need for services and a fear that there is nowhere else to turn. Knowing that hormone therapy is essential to transgender individuals and is a great need of the community, the WHNP considers whether it would be appropriate to offer this service through the clinic. However, she is conflicted about this choice. Offering hormone therapy to trans individuals is not as simple as incorporating some other more established healthcare options into practice. Transgender health is a new specialty that has been developing in the few past years. As such, the research is sparse. There currently exist no large-scale research studies evaluating the long-term risks of a lifetime of contra-hormone therapies. The WHNP asks herself if she begins to offer this service, will the informed consent of her patients be enough to ethically justify prescribing medical treatment that may have unknown future health risks?

Questions to Consider

1. Is it appropriate to override a patient's autonomy in order to avoid possible future harms?
2. Are the known pressing risks to the patient of not receiving treatment more important than the possible unknown future risks?
3. Is informed consent enough?

The *main problem* prominent in this case is a conflict between autonomy and nonmaleficence. As a reproductive health specialist, it is not unlikely that a WHNP would be faced with transgender clients requesting trans health services. In the current healthcare environment, the clinician may be conflicted about offering such services. Depending on the geographical location, there may not be a community of providers available to discuss practice guidelines and protocols. Additionally, without conclusive evidence regarding the long-term health risks and benefits of contra-hormone therapies, the clinician may not know if offering services would ultimately cause harm to the patient. Yet considering the current statistics on the health disparities and risks associated with the experiences of transgender individuals when they do not have access to affirming communities and comprehensive health care, the short-term risks of not offering treatment are clear. Hence the question, "Is informed consent enough?" Is it ethically enough to inform transgender clients of the state of the science, what is currently known and not known about long-term contra-hormone therapy, and allow them to make the decision for themselves? Or are the unknown health risks enough to deny services?

Researching the practice guidelines followed by some providers may fill some *information gaps*. Current recommendations do exist for the care of transgender patients. The World Professional Association for Transgender Health (WPATH) has put forth general practice guidelines for clinicians who care for trans patients. These recommendations suggest guidelines for holistic care including mental health, psychological care, and surgical and hormonal treatments (Bockting et al., 2011). In a similar manner, the American Endocrine Society has provided practice guidelines for clinicians who offer hormone treatment to both male-to-female and female-to-male transgender individuals (Hembree et al., 2009). Although these practice guidelines represent significant progress in the effort to provide access to safe and comprehensive care for transgender individuals, the research on transgender health is still in its infancy. The long-term health effects of a lifetime of contra-hormone therapy are not currently known, because up-to-date research has not yet been conducted following trans individuals throughout their lifespans. Additionally, transgender healthcare training is just beginning to be offered in medical and nursing schools. Thus, at this time many senior clinicians are not familiar with these services. Depending on the community in which a WNHP may work, there may be other providers with whom to consult and train; she or he may be able to travel to learn from another provider, or communicate through phone or Internet to receive invaluable consultation advice.

The WHNP, her professional setting, the patient requesting services, and the local trans community are all *players involved* in this case. Research has shown that there are drastic health disparities affecting the trans community. In a recent study, an alarming 30% of transgender participants reported at least one past suicide attempt. When compared to the .002% national average for all peoples, this statistic is overwhelming. Additionally, higher levels of domestic violence and abuse have been reported in the transgender population. Large disparities in healthcare access also exist, with only one-third of studied transgender individuals reporting that they have a primary care clinician. This number decreases significantly when looking specifically at transgender people of color. Finally, many transgender individuals have reported experiences of discrimination in the healthcare setting based on their gender identity (Kenagy, 2005). The American Psychological Society, as well as WPATH, has suggested that hormonal and surgical treatment for trans patients may greatly decrease these disparities (Bockting et al., 2011; Drescher, Haller, APA Caucus of Lesbian, Gay, and Bisexual Psychiatrists, 2012). Additionally, providing trans health services will benefit the community beyond the patients served. It will communicate to the local lesbian, gay, bisexual, and transgender (LGBT) community that they are a valid and unique group of individuals who have particular needs within the healthcare system. It will work to decrease a culture of silence that exists among clinical practice and research surrounding the health needs of LGBT individuals (Eliason, Dibble, & DeJoseph, 2010). Yet, at the same time, the clinician in this case has a duty to prevent further harm to the patient and protect her own practice from liability. Similarly, the clinic for which she works must also protect itself and be sure that it is servicing the community in a safe manner.

Prevalent values may have an effect on a clinician's willingness to provide trans services, especially in the form of personal or cultural biases. It is also important to consider, on a larger scale, how the stereotypes and assumptions present within a WHNP's practice affect vulnerable populations, such as LGBT-identifying persons, and can lead to population-based health disparities. Three-step strategies for healthcare providers to decrease the healthcare barriers faced by clients who are members of marginalized populations have been suggested. First, healthcare providers need to examine their own beliefs and values regarding the specific population of patients and compare these with current understandings available from research and philosophical inquiry and documented in professional literature to identify false assumptions that they may hold. Second, professional education should be used as a necessary tool to increase awareness and sensitivity to issues of stigmatization and marginalization. Finally, healthcare providers should work to communicate a validating and nonjudgmental attitude to all patients (Spinks, Andrews, & Boyle, 2000).

As the WHNP moves forward in this case, she first works to understand her particular patient's narrative. Her patient informs her that he has been on testosterone and living as a male for over a year. He explains to her that he once suffered from significant depression; however, since beginning hormone therapy and counseling, his depression has greatly improved. He associates this change mostly with his physical gender transition and expresses that for this reason continuing testosterone therapy is critically important to him. Knowing that the patient is in obvious need of this care and that he has nowhere else to access such therapy, the WHNP decides to move forward with providing care. She does the necessary research over the Internet, with professional groups, and consults with colleagues to develop a safe protocol for implementing hormone therapy. Before prescribing hormones for her patient, she discusses in depth with him the lack of research and clinical knowledge regarding the possible long-term effects of testosterone therapy in order to ensure that he is making an informed decision to consent to treatment. Finally, once a safe protocol has been developed within her clinical practice, she offers to serve as a consultant to other practitioners, knowing that this will allow her to serve as a change agent in her community, educating other practitioners about the specific needs of transgender patients.

Summary

Women's health issues continue to be of concern internationally. Among the reasons for this are power imbalances, women's historical roles as caregivers, and a historical lack of self-agency. The existence of a women's health specialty provides one avenue for addressing injustices by focusing on the special needs and concerns of women while also acknowledging their inevitable interrelationships with others in their lives.

Discussion Questions

1. What are the laws and resources in your country related to human trafficking?
2. A young woman named Miya is brought to your clinic/emergency department by an older woman who mostly speaks for her. She appears to be around 15 years old and speaks in broken English. She

is tearful, has old bruises on her neck and arms, and based on your immediate assessment, has a broken arm. Her companion claims Miya is her niece, but on questioning them both further about Miya's health history it becomes apparent that the "aunt" does not know her niece very well. Moreover, Miya seems afraid of her aunt.

Explore this case using a decision-making framework such as the one provided in Chapter 2 (Table 2-6).

1. How would you go about discovering what is going on with Miya?
2. If Miya seems at risk from her protector (whether this is a case of abuse or trafficking), what steps might you take to protect her?
3. What are the regulations in your country related to minors, abuse, and trafficking?
4. What are the resources?

Consider these additional questions related to the chapter's content:

1. What are the pros and cons related to mandating the reporting of abuse in adults?
2. IPV is prevalent in certain countries and cultures where women are not treated as the moral equal of men. What is the APN's responsibility in the case of a Middle Eastern woman whose husband speaks for her? What are the dangers of trying to empower her? Should an APN try to change such practices when they occur in a country where human rights are at least in principle accorded to everyone?

References

American Society for Reproductive Medicine. (2012). Practice committee report. Definitions of infertility and recurrent pregnancy loss. Retrieved from http://www.asrm.org/uploadedFiles/ASRM_Content/News_and_Publications/Practice_Guidelines/Committee_Opinions/Definitions_of_infertility.pdf

Association of Women's Health, Obstetric and Neonatal Nurses. (2007). Mandatory reporting of intimate partner violence: Position statement. Retrieved from http://www.awhonn.org/awhonn/content.do?name=05_HealthPolicyLegislation/5H_PositionStatements.htm

Bockting, C., Botzer, M., Cohen-Kettenis, P., CeCuprere, G., Feldman, J., Fraser, L., . . . Zucker, K. (2011). Standards of care for the health of transsexual, transgender, and gender-nonconforming people, version 7. *International Journal of Transgenderism, 13,* 165–232.

Caulfield, P. (2013, January 9). Defense lawyer in India rape case blames victim, says "respectable" women in India are not raped: Report. *New York Daily News.* Retrieved from http://www.nydailynews.com/news/world/tk-article-1.1236369

Centers for Disease Control and Prevention. (2010, September 20). Intimate partner violence: Definitions. Retrieved from http://www.cdc.gov/violenceprevention/intimatepartnerviolence/definitions.html

Centers for Disease Control and Prevention. (2011). Preliminary data – clinic tables and data dictionary (ARTs). Retrieved from http://www.cdc.gov/ART/

Centers for Disease Control and Prevention. (2013a). Assisted reproductive technology (ART). Retrieved from http://www.cdc.gov/art/

Centers for Disease Control and Prevention. (2013b). Reproductive health. Retrieved from http://www.cdc.gov/reproductivehealth/

Crozier, G. K. D., & Martin, D. (2012). How to address the ethics of reproductive travel to developing countries: A comparison of national self-sufficiency and regulated market approaches. *Developing World Bioethics, 12*(1), 45–54.

Davies, D. (2001). *Genetic dilemmas: Reproductive technology, parental choices, and children's futures.* New York, NY: Routledge.

Drescher, J., Haller, E., APA Caucus of Lesbian, Gay and Bisexual Psychiatrists. (2012). Position statement on access to care for transgender and gender variant individuals. American Psychiatric Association.

Dutton, M. A., Kaltman, S., Goodman, L. A., Weinfurt, K., & Vankos, N. (2005). Patterns of intimate partner violence: Correlates and outcomes. *Violence and Victims, 20*(5), 483–497.

Eliason, M., Dibble, S., & DeJoseph, J. (2010). Nursing's silence on lesbian, gay, bisexual and transgender issues: The need for emancipatory efforts. *Advances in Nursing Science, 33*(3), 206–218.

Frith, L., Jacoby, A., & Gabbay, M. (2011). Ethical boundary work in the infertility clinic. *Sociology of Health and Illness, 33*(4), 570–585.

Gendzel, G. (2011). What the progressives had in common. *The Journal of the Gilded Age and Progressive Era, 10*(3), 331–339.

Global Alliance for Women's Health. (2007). Report on GAWH involvement at the UN. Summary prepared by A. DeKalb. Retrieved from http://www.gawh.org/strategy/un_more.php5

Hembree, W., Cohen-Kettenis, P., Delemarre-van de Waal, H., Gooren, L., Meyer, W., Spack, N., . . . Montori, V. (2009). Endocrine treatment of transsexual persons: An endocrine society clinical practice guideline. *Journal of Clinical Endocrinology & Metabolism, 94*(9), 3132–3154.

Hershberger, P. E., Gallo, A. M., Kavanaugh, K., Olshansky, E., Schwartz, A., & Tur-Kaspa, I. (2012). The decision-making process of genetically at-risk couples considering preimplantation genetic diagnosis: Initial findings from a grounded theory study. *Social Science & Medicine, 74*, 1536–1543.

Jacobs, M. (2009). *White mother to a dark race: Settler colonialism, maternalism, and the removal of indigenous children in the American west and Australia, 1880-1940.* Lincoln, NE: University of Nebraska Press.

Kenagy, P. (2005). Transgender health: Findings from two needs assessments studies in Philadelphia. *Health and Social Work, 30*(1), 19–26.

Lippman, A. (2001). Worrying—and worrying—about the geneticization of reproduction and health. In W. Teays & L. Purdy (Eds.), *Bioethics, justice and healthcare* (pp. 635–643). Belmont, CA: Wadsworth/Thomson Learning.

Lombardo, P. (2011). *A century of eugenics in America: From the Indiana experiment to the human genome era.* Bloomington, IL: University of Indiana Press.

Lynn, R. (2001). *Eugenics: A reassessment.* Westport, CT: Praeger.

Marcellus, L. (2004). Feminist ethics must inform practice: Interventions with perinatal substance users. *Health Care for Women International, 25,* 730–742.

Meyers, D. (2001). The rush to motherhood: Pronatalist discourse and women's autonomy. *Signs, 26*(3), 735–773.

Northwest Association for Biomedical Research. (2011). BRAC1: Is it dominant or recessive? Retrieved from http://www.nwabr.org/sites/default/files/learn/bioinformatics/BRCA1_Dominant_or_Recessive.pdf

Patterson, S. (2009). (Re)Constructing women's resistance to woman abuse: Resources, strategy choice and implications of and for public policy in Canada. *Critical Social Policy, 29*(1), 121–145.

Peddie, V. L., van Teijlingen, E., & Bhattacharya, S. (2005). A qualitative study of women's decision-making at the end of IVF treatment. *Human Reproduction, 20*(7), 1944–1951.

Quist, N. (2008). Clinical ethics and domestic violence: An introduction. *The Journal of Clinical Ethics, 19*(4), 316–320.

Raine, S. (2012). Federal sterilization policy: Unintended consequences. *American Medical Association Journal of Ethics, 14*(2), 152–157.

Sabella, D. (2011). The role of the nurse in combating human trafficking. *American Journal of Nursing, 111*(2), 28–39.

Sandelowski, M. (1991). Compelled to try: The never-enough quality of conceptive technology. *Medical Anthropology Quarterly, 5*(1), 29–47.

Sanger, M. (1920). *Woman and the new race* (p. 94). New York, NY: Bretanos.

Schumacher, A. E. (2007). Mandatory report of intimate partner violence: An ethical dilemma for nurses. The John M. Rendes Ethics Essay Competition. Retrieved from http://www.honors.umaine.edu/files/2009/07/2007-schumacher.pdf

Sherwin, S. (1992). *No longer patient: Feminist ethics and healthcare.* Philadelphia, PA: Temple University Press.

Spinks, V., Andrews, J., & Boyle, J. (2000). Providing health care for lesbian clients. *Journal of Transcultural Nursing, 11*(2), 137–143.

Tower, M., Rowe, J., & Wallis, M. (2011). Normalizing policies of inaction: The case of healthcare in Australia for women affected by domestic violence. *Health Care for Women International, 32*(9), 855–868.

United Nations Office on Drugs and Crime. (2003). United Nations convention against transnational organized crime and the protocols thereto. Retrieved from http://www.unodc.org/unodc/en/treaties/CTOC/index.html

United Nations Population Fund. (2005). Ending violence against women (Resources). Retrieved from http://www.unfpa.org/endingviolence/html/index.html

U.S. Preventive Services Task Force. (2013). Screening for family and intimate partner violence: Recommendation statement. Retrieved from http://www.uspreventiveservices-taskforce.org/3rduspstf/famviolence/famviolrs.htm

Warshaw, C. (1998). Domestic violence: Changing theory, changing practice. In J. F. Monagle & D. C. Thomasma (Eds.), *Health care ethics: Critical issues for the 21st century* (pp. 128–137). Gaithersburg, MD: Aspen.

World Health Organization. (2009). The International Committee for Monitoring Assisted Reproductive Technology (ICMART) and the World Health Organization (WHO) Revised Glossary on ART Terminology. Retrieved from http://www.who.int/reproductivehealth/publications/infertility/art_terminology.pdf

Yee, L., & Simon, M. (2011). Perceptions of coercion, discrimination and other negative experiences in postpartum contraception counseling for low-income minority women. *Journal of Health Care for the Poor and Underserved, 22*(4), 1387–1400.

CHAPTER 10

Nursing Ethics and Advanced Practice: Adult-Gerontologic Health

Jane Flanagan

The longest journey of any person is the journey inward.
—DAG HAMMARSKJÖLD, 1961

Introduction

The role of the advanced practice nurse (APN) in many countries has developed out of a need to improve healthcare system efficiencies such as decreased length of stay, more rapid turnover time related to procedures, and economic interests. An example of an economic driver is the move in the United Kingdom and elsewhere to substitute nurses for residents in institutions as a result of mandated in-hospital resident work hour reductions. This has led to a weakening of the nursing perspective as the development of APN roles and objectives becomes subject to the influence of medical models or healthcare administrators. These factors have all contributed to confusion about APN roles and their objectives, which in turn has implications for the population that nursing serves related to nursing's practice goals. Complicating this problem further is the proliferation of specialties within the broader APN role. This chapter discusses ethics within the context of the adult-gerontology APN role, a newly designated credential in the United States. The role is discussed in the context of the overarching purposes of advanced nursing practice and exemplifies the foundational need to maintain a nursing perspective that is in the interests of individuals and society. Later in the chapter, cases will be presented that highlight both the ambiguity of and the potential for the role when it is guided by a nursing framework.

Although the role of the APN has been around since the 1960s in the United States and internationally for nearly 30 years, there is a general lack of understanding globally about what it means to be an APN (Duffield, Gardner, Chang, & Caitling-Paull, 2009). Misunderstandings abound among nurses, but more concerning is the fact that this lack of clarity about the role extends to and includes other healthcare providers and the public. In the United States, the American Nurses Association's (ANA's) *Social Policy Statement* outlines nurses' contract (2010). This contract is a public agreement that nurses will provide care that is autonomous, accountable, trustworthy, and grounded in nursing disciplinary knowledge. The International Council of Nurses (ICN, 2012), with over 130 member countries, also has a code of ethics that endorses a specific nursing perspective on health care as well as areas of disciplinary overlap and maintains that nurses are charged with understanding the boundaries.

In the United States, nursing is consistently rated as the most trusted profession (Gallup Poll, 2013), suggesting that the public trusts nurses to provide care that is in line with the ideas of the ANA's *Social Policy Statement*. In other countries such as the United Kingdom, trust in nurses is in danger of eroding as a result of media reports of nursing becoming an "uncaring" profession (Cummings, 2012).

Much of the confusion about what it means to be an APN is rooted in the reason why the role was developed, which varies globally. In certain countries such as the United States, United Kingdom, and Canada, some APN roles such as the clinical nurse specialist (CNS) were developed to provide expert care and consultation for a subset of patients, to improve outcomes, and to decrease complications related to illness (Kring, 2008).

In other cases, APNs such as nurse practitioners (NPs), certified nurse anesthetists (CNAs), and certified nurse midwives (CNMs) were developed to provide care in response to physician shortages (Bryant-Lukosius, Dicenso, Browne, & Pinelli, 2004). Consensus about why APN roles are needed, how APNs should be educated, and what the grounding focus, roles, and responsibilities are is not discernible in the literature. The various roles seem to have developed somewhat randomly and as a reaction to existing problems such as cost containment or physician shortages. In short, development of APN roles did not always occur in anticipation of a need for advanced "nursing" care.

Internationally, there is no consensus over the varying APN roles and to what extent they are "nursing" roles grounded in nursing's goals, perspectives, and responsibilities. For example, in many countries, midwifery is not considered a nursing role and in countries other than the United States, the CNA is a registered nurse with advanced training and education

(International Federation of Nurse Anesthetists, 2012), but CNAs are not included in the APN category. Countries such as the United Kingdom include as APNs both the CNS and nurse consultant (NC). The NC role, as developed in the United Kingdom, was envisioned as one of high-level leadership to improve nursing services in a variety of settings and specialties (Redfern, 2006). It does not translate well internationally, is not akin to the CNS role, and perhaps adds further ambiguity and confusion about APN roles, whether there is a unifying core to these roles such that their linkages to the nursing profession are clear and goals are shared with the broader discipline. Even in the United States, where some consensus has recently been reached about four APN roles—the CNM, CNA, NP, and CNS (APRN Consensus Work Group & National Council of State Board of Nurses Advisory Committee, 2008)—and commonalities among them, the scope of practice for each is regulated at the state level and therefore the actualization of any given role can vary widely from state to state (Institute of Medicine [IOM], 2010). Complicating the situation in the United States was the American Association of Colleges of Nursing's (AACN, 2004) assertion that the educational preparation of advanced practice nursing should be at the doctoral level. The AACN originally set a target date of 2015 for realization of this goal. However, there have also been calls to reexamine the mandate because of a lack of focus on the nursing discipline within and/or across programs (Fulton & Lyon, 2005; Meleis & Dracup, 2005).

Reaching Consensus Internationally: What It Means to Be an APN

Despite confusion about what it means to be an APN, several recent initiatives have provided clarity about the roles and population foci of APNs. This is particularly true for the NP role, the most clearly defined role worldwide. In 2000, the ICN created its International Nurse Practitioner/Advanced Practice Nursing Network in order to reach consensus globally on the roles, responsibilities, and education of APNs/NPs. The ICN determined that education should be at an advanced level and recommends a master's degree. Further, the ICN recognizes that the APN/NP is a registered nurse with advanced knowledge and expertise whose credentialing is shaped by the context/country in which he or she practices. The ICN recommends that APNs/NPs possess certain characteristics. These characteristics include the ability to be a first point of contact for patients, carry their own caseload, have advanced clinical competencies, provide consultative services, and perform advanced health assessment and diagnostic reasoning skills. Last, although the regulation may vary from country to country, in general the APN/NP role is supported by the following:

- The right to diagnose
- Authority to prescribe medication
- Authority to prescribe treatment
- Authority to refer clients to other professionals
- Authority to admit patients to hospital
- Legislation that confers and protects the NP and APN titles
- Legislation or some other form of regulatory mechanism specific to APNs
- Official recognition of titles for nurses working in advanced practice roles (ICN, n.d.).

In the United States, the APRN Consensus Work Group and National Council of State Board of Nurses Advisory Committee's report (2008) reached consensus on the roles of APNs and six population foci. CNAs, CNSs, NPs, and CNMs focus on one or more of the following: (1) family/ individual across the lifespan, (2) adult-gerontology, (3) neonatal, (4) pediatrics, (5) women's health/gender related, or (6) psychiatric mental health. In addition to a basic minimum of practice hours and other courses pertinent to the specialty or role, there are three essential courses that all APNs must complete. These are in pathophysiology, pharmacology, and advanced assessment. The pediatric or adult NP or CNS is prepared in either the acute care or primary care role. It is important to note that the scope of practice is not defined by the practice setting, but rather is based on patient care needs. This consensus model also provides clarity on APN specialty practices and certifications. Specialty certifications are awarded as a result of gaining supervised practice as an NP or CNS in a defined area after completion of a nursing master's degree and may or may not include additional coursework.

Post-master's specialties include holistic care, orthopedics, oncology, palliative care, and others. These post-master's specialties are ethically concerning because they add further to the ambiguity of what it means to be an APN with specialized knowledge. For example, for an APN in oncology or orthopedics, is their advanced knowledge rooted in advanced nursing knowledge or substitutive medical care? Further, if all nurses are grounded in a science concerned with caring for patients from a holistic perspective, which includes but is not limited to knowing the persons and journeying with them across the lifespan from birth through the dying experiences, why is there a need for holistic and/or palliative care post-master's specialties? The answer is likely grounded in the fact that nurses "lose their way," or worse, were never grounded in this nursing knowledge initially and therefore seek out this "additional" knowledge. Yet in some cases it is not nursing knowledge that is gained, and in other cases the specialty knowledge should have been core to both an initial and advanced practice nursing curriculum. Some argue that the APN education within nursing framework certifications that are considered post-master's specialties would in fact be a part of the knowledge gained within a basic nursing education and further explored in an APN curriculum. If what distinguishes nurses from other providers is their holistic perspective about health and the focus on caring for people through a trajectory of wellness through illness, a post-master's specialty in holistic nursing and/or palliative care should in fact be redundant of knowledge gained as part of an entry-level and certainly an advanced-level academic program, and yet, sadly the holistic and palliative perspectives are often set aside in order to focus on non-nursing skills and knowledge.

The initiatives of ICN and the APRN Consensus Work Group do provide some clarity about the APN role, but there are also concerns related to these position documents. That is, there is an assumption that there is clear consensus (1) on what it means to be a nurse who is gaining advanced skills and knowledge to provide improved and advanced nursing care, and (2) that these graduate-level programs build upon nursing knowledge and advance the knowledge related to the disciplinary perspective of nursing. While it is clear why nurses take pathophysiology, pharmacology, and advanced assessment courses, the relevance for achieving nursing goals of content in other required coursework is less obvious, often vague, and housed under the ambiguous category of "role preparation" courses.

Research indicates that the care provided by NPs, for example, is accessible, efficacious, and less costly, and that it is "as good as" the care provided by medical providers (Hoffman, Tasota, Zullo, Scharfenberg, & Donaue, 2005; Horrocks, Anderson, & Salisbury, 2002). The challenge, however, is for APNs is to provide care that fills gaps in healthcare services from the nursing perspective, which is complementary to but different from the focus of medicine. What is housed in U.S. curricula under the label "role preparation" can be quite variable across programs and schools. Preparation for advanced nursing roles should (an ethical imperative for the discipline) have some uniformity in and around what it means to have advanced nursing knowledge so that all nurses are practicing from the nursing perspective and striving to meet nursing goals. Curricula content, though, would vary to reflect practice environments, and a college or school of nursing's mission and philosophy.

The IOM, "an interdisciplinary nonprofit institution that works outside of government to provide unbiased and authoritative advice to decision makers and the public" about healthcare (2013), released a report entitled *The Future of Nursing: Leading Change, Advancing Health*. The report called for nurses to practice to the fullest extent of their education and to be equal collaborators with other healthcare providers in the delivery of patient care (IOM, 2010). Several nurse scholars have described the core of nursing practice to be embedded in the nurse–patient relationship, and in summary they suggest that the role of the nurse is involved in mutually engaging in dialogue with the patient to explore meaning, provide caring, offer a healing presence, and facilitate human betterment (Cowling, Smith, & Watson, 2008; Newman, Smith, Pharris, & Jones, 2008; Willis, Grace, & Roy, 2008). For the reasons given earlier and as evidenced in the credentialing and associated literature, the nursing part of this APN role is in danger of being lost in the push to advance healthcare agendas. Neither the ICN nor the APN Consensus Work Group literature explicitly identifies the disciplinary knowledge that guides the role development of the APN. This literature reads like a list of new skills to be obtained rather than skills needed to actualize nursing knowledge in practice. APNs should provide care that is uniquely different from, complementary to, and in collaboration with other healthcare providers. If APNs are not educated in this way, they are not able to distinguish themselves from others and hence they do not practice to their fullest extent possible, but rather practice advanced skills devoid of the core values embedded in nursing knowledge. Although recent documents provide clarity about what advanced practice roles and population foci are, what is less clear is the *nursing* foundations underlying the roles and foci.

The Role of the Adult-Gerontology Advanced Practice Registered Nurse

In line with the U.S. move to denote the advanced practice nurse as an APRN, this section relies on that acronym in describing the new U.S. adult-gerontology role. In the United States, several APRN roles are evolving as a result of shifting societal needs. The adult-gerontology NP and CNS roles have evolved from two individual specialties: adult *and* gerontology advanced practice nursing. The adult-gerontology APRN role has been developed in response to two facts: (1) that globally more people at younger ages are living with multiple chronic illnesses, and (2) people in general are living longer. The primary and long-term care these vulnerable patients need, both in times of wellness and illness, can be fully met by adult-gerontology APRNs, but if that care lacks a nursing perspective, it will fall short of meeting the demands of individuals or families in terms of addressing preventative and education needs and providing holistic, continuous, and transitional care.

Most ethical problems for adult-gerontology APRNs do not revolve around knowing what constitutes good nursing care, but rather an inability to deliver that care in the face of many obstacles. This includes APRNs not being able to (1) articulate what it is about their practice that makes it unique, (2) practice to the fullest extent that they are educated, and (3) be considered an equal voice or collaborator in the process of planning for or providing care.

Adult-gerontology APRNs care for adults in both the acute care setting and in primary care settings where the overall issue of good care is pressing and includes decision making around all aspects of health care. There are many ethical issues of concern for adult-gerontology APRNs across settings. A primary concern is whether APRNs are able to articulate what it is that is different and unique about their practice. Through their words and actions, APRNs must be able to distinguish their practice from that of other health-care providers in the interests of their populations. APRNs should be able to describe what is advanced about the nursing care they deliver and why it is needed. This distinction should not merely be about technical aspects that are incidental to the provision of holistic care. For example, it is not enough to state that an NP "can perform physicals and write prescriptions just like a doctor." The knowledge needed to appropriately perform these skills again is an adjunct to the need and ability to attend to the whole person as a contextual being. The distinctive role of nursing means that an adult-gerontology APRN focuses on the integration of advanced nursing knowledge; additional skills such as being able to complete a thorough patient history and physical exam are facilitative of the holistic care.

Another concern is related to the hierarchical structure that exists within health care. This still predominant model is a disease-oriented one. Due to this orientation, the medical doctor or physician is viewed as "in-charge" and directs all others in defining what is "good" care and how it should be delivered. Within this structure, APRNs struggle to be seen as "as good as" a medical doctor instead of recognizing that they have their own disciplinary perspective that is not the same as, but rather complementary to, the medical model. Viewed from the medical or disease-oriented perspective, the issues APRNs face are seen as somehow different from ones faced by point-of-care or bedside nurses. Additionally, according to the medical perspective, APRNs have a greater depth and understanding of the discipline than do other nurses that they then bring to their practice, but it is questionable if this is actually the case.

Another ethical concern results from the specialization of APRNs. Northrup and Purkis (2001) suggest that it is the compartmentalization of specialties such as adult-gerontology, family, pediatric, and psychiatric mental health, and the post-master's specialties that cause nurses to lose sight of the philosophical and theoretical underpinnings of nursing. This results in that which is essentially *nursing* being forsaken by many APRNs in the practice setting. For example, within the specialty of adult-gerontologic health nursing, the institutions that employ APRNs are concerned with disease and disease management. From a nursing disciplinary perspective, this focus on disease, cure, and the reliance on efficiency models does not reflect the perspective of nursing. Indeed, it may even divert attention away from patients' needs for good nursing care using a holistic perspective. Further, the constraints of practicing within medical institutions include the invisibility of APRNs in terms of economic contributions to an institution. As providers who do not bill for services, the tendency is not to be able to practice to their fullest potential, and not to have an equal voice in structuring how care should be delivered. All these factors militate against the delivery of good patient care from the nursing perspective.

What all U.S. APRNs do have in common, however, is the fact that they all must take required core courses that provide them with greater contextual understanding of the nursing discipline than what they may have received in an undergraduate program; therefore, these courses may contribute to APRNs being advanced in the discipline. The key here is whether these courses (1) are treated as nursing courses and taught from the disciplinary perspective; (2) are regarded as perfunctory, in which case the courses may not shape nurses' thinking of how they practice as APRNs; or (3) are integrated throughout the curriculum so that they do provide the APRN with greater disciplinary perspective. If the preceding is true and the APRN student has required courses in *nursing* ethics, research, roles, and concepts that are later integrated into courses on adult health *nursing* theory, then it is possible that students are advanced in their thinking about *nursing care* of the adult population. Because nursing academics are also responsible for good care of persons, it is their moral responsibility to design curricula and provide education that result in good nurses who will practice from a disciplinary perspective. Upon graduation, it is then crucial for APRNs to find a role that allows them to practice in the way they were educated. Even more critical, however, is the need for the employer to value the perspective of the APRN.

Contemporary forces affecting the nursing profession in the United States—literature supports that there are similar influences in other countries—and consequently its ability to further its goals include (1) interdisciplinary research as a mandate from the National Institutes of Health, which provides the majority of funding for healthcare research; (2) issues around the initiation of a doctorate in nursing practice, which would require many additional courses in the curricula that are not nursing discipline specific (see discussion in Chapter 2); and (3) suggestions that transdisciplinary healthcare workers should be educated and could "fill in" for a variety of professionals.

All nurses, especially nurse educators and APRNs, face a challenge—and have the ethical responsibility—to maintain nursing as a distinct and important discipline with a unique approach to patient care (the idea of educational preparation affecting the practice of the APRN is discussed in more detail later in the chapter). With so many concurrent debates in health care directly affecting APRNs, it is understandable that the focus of the nursing discipline can become murky, and this has important ethical consequences for patients and potential patients. It is for precisely this reason that throughout these ongoing debates the imperative is for APRNs to maintain their nursing focus.

A basic understanding of the adult-gerontology APRN role and the current thinking around it internationally and nationally is important, but the focus of this chapter is on issues of advocacy, health disparities, and health promotion in relation to the adult-gerontology APRN role. In earlier chapters, Grace provides a foundation for describing professional responsibility, disciplinary knowledge, and fiduciary relationships and has noted that the APRNs who practice in an ethical way use disciplinary knowledge. Building on this foundation, this chapter explores the historical perspectives of the nursing discipline, nursing knowledge development, and other concepts that will provide background for the case studies that follow. As Grace has pointed out in the earlier sections of this text, it is imperative that APRNs understand how the ANA's (2001) and the ICN's (2012) codes of ethics serve to guide their unique role in caring for patients, families, and communities in the healthcare system. The adult-gerontology specialty in advanced practice encompasses all persons from adolescence through the lifespan per the AACN and the nursing-focused care directed toward them during periods of both health and illness. The level of nursing care addressed is relevant to all nurses but is specifically within the realm of the APRN—both NPs and CNSs who practice within this specialty.

The chapter uses both a reflective approach in that questions are posed throughout the chapter and a case-based exploration of ethical issues that confront APRNs in adult-gerontology nursing care. The reflective questions are intended to help the reader pause and deliberate the ideas and issues that are being reviewed. The cases are designed to stimulate discussion about how adult-gerontology APRNs in practice can maintain a nursing disciplinary perspective in their practice. Questions aim to provoke the reader to delineate the unique role of the adult-gerontology APRN from other healthcare workers. The cases address the topics of autonomy, health disparities, and health promotion. Questions raised can help NPs, CNSs, and other APNs begin to articulate their own individual position about what they value as an APRN, what the role means to them, and how they meet (or do not meet) the needs of the public they serve. These discussions do not purport to answer the questions raised but rather are meant to increase the self-awareness of APRNs in practice so that they can recognize those constraints and issues in the healthcare system that affect practice. Further, APRNs have responsibilities both to provide leadership and to influence needed changes within their environments of practice and the broader healthcare system.

MORE NOTES ON NURSING, THE DISCIPLINE

To provide a foundation for the following discussion about how adult-gerontology APRNs should draw on nursing disciplinary knowledge to guide their practice, some of the writings of nurse scholars who have grappled with the issues of what nursing is, what nurses do, and what knowledge is needed for practice are briefly highlighted. Nursing knowledge development—that is, knowledge needed for good nursing practice—occurred by borrowing ideas and theories from other disciplines such as anthropology, sociology, biology, and psychology to inform nursing's understanding of the human condition and human health needs and thus facilitate appropriate actions. From a historical perspective, Dickoff, James, and Wiedenbach

(1968) proposed that nursing theory, practice, and research are all related and interdependent.

Nursing theory, which is the body of knowledge aimed at directing and supporting practice, is developed in a reciprocal fashion in that it is born from practice, tested in research, and brought back to practice for further theory/research progression. For example, an NP is working with a patient to educate him about care around diabetes. The NP begins by providing some general information about diabetes and basic information about what diet changes the patient must make until a referral appointment with a nutritionist is available. The NP uses a theoretical framework that includes stages of change as suggested by Prochaska and DiClemente (1983), but as she attempts to educate the patient, the NP notes that the patient is disengaged and that often this is the case with some of her newly diagnosed diabetic patients. Recognizing that the stages of change theory are not helpful in these situations, she begins to test a new intervention in which she allows the patient to dialogue about his life and what is most important or significant to him, as suggested by Newman (2008). The NP recognizes that this makes the patient feel known by and connected to the nurse and that this simple strategy allows patients some control over a situation in which they have little. The NP further tests this "intervention" and, in doing so, continues to inform the original theory or may develop another theory altogether if the theory does not seem to be working for patients. By virtue of the fact that nursing is a practice discipline, theories are intended for practice situations, and the testing and revising of theories is a natural and reciprocal process.

Dickoff and colleagues (1968) identified four kinds of theories that were in existence in the literature during the 1960s: (1) factor isolating, (2) factor relating, (3) situation relating, and (4) situation producing. They suggest that situation-producing theory is the highest level of theory construction. Situation-producing theory allows for the production of outcomes of a desired type that are in line with the goals of nursing theory such as improved health. Situation-producing theory is the most desirable for nursing if theory is to affect practice, but the perspective is paternalistic in that the patient's goal(s) or desired outcome(s) are not known but presumed. There are three essential ingredients of situation-producing theory: "a) goal-content specified as aim for activity; b) prescription for activity to realize the goal; c) a survey list to serve as a supplement to present prescription and as preparation for activity toward the goal content" (Dickoff et al., 1968, p. 421). Clearly, this approach stems from a medical model that is both paternalistic and prescriptive. It assumes that the provider knows what is best for the individual and all that is necessary for a desired outcome is the correct remedy to achieve the goal.

This prescriptive model of thinking was and is important to nursing. APRNs are easily able to recount the things that they do for patients—listening to heart and lung sounds, taking health histories, teaching about disease and disease management, and planning for transitions to other care environments. No doubt these activities are important, and often this is exactly what the public expects from APRNs. But is it different from the approach of medicine? If this is true, how is it so?

It could be said that nurses utilize nursing theories to guide their practice. Historically, this is supported by the work of Johnson (1974), who suggested that nurses develop a theoretical body of knowledge from which practice emerges. She suggested that for nursing to develop as a profession, nurses must be able to engage in research activities that further develop and enhance the nursing discipline's theoretical body of knowledge. If a nurse engages in research about whether patients understand written hospital discharge information they receive and what impact adhering to the instructions has on the overall recovery experience, and a nursing theoretical framework guides the research, then this is nursing research that is intended to answer the questions of the discipline. Nursing conceptual models serve as a guide for this type of research.

Today it is often said and understood that there is a reciprocal relationship among nursing theory, research practice, and education—that is, the theory guides the research, but the results of the research may lead to the development of new concepts in the theory or practice changes. Donaldson and Crowley (1978) initially proposed this idea in their seminal work that synthesized the work of nursing science up to that date. Through their review of nursing research, they unveiled three themes that today continue to serve as the essence of nursing:

1. Concern with principles and laws that govern life processes, well-being, and optimal functioning of human beings—sick or well.
2. Concern with the patterning of human behavior in interaction with the environment in critical life situations.
3. Concern with the processes by which positive changes in health status are affected (Donaldson & Crowley, 1978, p. 113).

These themes suggest that nurses are involved in more than just the things that they do. They are also involved in being with their patients in a dialogue and assisting in processing the goals of the patient. The work of Peplau (1952), Rogers (1970), and others is reflected in this perspective.

As theories of nursing have developed over the last four decades, the essence and goals of nursing have essentially remained unchanged, and the notion of the relationship between nursing research, practice, and education as reciprocal remains supported today (Fawcett, 2005). Thus, it is clear that nurse scholars and philosophers have traditionally been engaged in developing and clarifying ideas about nursing practice that reveal nursing to be distinguishable from other healthcare practice professions by its holistic focus and interests, as well as its knowledge development endeavors. This is important in light of the recent move of others in health care to claim holistic care and narrative inquiry as their specialty. Nursing has much to add to the discourse on transdisciplinary and interdisciplinary health care but needs to continue to anchor its endeavors in its own unique knowledge base.

As mentioned earlier, nursing science, which involves the research aimed at nursing knowledge development, has emerged by integrating ideas from other sciences. Pearson and Vaughn (1996) state that there are three major "borrowed" theories relevant to nursing models: (1) systems, (2) developmental, and (3) symbolic interactionism. Nursing models that have emerged from these theories agree on several concepts of importance that together are uniquely nursing related. They include assumptions of health, the holistic view of people, the humanistic view of people, the autonomy of patients, and the need for a therapeutic relationship to develop between the nurse and those who are nursed. As a discipline, nursing remains focused on developing a specialized body of knowledge that uses these assumptions (Flanagan, 2009). Attention to these concepts helps to distinguish nursing from other professions, which in turn facilitates attention to the whole patient within the contexts of his or her life. The nursing perspective is integrative in this sense. It permits the meanings of a person or group's health status to be accounted for. A crucial idea drawn from these assumptions is that nurses seek to partner with patients. Within this relationship, the nurse openly explores possibilities with the patient and helps him or her make choices based on an understanding of personal life experiences and consequences of interventions related to that person's life. The focus of the discipline of nursing has been described as the partnership between the patient and nurse that seeks to understand the human health experience (Cowling et al., 2008; Newman et al., 2008; Willis et al., 2008).

Donaldson and Crowley suggested in 1978 that nursing theories have historically been directed at practical aims to be utilized in practice, prescriptive aims that seek to predict, and descriptive aims that seek to know. If this has been so for 40 years, why do nurses still struggle to explain to the public (and each other) what this means, how it looks in practice, and how it is philosophically different from others in health care? How to actualize this partnership with the patient in a way that the public recognizes and expects from nursing is a challenge that remains today.

Using an approach such as Newman's (2008), which suggests nurses should ask patients a broad question about significant people and events such as, "Tell me about the significant people and events in your life" while grounded in nursing, can be difficult for nurses to incorporate into practice. In developing a model of care in which nurses used Newman's methodological approach to "come to know" their patients, Flanagan (2009) reported the nurses often described that this question caught patients off guard because this was not something they expected a nurse to ask or viewed as the work of nursing. Additionally, the nurses described that they initially found it challenging to practice nursing in this way because they worried peers would think they were socializing, rather than working.

In another study that used Newman's (2008) framework, Flanagan (2010) found that while some patients paused and then readily begin to share, others asked, "Are you a psychiatrist?" Clearly, these patients were not familiar with the nursing theoretical link to practice that suggests that nurses partner with patients in a way that explores meaning and purpose, which seems to be in conflict with the ANA's (2010) *Social Policy Statement* that suggests nurses have a dynamic relationship with the public they serve. As a professional practice, nursing has a public it serves, and it is the actions nurses take that are the phenomena of concern, such as safe medication administration, provision of comfort, and alleviation of suffering. As a practice discipline, nursing is concerned with philosophical and theoretical knowledge, methodologies, and ethics. The discipline encompasses research, practice, and education. The process among the three is dynamic and reciprocal in that they inform each other, but all are ultimately concerned with facilitation of the goals of the discipline with regard to the good of individuals and society.

Donaldson and Crowley (1978) concluded that nursing as a discipline and profession are linked and influence each other, but the discipline of nursing must guide the practice rather than be defined by it. This raises the question of what that practice is—is it one that is task based and devalues relationship-centered care, or does it value the nurse–patient relationship in the process of delivering skilled, safe, and competent care?

Nursing—Is It So Unique?

In health care, professional practice disciplines have various styles of learning. In medicine, teaching/learning often occurs in groups during teaching rounds. The process is that the more experienced, "expert"-level physician asks the novice (who is not necessarily younger) a series of questions that logically flow with the intent to flush out all the extraneous data and come to a conclusion or diagnostic evaluation. When a label does not fit, a cure is not effective, other anomalies arise, or something crucial is not known, questions for research are generated. Many other disciplines in health care utilize this clinical decision-making model for teaching, learning, and generating new knowledge.

Nursing also uses this clinical decision-making model in caring for patients. Nursing, however, is unique among professional disciplines in that it also uses a self-reflective, intuitive model to examine patient care situations, ethics of good care, the nurse–patient dynamic, and gaps in nursing knowledge. This process allows both the individual nurse and the practice as a whole to question situations, raise other possible solutions to problems, advance ideas, generate new knowledge, and think in a way that encourages diversity of opinion. APRNs do not toss aside medical and empirical evidence in patient care situations (or while conducting research), such as using an antihypertensive to control blood pressure. However, they also utilize an intuitive, reflective process and concurrently apply it while questioning the potential that one medical treatment, such as a pill, is the answer to the entirety of a person's health. APRNs also consider the impact of a new diagnosis, the medical plan of action, the patient's story, and other life circumstances that contribute to the situation, as well as observe for aberrations from expected responses to therapeutic actions and partner with their patients to revise plans of action or develop new ones.

Nursing as a discipline is also unique in that both practicing nurses and scholars are able to exemplify through their actions care that is often at the same time and in the same situation derived from several paradigmatic models: problem solving, process oriented, and aesthetic knowing

(Roy, 2006). In the problem-solving approach, the nurse assesses the patient and discovers an issue, such as impaired mobility, and plans strategies to assist the patient. In the process approach for this same patient, the nurse recognizes that this person is unique and has a story to share not only about the overall change in physical status but the patient's life as a whole. The nurse provides time for the patient to share the story of his life. The aesthetic approach suggests the nurse both uses intuition to act on a feeling that something more is going on than may initially appear and faciliates ways for the patient to creatively express (for example, through poetry, art, or music) what the experience has been like. Differences in these perspectives are addressed in the next section, but no one paradigm can be relied upon to resolve or answer all patient care dilemmas or questions for nursing.

From a nursing point of view, people are unique and complex; thus, one type of solution, or a solution to one type of problem, will not fit all cases. For example, even if a treatment does work, this does not necessarily mean that a person's quality of life is improved. Thus, an even more important question for nurses is what defines quality of life for an individual. Many people may in fact benefit from a treatment, but it is just as likely that patients may choose not to take a treatment, or that a treatment may cause hardship or simply not work. It is these unique situations that are phenomena of concern for nursing.

Philosophically, nurses do not view people from a perspective that reduces them to parts and solitary functions only, but rather act from a holistic viewpoint. This is not to say that nurses cannot or will not treat the particulars or use the deductive process to inform their decisions, but rather it is not the only process used—it is part of what is necessary to get the whole picture. Nurses will, for example, provide a patient with information and educate him or her about how to use a medication that best evidence suggests will work for a particular problem. However, nurses will use the context of a patient's life in choosing the medicine that best fits the patient's lifestyle and needs. Further, this holistic perspective may cause the nurse to ask pertinent questions such as: "Can this person afford the medication once discharged?" "Will he or she be able to get to a pharmacy?" "Can the person see well enough to distinguish this medication from the one that looks like it but that is taken on a different schedule?" "Does this person even have a desire to treat the problem in a way that is recommended?"

Changes in Health Care and the APRN

Rapid changes have been occurring in health care over the past two decades that have greatly affected patient care delivery for all healthcare providers. A healthcare system emphasis on economic concerns has led to shortened time for all primary care visits with providers, early discharge from acute care settings after procedures or events, and less follow-up by nurses as patients transition to home care. As a result, more questions are raised for nursing to address: Do nurses in general, and APRNs in particular, really practice holistically? Are there really differences in the care delivered by nurse providers and other healthcare providers? Is care adequate to meet a patient's real needs in either case? Do nurses on all levels, more realistically, adapt to a system that collectively has silenced the voice and perspective of nursing? If this is so, are nurses practicing nursing or some modification of it? Have the lines between what is a nurse and what is another type of healthcare provider become blurred? If so, is there a need for nursing to exist as its own unique entity? The discipline's self-reflection and the reflection of individual practitioners and scholars allow nursing to question its current purpose, its knowledge development, and its future. Ultimately, this is necessary to continue to meet the needs of patients related to health and well-being.

Nursing Knowledge and Nursing Practice

Nursing Practice, Philosophical Perspectives, and Theory-Guided Practice

As mentioned previously, nursing is both a practice profession and a practice discipline (Northrup et al., 2004). Nursing knowledge development is derived from three different perspectives: problem solving, process oriented, and cosmic imperative (Roy, 2006). Although each perspective is unique, nurses in practice often use all three approaches with patients in an effort to come to know them as unique, complex beings. Knowing the patient as a contextual and relational individual has been identified as essential to nursing practice (Radwin, 1995). How nurses come to know their patients (through problem-solving, process-oriented, or cosmic-imperative approaches) can vary, but ideally this is always done within a nursing disciplinary perspective. The next section describes the various approaches to nursing knowledge development and knowing the patient from a nursing disciplinary perspective.

THE PROBLEM-SOLVING APPROACH

A very rudimentary explanation of the problem-solving approach to knowledge development is that problems exist that need to be solved and that scientific inquiry that includes research is aimed at doing so. For APRNs who see problem solving in this way, the approach to care of a patient is problem oriented. From a nursing perspective, a systematic approach using a functional health pattern (FHP) assessment, which is composed of 11 areas of concern, is reviewed with the patient to determine the presence or absence of problems (Gordon, 1994). NPs, though, often forgo the FHP and utilize a medical model to assess patients. This is a system model that focuses on body functions and disturbances. In either case, parts of a person are separated out and evaluated individually. The APRN, using either method, seeks to understand the person through knowing how each part of that person functions or does not function and what requires assistance or fixing. Once the problem is understood, a plan is formulated that is aimed at correcting the situation.

In describing the problem-solving approach and its relationship to nursing, Rodgers (2007) suggested that this does not mean that this attempt to "solve the problem" is as simplistic as it may initially seem (or as many nurses have been taught or think that they were taught to approach it). Rodgers countered that the values, philosophy, and various approaches of nursing cannot be ignored by a nurse using disciplinary knowledge and are therefore inherent in the problem-solving approach. An underlying assumption of the problem-solving approach is not exclusive of the disciplinary perspective, which is that people are whole beings with physical, emotional, spiritual, and social dimensions. Rodgers suggested that to come to know and understand a patient or a problem, a nurse must use multiple ways of knowing—for example, aesthetic, personal, and scientific.

This willingness to use not only the hard, objective data from a patient or personal experience but also subjective information and perception to formulate ideas about what is a problem and how to intervene and measure the outcome of interventions is unique to nursing knowledge development. Classifying and grouping problems into phenomena of concern is a goal of groups concerned with nursing language development such as NANDA-I. Rodgers (2007) suggested that this work is important in that it identifies nursing problems as specifically nursing related and delineates how nurses think to improve or stabilize a problem.

THE PROCESS-ORIENTED APPROACH

Knowledge as process in nursing involves the nurse engaging over time with the patient in an open, undirected dialogue about meaning and purpose. Within this nursing disciplinary perspective, it is accepted that people are irreducible in that they cannot be broken down into parts or disease entities such as a person with cancer. Another underlying assumption of this perspective is that definitions of health or disease are arbitrary, value laden, and culturally infused and that any perception of disease or ill health is inseparable from a person as a whole. The process-oriented approach to nursing knowledge development can be focused on the individual or, from a post-structural feminist perspective, on groups, particularly oppressed groups.

In the process approach to knowledge, nurses come to know patients within their experiences of health and illness. There are several approaches described in the nursing literature, but in each the nurse mutually dialogues with the person (or if the person is unable to communicate, his or her designee) in an undirected fashion. The approaches, generally qualitative in nature, also assume openness to the potential of what may be and the possibility of transformation. Some approaches to the nurse–patient relationship include narrative analysis, reflective nursing practice, and aesthetic approaches such as storytelling, art, and music (Jones, 2006).

COSMIC KNOWING

A third perspective on nursing knowledge development is Roy's cosmic imperative (2006). There are three characteristics of this perspective: unity, purposefulness, and promise. Based on principles from quantum physics, unity suggests that as humans, we are one with the universe and our being is a microcosm of the cosmos. That is, the particular—individual human beings—are made up of the same materials as the universe, so it is reasonable to conclude that there is unity or oneness with that universe. Purposefulness within this perspective implies that there is creative yet intentional and increasingly complex unfolding of the universe through which a higher power is revealed. Last, promise evokes the ideas of timelessness and expansiveness of the universe within the context of a convergence of one point, the omega point, in which human meaning is rooted. The underlying assumption of the cosmic imperative is that the principles of unity, purposefulness, and promise compel nurses to practice well.

Blurring of Lines in the APRN Role: The Good APRN

Each approach to knowledge development discussed previously has methods applicable for nursing research and theories applicable in nursing practice. For example, the FHP assessment is appropriate to use in the problem-solving style, and a narrative analysis such as Newman's (1994) is appropriate in the process approach. Often nurses utilize a combination of approaches to come to know their patients. But APRNs too often state that they do not have enough time to do this work. This begs the question of what type of nursing they are practicing. Earlier in this text, Grace identifies several components of good care, which include drawing on previous experiences, utilizing nursing knowledge including ethics, an ability to reflect and clarify, and personal characteristics.

As discussed earlier, there are several reasons that many practicing APRNs do not practice nursing from the disciplinary perspective espoused by the scholars. Because nurses enter the profession at different levels of educational preparation, many APRNs have never been acquainted with the philosophical and theoretical foundations of their discipline. Even when academic programs in nursing require courses or modules in nursing theory and nursing ethics, there are differences in the depth of commitment to these goals on the part of instructors. This can result in students not understanding the basis of their practice in nursing theory and nursing goals, and so many nurses have only a cursory grasp of nursing theory and do not understand its relevance to practice, research, or even their own education.

Nursing education on both the undergraduate and graduate levels is often focused on tasks and skill acquisition. Basic sciences predominate the initial curriculum, often followed by courses that are disease focused with emphasis on tasks and clinical reasoning with theory and research as additional courses separated from patient care situations. Early in the career process, nurses complete nursing assessments, develop plans of care, and determine the effectiveness of outcomes, but this is when things begin to blur. The AACN (1995) delineated a "doer" role—the nurse who does things for the patient—from the "insider" role—the nurse who knows the human health experience. The AACN task force suggested that nurses on all levels be accountable for both dimensions and acknowledged a need to balance "doing" with "being with." But this suggests a dualism that is concerning to many nurses who philosophically engage in an ethic of caring and being with patients in a mutual, intentional process. It suggests that the tasks are performed adeptly and proficiently, and that the standard of measuring this is based on doing the procedure correctly. To be considered competent, a nurse must be able to perform the tasks. This type of caring by doing permits an easily measured outcome—either the nurse can safely do the task or not.

Measuring a nurse's ability to care in the sense of "being with" includes compassion and intentionality, but measuring this is more nebulous, and by virtue of the fact that they chose to enter a "caring" profession, it is often assumed that nurses are able to be caring in this way. If conducted in a task-oriented way, care that does not consider the person in a holistic way is done without attention paid to "caring for and with" the patient (DeRaeve, 2002). This type of care may include carrying out tasks with great attention paid to the details of the task—such as changing a dressing and using good sterile technique—but with no attention paid to the person and what it may mean to her to have a wound. Care that is merely task oriented does not assess for or necessarily address the contextual contingencies of a patient's situation. Thus, a person may not be willing to follow what is suggested as a plan for health or well-being. Although the nurse's stated goal may be to assist and care for a person through a process of restoring wellness, main-taining health, actualizing the person's potential, or alleviating suffering, the process is limited and "tunes out" other ways to come to know and care for the patient.

As Christensen and Hewlett-Taylor (2006) suggested, such patient care is lacking in expertise. They pointed out that expertise does not equate with experience. An experienced nurse may be caught up in the ritual of the act of doing or performing a skill in a proficient way rather than being an expert nurse who mutually engages and interacts with a patient while in the process of completing a task. The expert nurse uses the theoretical knowledge that defines and facilitates expert nursing care and in the process attends to all of a patient's needs. That is, the nurse provides care that is both proficient and completed in such a way that includes intuitive knowledge. Do APRNs ever practice in a way that is proficient, yet lacking in care? If so, how would their performance appraisal differ from an APRN who took time to talk to his or her patient about the overall care experience? Would the work of these APRNs be valued equally by an administrator?

Too often the distinction between what makes a "good" APRN (depending on the definition of good) and what makes a proficient APRN is based not on nursing knowledge but on skills, ability to work with fast patient turnover rates, and modeling of physician language and assessment skills (Rashotte & Carnevale, 2004). For example, at NP conferences, the presentations are often given by physicians, and the topics are oriented to diagnosis and treatment of disease and to efficiency models. As noted earlier, although these are important skills and necessary for good holistic care, they are inadequate (necessary but not sufficient for good care). The question is who benefits from nurses functioning in this "mini doctor" capacity. How is the NP practice different from that of a physician? At these NP conferences, there is little to no attention paid to functional health patterns and certainly none to health in the human experience. But when an APRN functions from a pure medical model, as is often encouraged by employers, physicians, and other APRNs, the APRN is at risk of abandoning the professional responsibility entrusted to him or her—being a nurse first and foremost.

Both the education and the practice environment of the nurse influence a nurse's ability to practice good nursing. Nurses who understand the bases of their professional responsibilities in nursing are more able to resist becoming indoctrinated into some other discipline's practice model. As discussed earlier, not all nurses are educated in core courses that reflect the essence of the discipline, and as a result there is a tendency in practice to devalue that which is nursing. Educational preparation and the environment of the practice setting are, of course, not the only influences on good nursing care; personal knowing, an ability to be reflective, and professional accountability are some other factors that are equally important. As argued earlier in the text and in this chapter, APRNs are nurses and their practice should reflect that. A blurring of the lines of distinction among healthcare professions is dangerous to the development of nursing knowledge, the profession, and thereby the public that nursing serves.

A good APRN has a capacity for self-reflection, is able to reflect on practice, and is willing to raise questions about what is good nursing care (Christensen & Hewlett-Taylor, 2006; Hardingham, 2004; Tarlier, 2004). Benner, Tanner, and Chelsea (1996) maintain that the ability and willingness to reflect are what distinguish an expert-level nurse from peers. Reflection is a more complicated idea, though, than it may initially seem. Even a nurse who is able to reflect on a practice situation and envision what good practice requires may be confronted with situations that he or she has no idea how to process and where mentorship or other resources are not readily available. An APRN may sense that something is wrong, but raising either personal awareness or group awareness can come at great cost because it may be seen as challenging the status quo. In other situations, a nurse may not be mature enough as a person, in the sense of having life experiences that have challenged personal knowing, to recognize the ethical content of a particular situation.

That is, a variety of factors can obstruct good practice even when the APRN understands the holistic nature of nursing practice and possesses the knowledge, skills, and characteristics necessary for good care. In these situations, the nurse's accurate perception of the issue, ethical decision-making capacity, and/or motivation for action may all fall short. This problem is explored further in the later case studies. First, however, it is important to address autonomy in practice and bring clarity to the issue. This awareness and discussion may help to initiate improvements in practice at all levels, but especially in advanced roles. The next section highlights some of the problems for nursing in fulfilling professional goals.

Threats to Autonomy

In this section, autonomy is discussed on two levels: personal and professional. Personal autonomy and professional autonomy are in one sense two very different things, but in reality they are intrinsically linked. As described in Chapter 1, *autonomy* is a word that has many meanings. For the purpose of this discussion, *personal autonomy* is defined as an individual's right to self-determine his or her own actions. *Professional autonomy* is discussed in terms of nursing as a profession and focuses on the fiduciary relationship between nursing and the public.

Nursing: A Trusted Professional Discipline

Academically, nursing is a young discipline, but it is generally accepted that nursing is a professional and practice discipline that has a unique body of knowledge and perspective that shapes practice, research, and education (Northrup et al., 2004; O'Shea, 2001). Both the ANA's (2001) and ICN's (2012) codes of ethics for nurses suggest that as a professional discipline, nursing is both responsible and accountable to the society it serves. The ANA's (2010) *Social Policy Statement* suggests that the relationship between nursing and the public is intended to be dynamic and that there is dialogue between the public and nursing as an organization. Grace (1998) discussed the fact that because the profession is responsive to societal changes and needs, the goals and the good of the public are reflected in the formulation of the ANA's code of ethics, but the reality is that the public is only indirectly involved in this dialogue. Further, Neale (2001) suggests that without knowing and understanding the public, nurses are not directing care at patient-sensitive outcomes.

Although it has been argued that many in the public are unclear about what nurses do, in surveys nurses consistently rank highly as trusted professionals (DeRaeve, 2002; O'Shea, 2001). Practicing nurses may agree with the idea that nursing is a discipline unique from other healthcare disciplines and may take pride in and agree that, as a profession, nurses are trusted. They may, however, not be able to say what underlies this trust, or why it is even relevant to their everyday practice. What is worse is that many will more readily point to times of moral distress or times when they felt their voice was not heard than agree that they can be trusted to fulfill professional goals in the face of environmental barriers. Of course, the implication is that nurses should not be trusted because they do not have the knowledge or power to do what is needed to fulfill professional goals. A further implication is that nurses could be held accountable for professional promises if the code was readily accessible to the public. No doubt the inability of many nurses to articulate the perspective of the discipline is a result of varying educational preparation, the failure of some academic curricula, and current healthcare economics (O'Shea, 2001). Traditionally nurses have been for the most part employed by and therefore embedded in a system with a historical tradition that values nurses for the tasks that they do to support the functioning of that system rather than for the questions they raise or the perspective they contribute. Nurses are paid by this system and it is therefore at great personal risk that nurses counter it (Grace, 2001).

This reality is contrasted with the notion that nurses are trusted by the public to collaborate with peers and to be advocates of patients in a shared decision-making process that permits a patient's real needs to be uncovered and addressed. Because, however, what nurses really do is unknown to most consumers of health care, and because many nurses report moral distress resulting from conflicts of varying sorts, questions can be raised about the professional responsibility of the nurse and how the public is both served and informed by nursing (Corley, 2002; Corley, Minick, Elswick, & Jacobs, 2005; Jameton, 1984). This situation is more complex in light of advanced practice nursing, especially when CNSs and NPs are not educated about and/or do not value the particular disciplinary perspective of nursing. For this reason, many either do not understand what good nursing care is or find it difficult to practice. The result is that they practice in a blended capacity, that is, a medical model with a few undertones of nursing. Consequently, the public often suffers from nurses who do not understand what nursing is. A core value of good nursing practice is the ability to be reflective, and as Grace points out earlier in this text, this process allows nurses to consider ways that practice can be improved.

Therefore, this text and especially this chapter highlight questions that can and should be raised about APRNs' professional responsibilities and the nature, scope, and limits of APRNs' capacity as a group to advocate for patients within the current healthcare system or effectively work at the societal level to change inadequacies in the system. For example, patients who undergo procedures are increasingly rushed through a given institutional system and sent home inadequately prepared to care for themselves during their recovery and without transitional homecare.

Further complicating this picture is the fact that many procedures could be avoided altogether if the appropriate preventive nursing care were incorporated into the care delivery model. Additionally, perhaps there would be a decrease in complications from procedures or recidivism if nurses were part of a transition model caring for patients at home. If nurses are really to serve as trusted advocates for the public, they must understand their own disciplinary perspective so that the voices of nursing and those who are served by nursing are heard.

Tarlier (2004) suggested that respect, trust, and mutuality are key elements of the process needed for nurses to form responsive relationships with their patients. She describes trust as being founded on personal morals and relates it to the ability of the nurse to be competent, skilled, and qualified. Prerequisites to trust are sincerity, genuineness, and acceptance. Implicit in this is a two-way dynamic of nurses being genuine, competent, and caring and patients trusting in nurses enough that they feel free to be open, honest, and trusting. This two-way dynamic is essential because patients spend a great deal of time with nurses while hospitalized and while in vulnerable situations (Grace, 2004). DeRaeve (2002) suggested that patients do not automatically place blind trust in individual nurses or in nursing actions. That is, they do not rely on nurses to do certain things such as advocate for them, primarily because they do not know what it is that nurses do and assume the role is limited to completing a series of tasks. Intentional individual inter-actions on the part of nurses with their patients are critical for therapeutic relationships to emerge. Implicit in this dynamic, though, is whether or not nurses can or will always strive to develop such therapeutic relationships. If a nurse is too busy to form such a relationship, patient care may suffer. It may suffer on two counts, one because important information needed to help a patient is not forthcoming, and two because a patient is in a susceptible posi-tion where he or she may be unable to address the feeling of being neglected because of worry about potential consequences. Further, if a nurse does not value being genuine, caring, and competent, a patient may be known and cared for in a way that is not consistent with the values of what it means to be a nurse. Patients, however, do place much trust in nurses as a group, and as a result of the ANA's *Social Policy Statement* (2010) and this trust, it is important that nurses both inform and enlist the public in the dialogue around what constitutes good nursing care and ways this can be achieved.

Autonomy

PROFESSIONAL AUTONOMY

Several years ago, *The New York Times* featured a piece entitled "Being a Patient: In the Hospital, a Degrading Shift from Person to Patient" (Carey, 2005) about several patients and their hospital experiences. Overall, the patients described their experiences as "degrading." Hopeful that these patients described an experience in which nurses would be viewed differently from other providers, it quickly became apparent that nurses were actually a part of the problem. Sadly, the report resonated with personal research (Flanagan, 2005, 2006, 2009; Flanagan & Jones, 2009) and experiences of family and friends, indicating that nursing action is not always caring.

The article suggested that nurses do not know their patients very well. In the article, one patient described having no idea who her nurses were; she did not know any of their names. Another patient described unhooking the intravenous line, getting dressed, and going across the street to have lunch—all without her nurse even knowing or realizing that she was missing. This patient wanted to feel more human, but the mere fact that she could carry out these activities unnoticed, be absent for so long, and not be missed is alarming, and nurses were complicit in this problem. This is a glimpse of the stark reality of certain contemporary healthcare situations. Patients are often left feeling lonely and abandoned in the process of being "cared for" in today's industrialized healthcare system. This problem is not isolated to the U.S. setting. The U.K. media has recently criticized nursing for being "uncaring" or losing its mandate to care (Odone, 2011; Weeks, 2012). The reasons are many and complex, but this is all the more reason for the profession via its membership to pay attention. Lack of caring or intention to engage with patients may impact patients at any point throughout their lifespans of care—from seeing a primary provider to episodic care including recovery. Nurses are often meshed into the system with all of its problems. In these situations, when the nursing care provided lacks a nursing disciplinary perspective grounded in knowing a person, caring, holism, and trust, nurses are viewed as part of the problem along with others in the eyes of patients.

Thus, although patients spend more time with nurses than they do with any other healthcare provider, it is questionable whether this time is spent coming to know the patient in a way suggested by those who discuss the focus of the discipline (Cowling et al., 2008; Newman et al., 2008; Willis et al., 2008). Rather, this time is often spent filling out required paperwork, which can make nurses feel disjointed from the disciplinary perspective of what it means to be a nurse. Further, it is not clear if nurses are prepared educationally and/or emotionally to actually care for patients on the level suggested by theorists and other scholars of the discipline.

PATIENT AUTONOMY

These questions of professional autonomy—the ability of the profession to fulfill its goals—affect how patients perceive or receive care. Intentional interactions with patients that ensure that they receive information tailored to their needs are needed to respect their autonomy (rights to self-determination about what care they will accept). In Chapters 1–3, several questions of informed consent were discussed in some detail. Contemporarily, many patients may not have or may lose decision-making capacity. Thus the question of how to ensure that they receive the care they would have wanted arises.

In the United States, the right to accept or refuse care receives legislative support from the Patient Self-Determination Act of 1991 (PSDA), as discussed in Chapters 3 and 13. Although not all countries have legislation that is supportive of patients' rights to accept or refuse treatment, this is increasingly understood to be a basic human right. Personal autonomy suggests that a patient has the ability to process the information provided and the freedom to make choices (Grace & McLaughlin, 2005). According to Faden and Beauchamp (2003), for consent to be considered voluntary three conditions must be satisfied: (1) the patient must have a considerable understanding of the procedure, (2) the patient must experience substantial absence of control by others, and (3) the patient must provide intentional authorization that allows the professional to carry out the intervention. The APRN must come to know the patient from a nursing disciplinary perspective before understanding patient readiness to make informed decisions about health care and what is required for that readiness. Moreover, APRNs in primary care settings are in an ideal situation to help patients to think through the issue of advanced care planning as a lifespan process, as discussed in other chapters.

Another article in *The New York Times*, entitled "Awash in Information, Patients Face a Lonely, Uncertain Road" (Hoffman, 2005), suggests that patients today are so inundated with medical information and choices that they are in fact in some ways less informed (and therefore less autonomous) than patients were a generation ago. In fact, some ethicists have called this "abandoning" patients to their autonomy (Loewy, 1989, 2005; Smith, 1996). Hoffman (2005) interviewed patients and physicians (the premise here is that APRNs often practice within the medical model, so they could also be included). The article described the many sources of medical information, which in the end overwhelm people who attempt to make an informed decision. The Internet, radio, television, newspapers, and healthcare providers bombard patients with many options, but with few conclusions or decisions. Often, "informed" patients will come to a healthcare provider asking for the tests they heard about via the media. Hoffman described healthcare providers who feel they should provide patients with a "maddening litany of medical correctness." In other words, they feel they must provide all the choices but avoid suggesting a preferred treatment in the name of autonomy. Additionally, Hoffman described that because of time constraints healthcare providers do not "know" their patients and therefore practice defensive medicine and resort to increased testing, which requires further interpretation or medical language that is incomprehensible to most laypeople.

Patients too often are previously unknown to their healthcare providers, have no one coordinating their care, are left to gather information where they can, must arrange for their own consultations, or are left to their own devices in interpreting medical jargon. Thus, they may well make decisions about their care that may not be the best choice for them.

The purpose of emphasizing the importance of autonomy as patient rights to self-determination is because in the past medical paternalism denied patients any involvement in deciding what was best for their individual and particular needs. However, today the pendulum may have swung too far in the opposite direction. Although in general people should be considered capable of self-determination, if they meet the criteria for being able to process information, to exercise their right to self-determination, they must possess the appropriate information, couched in understandable language and tailored to their particular needs. This all too often does not happen. As said by one patient Hoffman interviewed, at age 57 it was a little late for him to return to medical school so that he could understand the medical language being used in his care.

The following case studies exemplify the points made in this *New York Times* series of articles. They are based on real patient experiences (identifying characteristics have been changed to preserve anonymity).

CASE STUDY

Barbara is a new graduate of a master's program in nursing. Her prior nursing experiences were gained in various acute care settings. Most recently, she worked on a surgical unit that specialized in orthopedics, oncology, and general surgery. At the same time, she was undertaking part-time studies that culminated in a master's of science in nursing degree and prepared her for the role of adult-gerontology primary care NP. The university she attended had the reputation for graduating NPs who were "really strong" advanced clinical nurses.

She has just assumed her first NP position in a busy surgical oncology office. In this office, which is run by physician oncologists, visits are limited to 15 minutes per case. Most of her work involves seeing patients for any or all of the following purposes: consultation for surgical intervention for an oncology problem prior to surgery, testing, or procedures; postrecovery teaching; and obtaining presurgical consent. Barbara created templates for obtaining and documenting all of her patients' histories so that she could be more efficient. Her patient workup includes ascertaining the following: chief complaint, history of present illness, past medical history, a review of pertinent systems, and a focused physical exam.

Mr. S. is a patient who was referred to the clinic by his primary doctor for consultation. Mr. S. understands this visit to be related to the fact that he has an unresolved problem on his x-ray that could be either an infection or something more serious. He has arrived at the clinic with his wife and two sons. He is a 76-year-old white male.

From what she can tell from her schedule, Barbara notes that he has a new diagnosis of lung cancer that has yet to be staged. Barbara, who is already running behind schedule, assumes Mr. S. is aware of the reason for his visit and calls out his name, at which point Mr. S. and his entire family respond and ask if they can be present during the visit. Barbara is at first a little taken aback, but she does not want to appear cold, so she invites them all to come in and join the exam.

While obtaining the history of present illness and past medical history, she notices that Mr. S. is very quiet and that he defers all questions to his son, who is a dentist. The son answers each question intended for his father. The other son interrupts his brother periodically to clarify dates or share further details. Both Mr. S. and his wife sit quietly and offer very little information. From the information she has gathered, Barbara understands that Mr. S. is a nonsmoker and otherwise has been healthy. Because Mr. S. had a past chest x-ray and unresolved symptoms related to pneumonia, he was referred by his primary care doctor to this clinic for consultation. Again, she assumes that he has been notified by his primary provider that there is a question of lung cancer, and it is obvious to Barbara that the son who is a dentist is knowledgeable about the diagnosis. The history takes Barbara much longer than she planned, and Barbara becomes anxious that she is not moving along her patient schedule quickly enough. She fears being reprimanded by her program director for being too slow. Although she does so calmly and pleasantly, she asks the family to sit back in the waiting area, hoping that she can proceed more quickly while she examines Mr. S. alone. She assumes Mr. S. will provide her with quicker, more direct answers and that this will not only speed up the visit but will allow her to get to know him without interference.

Barbara begins the physical exam and asks Mr. S. some questions, but he barely speaks and appears to be angry. Again, taken aback by this, Barbara asks if he would like the family to rejoin them so that she can explain the available options, obtain an informed consent for a lung biopsy, and discuss various potential outcomes and options as well as other testing that will be required for staging the tumor. Mr. S. appears confused about all that Barbara has discussed, and he says that he would like to have his family present.

They rejoin Mr. S., but now they also appear angry and Barbara is not quite sure what she did wrong but proceeds to explain various options and procedures that are required for Mr. S. She then decides to check the scheduling program to determine options for dates for the biopsy. Because she must leave the room to do so, she decides that it would be good for the oncology nurse to come in and see Mr. S. and his family to provide teaching about the oncology center and services available.

The oncology nurse introduces herself to each member of the family. She then provides them with information about rides to chemotherapy, social work availability, nutrition services, support groups, and so on. The entire family is pleasant to the nurse, but they have no idea why she is providing them with this information. The family is still only aware that a chest x-ray and symptoms related to pneumonia were unresolved. The son who is the dentist suspects it is cancer, but no one has told them that in fact this is the actual or most likely diagnosis. No one has mentioned the word cancer. Having services described is perplexing, but they assume the nurse was sent into their room to stall for time.

Barbara has made and continues to make the assumption that the family is fully aware of the diagnosis, although she herself only mentioned that the biopsy would provide more information as to why this spot on his chest x-ray has not cleared. Barbara returns to the room and provides Mr. S. with a variety of options that are possible once the cancer has been confirmed and staged by biopsy, including "watchful waiting," surgery, chemotherapy and radiation, or a combination of these. She then mentions a variety of tests he can choose to undergo to get a more accurate diagnosis. These tests include a lung biopsy, and CAT and PET scans, along with further blood work; that is, if he chooses to have any at all.

Mr. S. is surprised to learn that he must undergo more tests and, potentially surgery, but more important, he does not understand why he has not been told exactly what is wrong and exactly which option is best for him. He looks to his sons for advice, and they suggest he get the biopsy. Barbara describes a procedure that will require anesthesia so that biopsies can be obtained and a litany of other tests to see if anything else is going on. Mr. S. admits later that he "never heard a word" Barbara said after agreeing to this, but he signed the informed consent anyway because he knew his sons thought he should. Mr. S. signs the consents and quietly the entire family walks away.

Questions to Consider

The following questions assist in reflecting on the case:

1. What information do you think the primary provider may have given Mr. S. or his family? How is continuity from the time of primary care through to home care after treatment ensured in the healthcare system?

2. What assumptions has Barbara made about Mr. S. and his family? Has Barbara made assumptions about the sons' knowledge and what information they may have shared with the parents? In the interest of time, have you ever felt rushed to just "get through the visit"? What has this been like for you? How has Barbara come to know her patient? Has she utilized disciplinary knowledge?

3. Do you believe all patients understand why they are referred to specialists? How does Mr. S.'s care reflect shared decision making? How do APRNs in practice ensure continuity of care? Do you think this type of efficient care is valued by Barbara's practice?

4. What would you do differently if you were Barbara? What nursing knowledge would guide your thinking? How does the APRN in this role distinguish what it is that she brings to this patient encounter that is different from other healthcare providers?

5. Have you ever heard patients describe this sort of experience? APRNs have a social mandate with the public they serve—how can APRNs assure the public that they are advocates for them through this sort of system of care?

6. What burden has been placed on the sons, especially the one who may have some sense of what is happening but who is certainly not an expert in this type of problem/care?

Case Discussion

In this particular case, the primary provider had told Mr. S. only that he was concerned about Mr. S.'s pneumonia not resolving and wanted this other doctor to look at the results. Mr. S. had no idea that there was any question of cancer and thought the referral was for an unresolved pneumonia, not cancer. His son, Michael (the dentist), knew they were being referred to an oncology practice and shared this information with his brother. Michael was still unclear if the diagnosis was definitive and assumed that if it was, the primary provider and/or oncologist would explain the diagnosis. Barbara assumed that Mr. S. and the entire family knew why he was there and that the primary provider had explained the situation. The note from the primary provider only mentioned that a referral was made and did not mention any discussion with the patient, but this is typical. Barbara and the primary provider never spoke to each other about the case.

Mr. S. now suspects more is going on than he was initially led to believe, but he has not yet been told he has cancer. Moving ahead in this case,

Mr. S. goes for all his testing, and the diagnosis is confirmed that this is an early stage lung tumor. It can be treated by surgery alone and no further treatment is necessary. Throughout follow-up visits, the healthcare team, including Barbara, now use the word cancer and tell Mr. S. how lucky he is to have such a treatable type of cancer. He goes through presurgery testing in a haze because he is so stunned with this new diagnosis, but he continues to hear he is "lucky." He is scheduled for surgery. The CNS on the unit he will go to is notified, and she promises to make sure things are coordinated for him. However, staffing is poor and the unit is going through a huge turnover period. The CNS is very busy orienting new staff to the unit and making sure the sickest of the patients are getting the best care possible.

Mr. S. is not nearly as sick as other patients on the unit, so his son and other family members make themselves more available to care for him throughout the hospitalization. They do this because other patients' family members on the unit tell them that this is the only way to ensure that Mr. S. is cared for during his stay. Mr. S.'s recovery is smooth, but he remains surprised at the diagnosis and is unable to integrate this new illness into his personhood. He describes feeling alone and abandoned while in the hospital. His sons have tried to explain the diagnosis and treatment, but their father remains too overwhelmed to comprehend this information. They are at a loss to explain it further. Mr. S. now considers himself a very sick person and worries constantly about a recurrence of cancer, which seems warranted given the repeat scans that are required over the next year. From a pure medical perspective of cure, Mr. S. is a success story, but from a nursing perspective of care, Mr. S.'s story is a dismal failure.

Further Questions to Consider

Here are some further reflective questions.

1. Has Mr. S. been abandoned by the medical system, medicine, or nursing? What is a goal of nursing care in the human health experience? Has this goal been met on any level for Mr. S. or his family?
2. The CNS agrees to coordinate things for Mr. S. but in reality is unable to because there are other more pressing issues on the unit. How do these issues factor into the reality of practice? How do they interfere with the CNS being able to function in the capacity of the role?
3. How has Mr. S.'s experience been reflective (or not) of "good" nursing care? What nursing intervention or strategy would you suggest for Mr. S. and his family to help them through the transitions that have occurred?

Models of Care

Another *New York Times* article, "Cancer Patients: Lost in a Maze of Uneven Care" (Grady, 2007), described patients as having to fend for themselves and "patch" information together. Patients interviewed for this feature described their experience as having no one healthcare professional who understood their whole story. Although each healthcare provider they saw knew his or her own role well, there was a lack of coordination of care. Further, patients were often left to their own devices to find what care they needed.

A nursing case management model of care used in Arizona at St. Mary's Hospital (Michaels, 1992) was set up so that primary nurses were assigned to patients at the time they chose a primary physician in the healthcare plan. Utilizing Newman's (1994) framework, the nurses came to know their patients and followed them over time. In doing so, they were responsible for and able to appropriately coordinate care and obtain necessary consultations for patients. This model of case management truly fosters the idea of nurses helping patients navigate the healthcare system, and it resulted in increased patient satisfaction and decreased healthcare expenditure. Flanagan (2009) described a model of care that includes nurses being mentored on how to incorporate nursing theory into practice. In addition, reflective rounds were incorporated into the practice setting to allow nurses to think not only about what did not go well in their patient/family interactions, but also what they could do to improve the individual situations and/or overall care environment.

Although there has not been further expansion of either of these models, if the series in *The New York Times* is any indication of public opinion, these types of models need to be more broadly implemented. There is hope that the IOM (2010) report on the future of nursing and the Affordable Care Act of 2010 in the United States, which will be fully implemented in 2014, will foster change that allows for such nursing models of care. At this time, however, insurance companies and funding sources such as the National Institute of Nursing Research do not support these types of bold initiatives, which include patients having a primary nurse along with a primary physician when they sign on for health insurance. Rather, the focus tends to be on an acute care medical model of treatment and prevention of disease—especially complex diseases. Although helping patients manage disease is certainly an interest of nursing, having most funding directed at this level of care is problematic for research and interventions directed at other areas of nursing concern. More rigorous studies describing patient experiences are needed to provide the impetus to change practice. To date, there is a lack of rigorous investigations aimed at care delivery that utilizes a model of care with APRNs practicing as equal partners and/or to their fullest extent. (See Chapter 4 to review other political strategies for implementing change.)

Health Promotion

Nurses as members of a profession are concerned with the core concepts underlying professional practice. These core concepts include health, holism, environment, person, and partnership. The question could be raised, however, whether nurses are unique in this perspective. A doctor who listens to a patient and encourages that person to share his or her concerns is also partnering with the patient to provide good care and is concerned with the whole person. Many physicians would argue that they are concerned with understanding the person and have a holistic approach to care. This raises anew the question of what is so unique about nursing. As Grace suggests in Chapter 1, different professions do share the same goals, but it is the knowledge of the discipline that shapes how the goal may be achieved or how outcomes related to the goal will be measured.

Nursing is unique from other disciplines in the way that nurses work together with patients to set goals and measure the outcomes related to those goals, yet not all nurses are aware of or choose to acknowledge that their disciplinary knowledge base is important and should underlie all patient care endeavors. The profession of nursing purports to have a unique focus on health, holism, and the nurse–patient relationship. If this is so, then nursing must develop and expand its own body of knowledge focused on health, holism, and the nurse–patient relationship to further enhance the quality of life of each individual and be true to the goals set forth by scholars of the discipline (Allan & Hall, 1988; Fawcett, 2005).

Health promotion has always been a key component of the NP role, and until the addition of acute care NP roles, it was a primary focus. CNSs tend also to focus on health and healing and use a holistic approach to care. CNSs have been instrumental in the development of screening, health promotion, and classes designed to educate and motivate people to improve their health. For example, they developed smoking cessation programs both for inpatients and outpatients. It is important to recognize that health promotion is not limited to prevention of problems such as diabetes, obesity, and smoking-related issues but rather is far more expansive. Health promotion also includes a nursing focus on the current situation a patient faces and partnering with a patient throughout the care journey—health in the human experience. Promoting health in this realm requires nurses to come to know their patients more fully than most standard nursing assessments or physical assessments allow. The next case study serves as an illustration.

CASE STUDY

J.S. is a 44-year-old female patient who presents to a preoperative clinic to be evaluated prior to surgery. J.S. is having surgery for a brain tumor. She has previously had radiation to shrink the tumor, and it is hoped that by having the surgery, much of the tumor can be removed, but it is doubtful that the surgeons will be able to remove it entirely. Her prognosis is uncertain.

In the clinic, she sees an anesthesiologist, who determines which anesthesia is most appropriate for the surgery and provides teaching according to the plan; a nurse, who performs a nursing assessment and provides pre- and postoperative teaching; and an NP, who provides the perfunctory presurgery history and physical. In this particular clinic, the CNS has successfully implemented a nursing model of care for patients who are seen by the nurse, although it is not integrated into the NPs' practice. The model includes interviewing patients using Newman's praxis methodology (1994). In this method, patients are asked to discuss the significant people and events in their life. In addition to being interviewed, patients are also offered therapeutic touch, meditation, and/or other relaxation techniques while they are in the clinic and throughout the hospitalization recovery process.

The first provider that J.S. sees is the anesthesiologist, who carefully reviews her previous history and discusses the anesthesia plan. J.S. finds talking with the anesthesiologist comforting. The anesthesiologist takes time to explain everything that will happen prior to and after surgery from the anesthesia perspective. Additionally, this anesthesiologist has gone through the spirituality fellowship at the hospital and has integrated this type of care into her practice. On ascertaining J.S.'s desire for this, she offers to pray with J.S., who agrees and is thankful for this opportunity. The anesthesiologist promises to follow up with J.S. on the day of surgery because coincidentally she will be scheduled for the neurology cases that day.

The next provider J.S. sees is the NP, Debbie, who appears quite harried. Debbie comes out to the waiting area to call J.S. and then asks her to have a seat in her office. Debbie then steps outside the office to complain to the other NPs about how busy she is and how distressed she is by the heavy schedule she has on this day. Debbie sticks her head back in the room and states that she will be right back because she needs to discuss the case with the anesthesiologist. Debbie leaves the room for 25 minutes, and during this time, J.S. hears other people calling her name for more testing, so she steps out to let them know that she is in Debbie's office. Debbie returns to her office and finds J.S. gone because the lab technician has decided to take her from Debbie's room to draw her blood. Debbie sees this and gets angry. She says to J.S., "I don't know if I can see you now. You might just have to wait until I am ready now."

J.S., not sure of what to say, asks if Debbie had a chance to talk to the anesthesiologist. At this point, J.S. is just trying to calm Debbie down because she sees that she is angry. Debbie responds, "No, I can't find her anywhere either. Today is just one awful day." Debbie then turns around and says, "Well, I'm off, I've got other things to do."

After her blood is drawn, J.S. goes back to the waiting area, but after waiting a long time, she wonders if she was supposed to just walk back to Debbie's office, so she goes to Debbie's office. Debbie is on the phone and says to J.S., "What, are you checking up on me now?" J.S. apologizes and returns to the waiting area. Eventually, Debbie takes her to her office and does a focused physical exam that takes about 10 minutes in total. Debbie barely speaks to her the entire time, and J.S. is feeling very vulnerable, so she says nothing either. Finally, Debbie says to J.S., "You are all set for surgery," and sends her back to the waiting area. At this point, J.S. is holding back tears.

Ideally no NP would act like this, but unfortunately this behavior is not uncommon. The reader might also question whether an anesthesiologist could be so "caring," but these cases are real as well.

Questions to Consider

The following questions are useful in understanding the case:

1. As a nurse, how would you say you care? Would this care be different from the care provided by the anesthesiologist?
2. Have you seen nurses act in the manner that Debbie did? What have you done when you have seen this behavior? If nothing, what has caused you not to deal with it? If you have confronted this, did it make a difference? Were you supported? By whom?

3. The way Debbie acted was certainly not "health promoting." Do you think that the average person would know what to do if he or she had a nurse who acted in this way? Is there in fact an effective way for a person to deal with this behavior? What impact do you think Debbie had on J.S.?

Effective Care

The next person to see J.S. is in fact the CNS, Ann. One of the technicians saw J.S. crying and thought Ann would be the best person to see her, given how upset she is. Ann calls J.S. into her office, which has soft lighting, plants, and a waterfall that makes soothing, musical noises. In addition, serene artwork adorns the walls. Immediately, J.S. senses something different, but she is still quite upset. Ann suggests that J.S. relax by taking some deep breaths, and J.S. does so. Ann begins to ask a few questions that are part of the standard nursing assessment: previous hospitalizations, medications, allergies, living situation, and pain and anxiety levels. Ann continues to address these perfunctory questions but instinctively knows that more in-depth questions need to be asked. She waits, though, until J.S. seems more relaxed and then says, "Tell me about you. Who are the significant people in your life? What are the significant events?"

J.S. begins with her childhood and describes it as an overall happy one until her mother died when she was 14 years of age. Her mother died of ovarian cancer, and J.S., who was the oldest daughter and child, began to care for her younger siblings. While her mother was ill, her father worked long hours, so J.S. essentially was the primary caregiver for her mother through her dying experience. J.S. lived at home during college so that she could continue to care for her siblings. She then described moving away from that life, getting married, and loving the first few years of marriage because "it was the first time I could just be free." She had children, an experience she thoroughly enjoyed, but gradually she and her husband drifted apart. They are now divorced. She has two children, 15 and 13, and her biggest fears and concerns are around how they will handle her illness. J.S. says, "I am not so afraid of death, but I am afraid for them. I know what it is like to care for someone who has cancer. I know what it is like to be left alone."

Ann and J.S. continue to dialogue about meaningful events and experiences. Ann is fully attentive to J.S. and engaged in her story. Ann is completely open, allowing J.S. to provide the details as she chooses and carefully listens without interrupting, yet shares ideas, thoughts, and reflections. Ann offers

J.S. therapeutic touch and says that she can visit her in her hospital room postoperatively. J.S. is grateful for this.

Her recovery goes smoothly, but her prognosis remains uncertain. Over the course of the next year, she continues to check in with Ann and share with her what is happening in her life. J.S. has made several changes, including incorporating yoga and a healthy diet into her regime. She has moved to a smaller, more manageable home and has planted a garden. She has found a new job that is less stressful, participates in a theater group with her two children, and has reconnected with old friends. J.S. describes the experience of meeting Ann as "a gift that was meant to be." Ann is gracious but states that this story is not unusual for her now that she practices nursing "in a way it was meant to be." Ann says that she loves her work, that it gives her life great meaning, and that through connecting with her patients in this way, she too gains from the experience.

Further Questions to Consider

Here are some further questions for discussion:

1. Would you describe the care Ann has provided as health promoting?
2. How is this different or not from your original ideas about health promotion?
3. Do you think it is possible for nurses to practice in this way?
4. What are the potential deterrents to such a practice?
5. What or who could act as the support for such a practice?
6. If this is true nursing care from a disciplinary perspective and yet it is unusual because of constraints placed on nurses in practice, how do nurses address this as part of the commitment to the public as outlined in the ANA's *Social Policy Statement* (2010)?

Access to Care

The issue of access to care is of utmost importance to nurses. Although many see access to care as an issue of the underserved and those without insurance, being poor and uninsured are not the only factors that relate to access to care. The issue of access to care is broader in scope and it also includes those who do have insurance. In a profit-driven or economically focused healthcare system, patients are left to their own devices to navigate the healthcare system or to inform themselves about available choices. This along with the plight of the poor and underserved is another aspect of poor access to appropriate care. The problems associated with a profit-driven healthcare system and what this means both for patient care and preventive care is considered under this broad umbrella of access to care.

In an economically driven healthcare system, emphasis is primarily on economic concerns and not primarily on trying to meet patients' needs, so it is important to discuss the implications of access to care in such a system. Understanding this issue permits APRNs to collaborate with others such as the public, lawmakers, and other healthcare providers in the interests of good patient care.

The numbers of short-stay surgeries and procedures continue to increase for several reasons, including improved anesthesia care, improved surgical technologies, and an aging population with more health problems. These procedures are highly profitable. Some surgeries and procedures that are increasingly used include bariatric, plastic, orthopedic, cardiac, and vascular. This is concerning on many levels. Most of these procedures require patients to spend little or no time on an inpatient unit. Inpatient care is, of course, expensive and can drive up the costs of procedures. But this also means that patients spend less time with nurses. Thus, the care that nurses provide such as partnering with the patient through the experience, teaching, and providing health promotion is missing.

The institutional emphasis can shift toward providing those procedures and interventions that are likely to be profitable. This means the system rewards those physicians who do a large number of these types of procedures. Further, nurses who work within this system are paid by this system, which raises an issue of potential conflicts of interest. The complexity of the system with the competitive nature of healthcare insurance companies and the fragmentation of services all tend to shift the emphasis of healthcare services away from attention to other types of care and the need to look at the social conditions that lead to health disparities. Thus, health promotion, public health, and the health needs of the underinsured and underserved populations tend to be neglected.

Also, the idea of health promotion has fallen so far out of favor as a result of profit-driven care that it is no longer a major focus of most care within this system. If a person with a health problem has insurance, there is a procedure to fix it. Are you obese? Have gastric bypass surgery. Are you aging? Many plastic surgery options are available. Are you stressed? Have a procedure and take legitimate time off from work. This may seem extreme, but this is the perspective of a profit-driven system. Nurses in this system are not partnering with patients to explore purpose and meaning so that they can understand individuals in the human health experience. They are caught up in this system of high productivity and turnover and do not have the time to provide "nursing" care.

There are practices within hospitals in which surgeons and other interventionists are pressured to keep up the actual numbers of surgeries or procedures they perform. Indicators of success are around the number of surgeries booked as well as the ability to "turn over" an operating room or procedure room rapidly. Physicians who are able to respond to this message with increased numbers and faster turnaround times are rewarded with prime operating schedules; those who do not respond lose operating and/or procedure room time.

Pressuring surgeons to do surgery places an unfair burden on them, and on patients and the nurses who in theory are trusted professionals who advocate on patients' behalf. Elective surgery or procedures are just that—*elective*—and important questions to consider include (but are not limited to) the following: Is this the best option available to this patient? Will the patient in fact benefit from this surgery? What is the patient's overall health status and how will it be affected by the surgery? Does the patient have the resources in place to enhance recovery from surgery? What if the surgery is not successful? Is there another option, perhaps one that is nursing oriented, that is less costly overall, and that will help this person instead of surgery?

Research indicates that patients do not fully understand that they have a choice about whether or not to have surgery and that in some cases they elect to have surgery to address other unmet needs. Patients described not feeling they could take time off work to deal with stresses such as caregiving, and they reported that surgery and a recovery period would allow for a much needed respite (Flanagan, 2005, 2006, 2009; Flanagan & Jones, 2009). Thus, although surgery is an expensive, risky way for people to take time for themselves, it is an allowable way—both according to society's norms and healthcare reimbursement. Surgery does not, however, address the underlying need for a less stressed lifestyle.

Perhaps, for example, as nurses look at the issues related to aging—people living healthier, longer lives and wanting to contribute later in life to the workforce—in addition to considering lack of planning for retirement and concerns about skyrocketing healthcare costs, one solution could be to offer working people adequate breaks or sabbaticals every 5 or so years. This would allow people to take time off while raising a family, pursuing advanced degrees, caring for elderly parents, or just to take a vacation, pursue interests, and rejuvenate. It would also allow people who would like to work later in life to do so, perhaps in roles as mentors and advisors to the younger workforce. Nurses, particularly APRNs who see the myriad health-related consequences and huge costs associated with not caring for individuals throughout various life stresses must work through their professional organizations such as the ANA to create, lobby, and implement innovative policies that affect the health of society. Policies that make this type of option available to people will take overhauling current health strategies and creativity to implement, but an option like this that allows people time away from a harried lifestyle could have an enormous impact on the overall health and well-being of individuals and society as a whole. Situations such as the one described previously—obtaining time off by having surgery—left nurses confounded. The following is a case study that exemplifies this situation.

CASE STUDY

W.D. is a 52-year-old man who presents to the office for a medical clearance for laparoscopic surgery. He had a gallbladder attack 6 months ago but has changed his diet so that he consumes much less fat. Since then, he has not had another gallbladder attack. Nevertheless, he plans to have the gallbladder surgery. While in your office, W.D. mentions that he also plans to have an arthroscopy of his knee that he says has "been bothering me forever." He is a teacher in a major urban school system and reveals that he has been under a lot of stress recently, both at work and at home. He has a second job working as an auto mechanic. As you talk further with him, he reveals that the principal of the school is after every teacher to improve standardized testing scores in the classroom. W.D. has always been interested in teaching the students with social and personal challenges and fears that this new mandate compromises his values as a teacher. Further, he has been caring for his wife, who has been quite ill with breast cancer, and although she is now doing well, he remains worried about her.

As you talk, and as more of his story is revealed to you, you begin to recognize that W.D. is completely stressed. He describes being unable to sleep and losing weight without trying (20 pounds in 6 months), and complains of feeling a constant knot in his stomach along with constant stomach irritation.

Later, he shares, "I need a break, so I'm just going to have this surgery and when I get better from that, I will have the other. I don't know what else to do." W.D. does have problems that may benefit from surgery, but these surgical procedures are not risk free. In addition, his stress is not being addressed.

Questions to Consider

The following questions are useful to consider:

1. What should you, as an APRN, do in this situation?
2. What biases do healthcare providers bring to this type of situation?
3. Although it is true that he may have underlying problems that could require surgical intervention, do you think it is necessary for him to have these surgeries to correct the problems?
4. In terms of access to care (as described earlier), how does a case like this contribute to the problem?
5. How can the public be informed about unnecessary surgery without violating the trust they have in the system?
6. How would you begin to address the stigma of a patient like W.D. taking time off to address the real problem of stress as opposed to the perceived legitimate time off that recovery from surgery allows?

A Flawed System

There are many other issues relevant to access to care that are related to underserved populations, but overwhelming (and increasingly so) an underlying issue is a healthcare system that does not work. One reason for the malfunctioning system is the emphasis on profits or cost savings and no attention paid to the real health needs of individuals and society (Mechanic, 2006). And although there may be some good things that result from this system, it is inherently unfair. It is unfair, for example, that members of the U.S. Congress have unlimited access to a universal-type health plan while millions in the country go without even basic health care. It is unfair to have a system that pressures surgeons to produce and turn over cases or lose surgical privileges. It is unfair for nurses to be either blinded by the system that exists or aware of it but silenced. And it is an apoplectic situation for patients to be so trusting of the system and the providers, including nurses, that they never question if in fact nurses have their best interest first and foremost in mind in the way care is delivered.

Summary

The purpose of this chapter is to review ethical issues that confront adult-gerontology APRNs in daily practice. Discussing these issues in light of the disciplinary perspective and knowledge development can provide context. All the case studies were derived from personal practice. Such cases will arise for adult-gerontology APRNs, raising the questions of if and how these situations can be handled differently. If so, what would be enough to make things right? Grace points out in earlier sections of this text that speaking up is not without risk, and no one person should stand alone. This does not mean that situations should be overlooked, and sometimes situations are more successfully addressed one person to another.

In reality, though, most of these issues are too big for any one person to tackle and address alone. Hopefully adult-gerontology APRNs have the opportunity to address such issues during nursing ethics rounds. At such rounds these issues can be brought to the table for discussion. If a facility does not have ethics rounds, nearby colleges with schools of nursing may, and alliances can be made to address these issues in that format. Other options include joining and actively participating in nursing organizations that address these issues of concern. Self-reflection on both the individual level and organizational level is unique to nursing, and it is imperative that adult-gerontology APRNs are aware of the issues, recognize how situations that may seem normal or routine conflict with the disciplinary perspective, and are able to raise the questions that the public expects of nursing—a most trusted profession.

References

Allan, J., & Hall, B. (1988). Challenging the focus on technology: A critique of the medical model in a changing health care system. *Advances in Nursing Science, 10*(3), 22–34.

American Association of Colleges of Nursing. (2004). AACN position statement on the practice doctorate in nursing, October 2004. Retrieved from http://www.aacn.nche.edu/publications/position/DNPpositionstatement.pdf

American Association of Colleges of Nursing, American Organization of Nurse Executives, & National Association of Associate Degree Nursing (1995). *A model for differentiated practice*. Washington, DC: American Association of Colleges of Nursing.

American Nurses Association. (2001). *Code of ethics for nurses with interpretive statements*. Washington, DC: Author.

American Nurses Association. (2010). *Social policy statement*. Silver Spring, MD: Nursebooks.org.

APRN Consensus Work Group & National Council of State Board of Nurses Advisory Committee. (2008). Consensus model for APRN regulation: Licensure, accreditation, certification and education. Retrieved from https://www.ncsbn.org/1623.htm

Benner, P., Tanner, C. A., & Chelsea, C. A. (1996). *Expertise in nursing practice: Caring, clinical judgment and ethics.* New York, NY: Springer.

Bryant-Lukosius, D., Dicenso, A., Browne, G., & Pinelli, J. (2004). Advanced practice nursing roles: Development, implementation and evaluation. *Journal of Advanced Nursing, 48*(5), 519–529.

Carey, B. (2005, August 16). In the hospital, a degrading shift from person to patient. *The New York Times.* Retrieved from http://www.nytimes.com/2005/08/16/health/16dignity.html?pagewanted=all

Christensen, M., & Hewlett-Taylor, J. (2006). From expert to tasks, expert nursing practice redefined? *Journal of Clinical Nursing, 15*, 1531–1539.

Corley, M. C. (2002). Nurses' moral distress: A proposed theory and research agenda. *Nursing Ethics, 9*(6), 636–650.

Corley, M. C., Minick, P., Elswick, R. K., & Jacobs, M. (2005). Nurse moral distress and ethical work environment. *Nursing Ethics, 12*(4), 381–390.

Cowling, W. R., Smith, M., & Watson, J. (2008). The power of wholeness, consciousness, and caring: A dialogue on nursing science, art, and healing. *Advances in Nursing Science, 31*(1), E41–E51.

Cummings, J. (2012, December 12). Nurses in drive for compassionate care. BBC News Health. Retrieved from http://www.bbc.co.uk/news/health-20583115

DeRaeve, L. (2002). Trust and trustworthiness in nurse-patient relationships. *Nursing Philosophy, 3,* 152–162.

Dickoff, J., James, P., & Wiedenbach, E. (1968). Theory in a practice discipline, part one: Practice oriented theory. *Nursing Research, 17*(5), 415–435.

Donaldson, S. K., & Crowley, D. M. (1978). The discipline of nursing. *Nursing Outlook, 26*(2), 113–120.

Duffield, C., Gardner, G., Chang, A. M., & Catling-Paull, C. (2009). Advanced nursing practice: A global perspective. *Collegian, 16,* 55–62.

Faden, R., & Beauchamp, T. (2003). The concept of informed consent. In T. Beauchamp & W. LeRoy (Eds.), *Contemporary issues in bioethics* (6th ed., pp. 145–149). Belmont, CA: Wadsworth.

Fawcett, J. (2005). Integrating nursing models, theories, research, and practice. In J. Fawcett (Ed.), *Contemporary nursing knowledge: Analysis and evaluation of nursing models and theories* (2nd ed., pp. 589–599). Philadelphia: F. A. Davis.

Flanagan, J. (2005). Creating a healing environment for staff and patients in a pre-surgery clinic. In C. Picard & D. Jones (Eds.), *Giving voice to what we know: Margaret Newman's theory of health as expanding consciousness in nursing practice, research and education* (pp. 53–63). Sudbury, MA: Jones and Bartlett.

Flanagan, J. (2006). The nursing theory and practice link: Creating a healing environment within the pre-admission nursing practice—an exemplar. In C. Roy & D. Jones (Eds.), *Nursing knowledge development and clinical practice* (pp. 275–286). New York, NY: Springer.

Flanagan, J. (2009). Post-operative phone calls after same day surgery—timing is everything. *AORN: The Journal of the American Association of Operating Room Nurses, 90*(1), 41–51.

Flanagan, J. (2010). Using Newman's Health as Expanding Consciousness (HEC) to explore the life patterns of individuals recently hospitalized for an exacerbation of chronic obstructive pulmonary disease (COPD). *Journal of Nursing and Healthcare of Chronic Illness, 2*(3), 204–215.

Flanagan, J., & Jones, D. (2009). High frequency nursing diagnoses following same day knee arthroscopy. *International Journal of Nursing Terminology and Classifications, 20*(2), 89–96.

Fulton, J., & Lyon, B. (2005, September 30). The need for some sense making: Doctor of nursing practice. *OJIN: The Online Journal of Issues in Nursing, 10*(3), 3.

Gallup Poll. (2013). Honesty/ethics in professions. Retrieved from http://www.gallup.com /poll/1654/honesty-ethics-professions.aspx

Gordon, M. (1994). *Nursing diagnosis: Process and application.* Philadelphia, PA: Mosby.

Grace, P. J. (1998). *A philosophical analysis of the concept "advocacy": Implications for professional-patient relationships.* Unpublished Dissertation. University of Tennessee Knoxville. Retrieved from http://proquest.umi.com. Publication number AAT9923287, Proquest Document ID No. 734421751.

Grace, P. J. (2001). Professional advocacy: Widening the scope of accountability. *Nursing Philosophy, 2*(2), 151–162.

Grace, P. J. (2004). Patient safety and the limits of confidentiality. *American Journal of Nursing, 104*(11), 33, 35–37.

Grace, P. J., & McLaughlin, M. (2005). When consent isn't informed enough: What's the nurse's role when a patient has given consent but doesn't fully understand the risks? *American Journal of Nursing, 105*(4), 79–84.

Grady, D. (2007, July 29). Cancer patients, lost in a maze of uneven care. *The New York Times.* Retrieved from http://www.nytimes.com/2007/07/29/health/29Cancer .html?pagewanted=all&_r=0

Hardingham, L. (2004). Integrity and moral residue: Nurses as participants in a moral community. *Nursing Philosophy, 5,* 127–134.

Hoffman, J. (2005, August 14). Awash in information, patients face a lonely, uncertain road. *The New York Times.* Retrieved from http://www.nytimes.com/2005/08/14 /health/14patient.html?pagewanted=all

Hoffman, L., Tasota, F., Zullo, T., Scharfenberg, C., & Donaue, M. (2005). Outcomes of care managed by an acute care nurse practitioner/attending physician team in a subacute medical intensive care unit. *American Journal of Critical Care, 14*(2), 121–130.

Horrocks, S., Anderson, E., & Salisbury, C. (2002). Systematic review of whether nurse practitioners working in primary care can provide equivalent care to doctors. *British Medical Journal, 324*(7341), 819–823.

Institute of Medicine. (2010). *The future of nursing: Leading change, advancing health.* Washington, DC: National Academies Press.

Institute of Medicine. (2013). About the IOM. Retrieved from http://www.iom.edu /About-IOM.aspx

International Council of Nurses. (n.d.). Definition and characteristics of the role. International nurse practitioner/advanced practice nursing network. Retrieved from http://international .aanp.org/DefinitionAndCharacteristicsOfTheRole.htm

International Council of Nurses. (2012). *Code of ethics for nurses*. Geneva, Switzerland: Author. Retrieved from http://www.icn.ch/images/stories/documents/publications /free_publications/Code%20of%20Ethics%202012%20for%20web.pdf

International Federation of Nurse Anesthetists. (2012). 120th National certification examination candidate handbook. National Board or Certification and Recertification for Nurses Anesthetists: Author. Retrieved from http://www.nbcrna.com/Pages/default.aspx

Jameton, A. (1984). *Nursing practice: The ethical issues*. Upper Saddle River, NJ: Prentice Hall.

Johnson, D. E. (1974). Development of theory: A requisite for nursing as a primary health profession. *Nursing Research, 23*(5), 372–376.

Jones, D. (2006). A synthesis of philosophical perspectives for knowledge development. In C. Roy & D. Jones (Eds.), *Nursing knowledge development and clinical practice* (pp. 164–180). New York, NY: Springer.

Kring, D. L. (2008). Clinical nurse specialist practice domains and evidenced-based practice competencies. *Clinical Nurse Specialist: The Journal for Advanced Nursing Practice, 22*(4), 179–183.

Loewy, E. (1989). *Textbook of medical ethics*. New York, NY: Plenum Medical Book Company.

Loewy, E. (2005). In defense of paternalism. *Theoretical Medicine, 26*(6), 445–468.

Mechanic, D. (2006). *The truth about health care: Why reform is not working in America*. Piscataway, NJ: Rutgers University.

Meleis, A., & Dracup, K. (2005, September 30). The case against the DNP: History, timing, substance, and marginalization. *OJIN: The Online Journal of Issues in Nursing, 10*(3), 2.

Michaels, C. (1992). Carondelet St. Mary's nursing enterprise. *Nursing Clinics of North America, 24*(1), 77–85.

Neale, J. (2001). Patient outcomes: A matter of perspective. *Nursing Outlook, 49,* 93–99.

Newman, M. A. (1994). *Health as expanding consciousness* (2nd ed.). New York, NY: National League for Nursing.

Newman, M. (2008). *Transforming presence: The difference that nurses make*. Philadelphia, PA: F. A. Davis.

Newman, M., Smith, M., Pharris, M., & Jones, D. (2008). The focus of the discipline revisited. *Advances in Nursing Science, 31*(1), E16–E27.

Northrup, D. T., Coby, L. T., Olynyk, V. G., Schick Makaroff, K. L., Szabo, J., & Biasio, H. A. (2004). Nursing: Whose discipline is it anyway? *Nursing Science Quarterly, 17,* 55–62.

Northrup, D. T., & Purkis, M. E. (2001). Building the science of health promotion practice from a human science perspective. *Nursing Philosophy, 2*(1), 62–71.

Odone, C. (2011, August 28). Nursing is no longer the caring profession. *The Telegraph*. Retrieved from http://www.telegraph.co.uk/health/8728849/Nursing-is-no-longer-the-caring-profession.html

O'Shea, H. (2001). The state of the discipline in nursing: Science, technology, and culture have stirred rapid change. Retrieved from http://www.emory.edu/ACAD_EXCHANGE/2001 /octnov/oshea.html

Pearson, A., & Vaughn, B. (1996). Common characteristics of nursing models—the patient or client. In A. Pearson, M. Fitzgerald, & B. Vaughn (Eds.), *Nursing models for practice.* (pp. 39–55) Oxford: Butterworth Heinemann.

Peplau, H. E. (1952). *Interpersonal relations in nursing.* New York, NY: G. P. Putnam's Sons.

Prochaska, J. O., & DiClemente, C. C. (1983). Stages and processes of self-change of smoking: Toward an integrative model of change. *Journal of Consulting and Clinical Psychology, 51,* 390–395.

Radwin, L. E. (1995). Knowing the patient: A process model for individualized interventions. *Nursing Research, 44*(6), 364–370.

Rashotte, J., & Carnevale, F. A. (2004). Medical and nursing clinical decision-making: A comparative epistemological analysis. *Nursing Philosophy, 5,* 160–174.

Redfern, S. (2006). Examining the effectiveness of the nurse consultant role. *Nursing Times, 102*(4), 23–24.

Rodgers, B. (2007). Knowledge as problem solving. In C. Roy & D. Jones (Eds.), *Nursing knowledge development and clinical practice* (pp. 107–118). New York, NY: Springer.

Rogers, M. E. (1970). *An introduction to the theoretical basis of nursing.* Philadelphia, PA: F. A. Davis.

Roy, C. (2006). Unity, diversity, conformism, and chaos: Applications of Roy's epistemology of the universal cosmic imperative. In C. Roy & D. Jones (Eds.), *Nursing knowledge development and clinical practice* (pp. 307–314). New York, NY: Springer.

Smith, G. (1996). *Legal and healthcare ethics for the elderly.* Washington, DC: Taylor & Francis.

Tarlier, D. (2004). Beyond caring: The moral and ethical bases of responsive nurse-patient relationships. *Nursing Philosophy, 5,* 230–241.

Weeks, S. (2012). Staff caring for my mother came across as cold and uncaring. *Nursing Standard, 26*(37), 33.

Willis, D., Grace, P., & Roy, C. (2008). A central unifying focus for the discipline: Facilitating humanization, meaning, choice, quality of life, and healing in living and dying. *Advances in Nursing Science, 31*(1), E28–E40.

CHAPTER 11

Nursing Ethics and Advanced Practice: Psychiatric and Mental Health Issues

Pamela J. Grace and Pamela A. Terreri

There was a change in Boldwood's exterior from its former impassibleness; and his face showed that he was now living outside his defences for the first time, and with a fearful sense of exposure.
—Thomas Hardy, *Far from the Madding Crowd* (2001/1874)

Introduction

The authors of this chapter collaborated on the content. One of us has expertise in ethics and adult health advanced practice, and the other is an experienced advanced practice mental health nurse, psychotherapist, and educator. We worked together to make the content as relevant and helpful as possible in the limited space available. The aim of this chapter is to provide the basis and resources for advanced practice psychiatric–mental health nurses (APPMHNs) to gain confidence in their ethical decision making. However, topics explored within this chapter have salience for all nurses and advanced practice nurses (APNs). There are certainly many areas of specific concern that have not been addressed here. Additionally, the scope of practice for psychiatric APNs varies among countries and the issues that arise may differ based on cultures, contexts, and types of healthcare delivery systems. However, the resources and strategies in this chapter can provide a basis for understanding the nature of professional responsibility in this specialty area and direction for action in difficult situations.

All specialty practice nurses benefit from collaboration and consultation with thoughtful and knowledgeable colleagues. Of course, it is best to have assistance when a problem is developing, but confidence in ethical decision making is also built by after-the-fact analysis of cases with peers, allied professionals, and when possible, an ethics expert. Maintaining patient confidentiality is, of course, a crucially important aspect of psychiatric and mental health care, including during the process of collaboration and supervision. There are few exceptions to this rule because of the harm that can be caused to patients by the careless exposure of their history. When exceptions are necessary, for example, when a patient or others are at serious risk of harm as a result of their uncontrolled behavior, a judicious sharing of only necessary information is warranted. Additionally, it is necessary to try to ameliorate any damage to the trust relationship that may be caused by this information sharing.

As has become the convention, the term *psychiatric* as used in this chapter means associated with a mental illness perspective, and *mental health* means concerned with restoring a person's sense of well-being and integration. Thus, the advanced practice of psychiatric–mental health nursing utilizes "a wide range of explanatory theories and research on human behavior as its science and the purposeful use of the self as its art" (Kneisl, Wilson, & Trigoboff, 2004, p. xix) in promoting the mental stability or well-being of persons or in reducing their suffering.

The current nature of healthcare delivery systems, associated economic problems, and the philosophies behind mental health system structures and facilities can cause some of the more difficult issues for APPMHNs. The International Council of Nurses (ICN) urges the involvement of nurses in the move toward good psychiatric and mental health policies. The ICN's position statement on mental health notes that "[G]reater attention should be paid to the developmental and mental health of vulnerable groups (women, young people, elderly, poor, abused, addicted, refugees, etc.); to securing sufficient financial and human resources for effective service delivery, and to the education and training of mental health specialists" (ICN, 2008). Addressing such problems requires the action of all professions and professional groups whose patient populations are negatively affected. Chapter 4 provides further resources and suggestions for addressing broader healthcare delivery or policy issues that are unjust. This chapter concentrates on analyzing and clarifying the nature of problems faced in direct practice while acknowledging that psychiatric APNs, like other specialty APNs, do have responsibilities to inform and influence policy where necessary for their populations.

Good Psychiatric Advanced Nursing Practice

Foundations

The warrant for psychiatric advanced nursing practice, like other nursing specialties, issues from the goals and objectives of the nursing profession. These objectives are to provide a good for individuals and society related to their health or well-being, as described in earlier chapters. They require viewing all persons as unique individuals, deserving of dignity and of equal moral worth with others (American Nurses Association [ANA], 2001). Historically, patients suffering from mental illness have been especially stigmatized. *Stigma* can be defined as a negative image held by society or groups within a society toward those who are perceived as different from the majority in some way. The problem with stigma is that it facilitates the poor treatment of such people by others—they are treated as less than fully human or less worthy of moral concern. Another problem with stigma is that it can prevent people from seeking mental health care. Some researchers have pointed out that it is not only those suffering from mental illness that are likely to be stigmatized but also associated others such as relatives and even psychiatric–mental health professionals themselves (Halter, 2008). Thus, the responsibility exists for APPMHNs both to treat each patient as an individual equally worthy of dignity with other individuals and to address the stigmatizing attitudes of others through raising public consciousness.

Difficulties

Decisions about which actions are appropriate often must be made under conditions of extreme uncertainty that add to the difficulty of providing good care. Additionally, APPMHNs may face pressures from colleagues, employers, or funding sources to abandon their professional goals for the purposes of expediency or to meet institutional or practice needs. Conflicts of interest are prevalent in psychiatric and mental health settings, as they are elsewhere, but the particular nature of mental health practice—concerned as it is with people who are made especially vulnerable by perceptual and reasoning difficulties—gives these problems their own particular nuances.

A firm understanding of what good nursing practice is in psychiatric and mental healthcare settings is crucial both for resisting pressures to make choices that are not ethically supported and for articulating the rationale for a nurse's actions and decisions to others. The next section provides background on the nurse–patient relationship and its importance in advanced practice psychiatric and mental health settings.

The Nurse–Patient Relationship: History

The process of knowledge development for nursing practice was discussed in earlier chapters. However, it is important to note that several early nursing philosophers and theorists derived their understanding of what nursing is and what it does from their practice in psychiatric settings. Hildegard Peplau (1952), Ida Orlando (1961), and Joyce Travelbee (1966) all practiced at one point in their careers as psychiatric nurses. Their writings and theoretical explanations of nursing and the work nurses do emphasize the therapeutic importance of the nurse–patient relationship in recognizing and identifying a person's needs and thus promoting that person's well-being or relieving his or her suffering. Their insights were recognized as important for all areas of nursing practice, not just for practice in psychiatric settings.

The implications of therapeutic nurse–patient relationships apply to all patients in need of nursing services. Their understanding of persons, nursing, environment, and health—nursing's *metaparadigm* concepts as elucidated by Fawcett (1984)—is congruent with the nursing discipline's focus on persons as complex and integrated wholes. Because human beings are understood as integrated wholes, a breakdown or threat of breakdown in any area of life—physical, psychological, or social—could negatively affect an individual's experience of well-being.

Disruptions in well-being can occur in multiple ways. The insights of these scholars, along with those of other nursing philosophers and theorists, have ensured a nursing perspective that, regardless of area of specialty practice, views persons as unique and contextual. This perspective necessitates engaged interaction with the person in question for the purposes of ascertaining that person's needs. More recently, Willis, Grace, and Roy (2008) identified a central focus of the discipline as discernible from historical nursing literature. The focus on "facilitating humanization, meaning, choice, quality of life, and healing in *living and* dying" *is especially* pertinent to mental health settings.

Current Trends

Some commentators note that there is a trend away from this traditional focus of psychiatric advanced practice nursing on the importance of the nurse–patient relationship. Perraud and colleagues (2006) attribute the "sweeping changes in mental health delivery" (p. 216) along with the inception of the psychiatric nurse practitioner role as being instrumental in diluting the "profession's core identity" (p. 216). Although biologic and theoretical knowledge developments along with an understanding of societal needs can provide an ever stronger basis for practice, they can also shift the emphasis of care away from the therapeutic alliance. Perraud and associates (2006) noted that "under the paradigm shift ushered in by the decade of the brain" (p. 216), neurobiologic advances, and a firming up of core curricula for psychiatric mental health nursing at the advanced practice levels, a new emphasis emerged. "PMH [Psychiatric mental health] graduate programs began teaching the primary care trio of physical assessment, pathophysiology, and pharmacology" (Perraud et al., 2006, p. 216), and these innovations may have accidentally served to lessen the perceived importance of nursing practice as being founded in the nurse–patient relationship. They argued that a shift back to the primacy of the nurse–patient relationship need not exclude the development of knowledge and skills related to pathophysiologic or neurobiologic advances.

Thus, it can be argued that APPMHNs may be differentiated from nurses in other specialties not by goal but rather by substance. They acquire, via theoretical knowledge and experience, an in-depth understanding of factors that influence mental health. This knowledge may come from within or outside of the nursing discipline. Knowledge from other disciplines such as psychology, biology, and the cognitive sciences when used in nursing practice is necessarily filtered through the lens of nursing goals. These are asserted in the preamble to the ICN's *Code of Ethics for Nurses* as being "to promote health, to prevent illness, to restore health and to alleviate suffering" (ICN, 2012) and are rooted in the ideal that the nurse–patient relationship is of primary importance in practice with individuals. The ethic of care with its emphasis on the importance of understanding contexts and relationships is a good way to conceptualize the APPMHN's relationship to individual patients.

Psychiatric and Mental Health Ethics: Importance for All APNs

APPMHNs become experienced in applying knowledge gained in their education and experience, via clinical judgment, to ameliorate a given patient's problem or suffering. However, the ethical issues that face advanced practice psychiatric nurses are not isolated to psychiatric settings and may well confront other nurses and APNs working in a variety of settings. For example, APNs who practice in emergency departments, in primary care practices, or with children are all liable to care for patients with concomitant mental health issues, whose physical symptoms have implications for their mental health, or whose mental health issues pose a threat to their physical well-being. Moreover, the complex and interwoven nature of human beings is such that any one of us can be susceptible to integrity disruptions that threaten our mental and physical well-being. Thus, all nurses benefit from understanding what constitutes ethical practice for those experiencing disturbances in health, whether this manifests in physical ways or in perceptual changes or some combination of both.

As discussed in Chapter 5, leadership, collaboration, and sharing expertise are responsibilities of advanced practice. APPMHNs may well be called upon to collaborate with, educate, or assist colleagues in situations that require their expert knowledge. Additionally, advisory supervision is accepted practice both for novice and experienced psychotherapists and has been proposed as important in other settings where difficult cases are encountered. Those working in large institutions often have access to an ethics expert or resource for assistance in resolving dilemmas or difficult issues. Those in primary care or smaller practices may have to develop their own discussion groups or resources. The discussion, cases, and analyses that follow focus on either especially difficult or frequently encountered problems in psychiatric settings; they can be helpful for other healthcare professionals as they attempt to provide good care under uncertain, dangerous, or difficult circumstances. The cases are presented and explored with the aim of separating out important aspects and providing some clarity. Pertinent strategies and resources for resolving problems are offered. Before moving on to the cases, though, some themes prevalent in psychiatric settings and those that historically have been seen as related to the particular nature of mental health problems are discussed for the purposes of comprehending why decision making and action are sometimes so tricky.

Psychiatry and Mental Illness: Goals and Ethical Principles

The Relationship of Goals of Nursing to Goals of Mental Health Care

THE GOOD OF THE INDIVIDUAL

The goals of nursing apply to advanced practice psychiatric nursing care no less than they do in other environments of nursing care. Disorders or disturbances of mental health, whatever the underlying cause, have effects that occur along a continuum: they range from relatively mild, causing slight altered experiences of health, perspective, or mood, to severe, causing distortions of reality that can be dangerous for a person or others in the range of that person's destructive behavior. However, even mild mental health problems affect people in complex ways, altering their relationship to their environment and the contexts of their daily lives. In the absence of a risk of harm to others from the person in question, the focus of therapy or the therapeutic relationship is to provide a good for the individual, to help him or her restore a prior sense of well-being or improve it. Although achieving this goal may be difficult given all sorts of constraints placed upon the APN by the healthcare environment and the status of contemporary knowledge, locating the idea of professional responsibility in the goals of the profession provides guidance about what constitutes ethical action.

MENTAL ILLNESS: AVOIDING HARM FROM MISUNDERSTANDING

Based on historical accounts, pervasive misunderstandings about mental illness have resulted in terrible atrocities. In ancient times, mental illness symptoms were taken as signs that a person was possessed by an evil spirit. In the Middle Ages, people showing signs of mental illness were imprisoned in mental asylums and often treated as animals, ridiculed, and even exhibited as entertainment. More recently, mental illness was viewed as a genetic problem curable by eliminating from the breeding population those who showed signs of imbalance or retardation (Kelves, 1999). To give one extreme example, the Nazi "euthanasia" programs of the 1930s were responsible for the deaths of thousands of mentally ill persons (Kelves, 1999). Nurses were among those who were complicit in these programs (Benedict, 2003). Ongoing studies in moral development, the cognitive and behavioral sciences, and psychology have provided explanations for why and under what conditions human beings may not follow a moral course of action (Doris & The Moral Psychology Research Group, 2010; Eagleman, 2011; Kahneman, 2011). Philosophers have also debated the issues of free will and choice. The debate is complex, centering on questions about what it means to be held morally responsible for actions. To be held responsible for actions two conditions have to be met—there must be two or more options and the person must be relatively free of psychological and physical obstructions to making a reasoned choice (Meynen, 2010). If no choices exist then a person cannot be held responsible. This is not the same as saying that healing, corrective, or restorative measures are not possible; rather it is about understanding that people are more or less responsible for their behavior. This knowledge permits professionals to develop mindfulness about the possible prejudices held by themselves and others. It helps them resist pressure not to do the right thing for their patients.

Despite advances in understanding the complexity of mental illness, contributing factors, and their interrelationships, stigma persists, and not infrequently those with mental illness are perceived as being or are held partially responsible for their illness (Halter, 2008; Meynen, 2010). Moreover, from culture to culture mental illness is viewed very differently. Some societies do not recognize the concept of mental disorder at all, and some critics in Western countries, where providing mental health services is an accepted practice, have called into question the purpose of the label "mental disorder" (Wakefield, 1992). It is beyond the purpose of this chapter to provide a philosophical discussion of the nature of mental illness. Controversies continue to be the subject of debate within mental health and philosophy circles. The interested reader is referred to Green and Bloch's (2006) collection of essays and articles for further information about these historical and ongoing debates.

The important point is that conditions continue to be ripe for misunderstandings about the nature of mental illness, which in turn cause further suffering for persons with mental illnesses. APPMHNs are well positioned to inform policy making and public discussions related to this problem for the purposes of promoting good patient care and the provision of adequate and appropriate services. Additionally, they understand the implications for patients of lapses in confidentiality, given that negative attitudes about mental illness persist.

Ethical Principles Plus the Goals of Nursing: Providing Direction

Ethical principles and considerations that have special salience in psychiatric/mental health settings broadly include autonomy, beneficence, and nonmaleficence. Justice is also an important factor because it provides the basis for addressing issues of needed change at the social or institutional policy level. In many countries, the level of healthcare services available for mental health and substance abuse issues does not parallel that of physical illness, in spite of the fact that mental health issues have been proven to underlie many chronic diseases. That is, the principle of justice as fairness is important in helping to see problems related to the inadequate or inappropriate healthcare service provision related to the population's need for access to mental health services. (See Chapter 4 for a more in-depth discussion of professional responsibility for social action.)

Each of these principles (autonomy, beneficence, and nonmaleficence) has important implications for the safety and well-being of persons experiencing mental health problems and places responsibilities upon professional providers of care. An in-depth discussion of these principles and their applications was given in Chapter 1 and later chapters; here their particular implications for mental health are discussed. As stressed previously, the principles are useful only insofar as they provide clarity. The main focus of ethical decision making is on trying to achieve a good for a patient, and in the process, to prevent harm to that person or others.

Perhaps the most problematic aspects of mental health disturbances are that they cloud judgment or alter a person's perception of the nature or meaning of their life, which in turn renders voluntary informed decision making difficult, if not impossible. This particular problem presents APPMHNs and other psychiatric mental health professionals with some of their most difficult challenges. Aligned with this issue is the problem that impaired judgment can lead to personal harm for a patient, harm to significant others or innocent bystanders, and sometimes harm to the professional caring for the patient. A further issue described by Sadler (2007) is that associated with the conception of "personal self." He notes that "the personal self is a Western common-sense concept which is characterized by five aspects: agency, identity, trajectory, history and perspective . . . the personal self has considerable psychiatric significance in moral, professional, research, and existential realms" (p. 113). The idea of a personal self is very much bound up with the idea of autonomy in ethical psychiatric mental health practice.

Autonomy

LIMITS AND PROBLEMS

In the discussion of autonomy earlier in the text, the question was raised, "Is anyone ever really capable of autonomous action?" The suggestion was made that all people are susceptible to subtle and not so subtle influences of various sorts; thus, no person can be truly autonomous. Moreover, physiologic influences also cause disruptions in cognition and perception. Diseases or conditions that alter cerebral perfusion, biologic changes that alter neurological functioning, and chemicals including pharmaceuticals can all contribute to perceptual or information-processing problems.

Conditioning influences from a person's previous life experiences and culture give rise to certain beliefs and values. These may change over time and with education, exposure to other viewpoints, and other life experiences. Some influences are external and derive from the expectations of others, the need to earn a living, the legal system, and so on. That is, all humans have conscious and unconscious drives that cause them to not always know what is in their best interests. Even if people do know what is in their best interests, they do not always know what actions are most likely to further these. Stated another way, a person's actions often do not have the effects that they desire or expect, even when they think that they have accounted for everything in their decision-making process.

Given that this is true, there are several questions to answer. If all persons have flawed decision-making processes, why is it thought that some people might make better decisions (those that are in line with their personal best interests) than others? If this question can be answered satisfactorily, the question can then be asked, "Is it ever permissible for a person to make a decision on behalf of another in the absence of that person's permission?"

HARM TO SELF OR OTHERS

Generally, it is accepted that if a person's actions are unlikely to cause significant harm to self or others, interfering on behalf of that person is not warranted. A person is expected to know what is best for him- or herself. Even if this knowledge, as noted earlier, is somewhat imperfect, it is still probably better than an outsider's knowledge of that person—as long as the subject is in possession of pertinent information. When significant harms to a person or others are certain or highly likely, then a more stringent evaluation is warranted and a responsibility to intervene may exist. The purpose of intervening when harm to a person is likely is to restore the person to his or her previous ability to exercise autonomy. For example, we would stop someone from jumping off a high bridge because this would result in certain death and, thus, no further opportunities for the person to exercise autonomy would exist.

Some of the following cases exemplify conditions of uncertainty where significant harm is possible. They are explored using points from the discussion here. Criteria for judging the ability of people to make their own informed decisions were given in Chapters 1 and 4. These include the ability to process relevant information, articulate how personal goals are likely to be met by given specified courses of action, and discuss the risks and provide reasoned explanations about why these risks are acceptable.

Buchanan and Brock's (1989) comprehensive look at decision making for those with impaired cognition has provided helpful insights in psychiatric–mental health settings. They note that decision-making abilities should be judged relative to a given task. In psychiatric–mental health settings, tasks might include such things as refusing medicines or accepting or refusing other therapies. Limits placed on a patient's freedom to make his or her own decisions are based either on that person's best interests (using what is known about the patient when possible) or on the likelihood that another will be significantly harmed by the person's actions.

Thus, a person's right to autonomy in choice of action may be limited because of lack of decision-making capacity and should be judged according to the degree of risk to self that is present. But a person's right to autonomous action may also be limited when that person presents a significant threat of harm to others. (This idea is discussed later in the chapter.) The serious and imminent threat of harm to others serves as a valid reason to limit a person's autonomy. When persons are prevented from following self-chosen courses of action because of worries that they may cause harm to themselves, the term used to justify the restriction is *paternalism*.

PATERNALISM

Paternalism is often used as a somewhat derogatory term to describe the imposition of the will of one person on another less powerful person. In healthcare ethics, the term is derived from the doctrine of *parens patriae* in medieval English Common Law and represents the responsibility of governments and states to protect those who cannot protect themselves (Payton, 1992). The intent of paternalistic actions is to ensure the safety and well-being of vulnerable persons such as children and the cognitively impaired. Paternalism also captures the idea that when a person's decision-making capacity is impaired such that the person may not be able to protect him- or herself from harm, efforts should be made to decide appropriate actions. *Appropriate actions* are those that are in line with what is known about a person's beliefs, values, and previous life trajectory. That is, the chosen action is not based on what the proxy decision maker would want, but rather what the impaired individual would.

Only when nothing is known about the individual in question is a best-interest or reasonable person standard used as the next best option. The reasonable person standard is self-explanatory: a decision is ethically warranted if it is what a reasonable person would want. Sometimes, of course, it is hard to determine what a reasonable person would want, but the standard does provide some guidance for action when it is not knowable what the person would wish. Although paternalism does permit the conceptualization of actions that are likely to further the specific interests of an incapacitated person, it is obviously not as good as being able to follow a person's own articulated directions. For such reasons, and as a result of ethics debates and discussions, the idea of having psychiatric advance directives arose in the 1980s (Green & Bloch, 2006).

PSYCHIATRIC ADVANCE DIRECTIVES

Many psychiatric illnesses cause fluctuations in a person's ability to make reasoned or informed decisions about acceptable care and therapeutics. Sometimes a person has decision-making capacity, and then at others times while experiencing a relapse, he or she does not. Examples of such problems are schizophrenia and bipolar disorders. In the 1980s, a revolutionary idea was proposed to help patients diagnosed with relapsing psychiatric illnesses retain control over what treatment would be acceptable to them in the event of decision-making incapacity (Culver & Gert, 1982; Green & Bloch, 2006; Howell, Diamond, & Wikler, 1982; Lavin, 1986; Winston, Winston, Appelbaum, & Rhoden, 1982). These are variously named psychiatric *advance directives, Ulysses contracts, self-binding contracts*, and *advanced treatment authorizations* (Green & Bloch, 2006, p. 183). Atkinson's (2007) book, *Advance Directives in Mental Health*, provides a detailed, comprehensive, and practical account of the use of this strategy to enhance autonomy for those with recurring or relapsing mental health problems. The advance directive can be either instructional or be realized by way of appointing a trusted proxy decision maker. For written directives, a discussion involving the person and his or her psychiatric–mental health provider occurs in which possible scenarios are articulated and acceptable treatments and interventions are agreed upon. The limitations of this are that not all possibilities can be anticipated. The appointment of a proxy can resolve this problem to a certain extent, although then the patient may need to be assisted in identifying a trustworthy and capable proxy. The combination of written instructions and an appointed proxy may be even more effective in providing what the patient would want. Psychiatric advance directives resemble advance directives as used in the broader healthcare setting; they differ only in that they are specific to the mental health needs of a patient. APPMHNs who work with such patients have an important role in assisting patients who are willing to prepare their own advance directives. This requires a careful process of decision making and information sharing.

Nonmaleficence

The principle of nonmaleficence captures the idea of a power imbalance in healthcare provider–patient relationships. The principle cautions healthcare providers to avoid doing harm in the course of their professional endeavors. In psychiatric mental health settings, harm to a patient can be caused in a variety of ways. A person can be harmed as a result of his or her illness-related actions, vulnerability to a condition, lack of knowledge about therapeutics and their aims, unethical practitioners, limits on freedom, or any combination of these. Some specific examples of particular harms include inappropriate referrals, misdiagnosis, boundary violations, restrictions on freedom, abandonment (Gutheil & Simon, 2003), and inappropriate dissemination of information gained in the course of the therapeutic relationship. Maintaining a focus on the fiduciary aspects of the nurse–patient relationship is important. The fiduciary relationship is based on trust. The patient should be able to trust that the healthcare provider maintains the patient's best interest as his or her primary concern.

When the problem is that the patient poses a risk to others, the trust versus safety issue presents tension for the APPMHN. The principle of nonmaleficence imposes a responsibility to lessen the harm that results from the necessary breech in confidentiality that results from the need to protect others from a patient's actions.

BREAKING CONFIDENTIALITY

Although the principle of autonomy underlies the idea that maintaining confidentiality is crucially important in healthcare settings, it is not an absolute value. Limits to respecting a person's autonomy occur when a person's action might cause danger to self or others. The idea behind confidentiality is that a person has a right to say what can be done with his or her information and who can have access to it. However, when information that has implications for the well-being of another person is shared with a healthcare provider, that provider is faced with the task of determining the likelihood and severity of the risk and making a judgment about whether that information should be shared and with whom.

At one time, the provider–patient privilege was understood to be as binding as that of the clergy or advocate. *Privilege* means that it is "shielded from exposure to the legal system" (Grace, 2005, p. 114). Several landmark legal cases changed ideas about providers' responsibility to break confidentiality and under which sorts of conditions they must do so. Healthcare providers have duties to warn others who do not know that they are in physical danger. This responsibility was acknowledged in the United States as a result of the highly publicized Tarasoff case.

> On October 27, 1969, Prosenjit Poddar killed Tatiana Tarasoff. Poddar was receiving psychiatric care during this period. He had informed his therapist two weeks earlier that he was going to kill a certain girl, easily identifiable as Tarasoff, on her return from Brazil. At the time his therapist tried to have him committed. The police detained Poddar briefly but decided he was rational so released him. (Grace, 2005, p. 115)

Tatiana was not informed that she was at risk and she was killed by Poddar shortly after she returned to the United States. The courts concluded that "once a therapist does in fact determine, or under applicable professional standards reasonably should have determined, that a person poses a serious danger of violence to others, he bears a duty to exercise reasonable care to protect the foreseeable victim of that danger" (*Tarasoff v. Regents of University of California*, 1976).

However, nonmaleficence also warns providers to limit the harms that can be caused by a possible loss of trust in the therapist, which in turn has implications for a patient's well-being. Loss of trust may mean that a patient holds back important information that can lead to effective interventions. Trust is also lost when a decision is made to hospitalize a patient against that person's will or without that person's permission. Additionally, while hospitalized (voluntarily or involuntarily), a decision may be made to use chemical or physical restraints to control a person's harmful behavior. Both the principles of nonmaleficence and beneficence apply to decisions to involuntarily hospitalize patients or to use restraints to control behavior.

Beneficence

INVOLUNTARY HOSPITALIZATION AND CHEMICAL AND PHYSICAL RESTRAINTS

Harm can also be caused in the course of trying to provide a good for a patient when the patient needs to be restrained to prevent harm to self or others. Beneficence, the ethical principle that best captures the healthcare provider's duties to provide a good for persons, is also relevant to the discussion related to behavior control.

Chodoff's (1976/1999) carefully argued defense both of the need for involuntary hospitalization and the criteria that should be applied to such decisions remains pertinent today. He presented a series of cases and then made an argument that the nature of mental illness is such that providers are warranted in involuntary hospitalization in certain instances on the grounds that it will further a person's good (note that this is not the issue of dangerousness to others as discussed earlier but is concentrated on the likelihood of personal harm). He argued that involuntary hospitalization may be warranted if "obvious disturbances that are both intrapsychic [for example, the suffering of severe depression] and interpersonal [for example, withdrawal from others because of depression]" (p. 108) exist. The criteria for such hospitalizations are that the institution has treatment available, there is a focus on the patient regaining control rather than on controlling the patient, and adequate surveillance exists. In the absence of the possibility of cure, the amelioration of suffering is the goal (Chodoff, 1976/1999).

Related Issues

The preceding discussion is far from a complete account of issues encountered in psychiatric and mental healthcare environments or in society in general. Other contemporary issues worthy of further discussion relate to managed care funding issues, parity in healthcare coverage by insurance companies, problems caused by profit-motivated health care and the pharmaceutical industry, direct-to-consumer marketing of drugs and treatments, and even the development of new diseases for which new drugs can then be developed and prescribed. Another issue is that of informed consent to enroll in research studies. (Issues of informed consent and research were discussed in more detail in Chapter 6.) Such topics can be given as class assignments to explore further. The next section presents cases with associated discussion and questions to stimulate further thought. The cases are composites and details have been altered to maintain confidentiality.

CASE STUDY 1: INADEQUATE CARE

Andrew is a graduate student in psychiatric nursing and has a clinical placement at a crisis intervention center of a local mental health clinic. Martha

Adams presents for an evaluation and states that she has not been able to contact her psychiatrist, who practices at a well-known teaching hospital, and that she is in need of a renewal of her antidepressant medication. In fact, she took her last dose of paroxetine 3 days ago and has been questioning whether paroxetine is the right medication for her. She has experienced a number of side effects that include a 30-pound weight gain and a decreased libido. Martha sees her psychiatrist once every 6 months for 10-minute visits, during which she feels that her doctor always seems rushed and more focused on other office issues. Martha has not felt that her doctor listens to her concerns, and after meeting with Andrew and his preceptor, she asks if there is another medication to try and if she could possibly return and be followed here at this clinic where she feels her concerns are heard.

Andrew notes Martha's symptoms of decreased concentration, lethargy, and lack of motivation coupled with her desire to quit smoking, and he thinks that a change of medication to bupropion might be beneficial to the patient because it is helpful in smoking cessation. In addition, he discusses the need for Martha to be in ongoing therapy to help with her self-esteem issues and depressed thoughts. When he reviews his plan with his preceptor prior to presenting it to the client, Andrew's preceptor instructs him that they will renew the paroxetine that she has been already prescribed and call and leave a message for her current psychiatrist. The preceptor is very aware of the need to maintain a positive rapport with the psychiatrist, who is a well-known lecturer in psychopharmacology. Andrew feels that this is letting the patient down because they have already heard from the patient her desire to seek more active treatment. He is mindful of the need to be an advocate for the patient in her efforts to obtain quality care.

Case Discussion

As a result of Andrew's advanced practice educational process and his previous nursing experiences, he knows that the primary goals of care for Martha are to establish a therapeutic relationship and use sound clinical judgment in assisting her to receive the care she needs. His holistic approach to her care has already unearthed some of the complexities of her case, including weight gain, libido problems, and the desire to stop smoking. If Andrew were the primary provider in this instance, he could use his judgment about how to address the issue of appropriate care. Various strategies could be tried, depending upon the patient's needs and Andrew's knowledge of the psychiatrist in question. For example, Martha could be empowered to decide for herself whether to change providers and how to go about this. Additionally, Andrew could persist in trying to contact the psychiatrist to discuss his concerns, including the fact that Martha stopped taking paroxetine and that he would like to try something that would work for both the depression and the smoking cessation.

Although there is a responsibility not to undercut a patient's trust in another provider, when APNs are sure that the other provider's care is not serving the patient well, they have a responsibility to help the patient figure out how his or her needs can be met. For U.S. nurses, the ANA's *Code of Ethics for Nurses with Interpretive Statements* (2001) provides guidance related to the practice of other professionals. Provision 3.5 clearly affirms that the nurse's "primary responsibility is to the health, well-being and safety of the patient" and this preempts loyalties to other professionals who are not serving the patient's interests.

Abrupt withdrawal from antidepressants also has negative consequences, and renewing the paroxetine is no guarantee that Martha will take it. In fact, when she has clearly stated her issues with it, persisting with the prescription is likely to undermine her trust both in Andrew, who has developed a rapport with her, and in his preceptor, who would presumably be the one to have an ongoing relationship with her. Thus, there is the possibility of harm to Martha both from the withdrawal from the antidepressant in the absence of a substitute and perhaps even more important from the loss of trust in providers.

However, Andrew is not the primary provider in this instance. He is faced with the tricky issue of working with a preceptor and as such being a "guest" in that environment. Preceptors often give their time with no obvious rewards except the fact that they are contributing to the discipline and think that they can have a positive influence on the development of good practitioners. Andrew does not have the power to override his preceptor's decision, and he must have strong rationale for his point of view; he should be willing to hear his preceptor and accept a reasonable decision. Failing this, he can try to articulate his concerns and find a middle ground that serves the patient's best interests while maintaining a rapport with his preceptor. If, however, Andrew has other concerns about his preceptor's philosophy of practice, then his next step is to talk to his supervising faculty about the possibility of a more suitable clinical placement.

CASE STUDY 2: SPLIT TREATMENT AND ALICE'S WELL-BEING

Alice is a 20-year-old single woman currently in her third year of college. She has struggled with symptoms of major depression and anxiety since early adolescence. At age 13, she began individual therapy with a social worker specializing in child psychiatry and a child psychiatrist who prescribed medications. She attended a therapeutic high school and during the last half of her senior year made an unsuccessful suicide attempt. She was admitted to a psychiatric hospital against her will.

When it came time for discharge planning, the hospital staff in consultation with her outpatient therapist began to form a treatment team of clinicians specializing in care of adults that could follow Alice over the long term. She was referred to an art therapist (AT) named Amy Bowen for individual therapy and to a clinical nurse specialist (CNS), Lynn Arnold, who would monitor her response to medications and her overall well-being. At that time, her diagnoses were bipolar disorder I —her most recent episode of this was severe and she exhibited psychotic features—and attention deficit disorder hyperactive (ADDH) type. As graduation approached, Amy Bowen, Lynn Arnold, and the social worker met with Alice to plan for her transition from therapeutic high school to college. This meeting offered Alice and all present the message that her treatment was a team effort.

Two years into Alice's college experience, Amy (the AT) reluctantly withdrew her services due to an ongoing family crisis that resulted in her closing her clinical practice. After consulting with Lynn Arnold, Amy informed Alice of the reasons for her decision and referred Alice to another AT, who unbeknownst to Amy did not share Amy's willingness to collaborate treatment with a prescribing clinician. Lynn attempted to leave messages for the new therapist after each visit with Alice but never received return calls. Alice reported feeling very comfortable with her new therapist and indicated the presence of a strong alliance, albeit not the same as the one she experienced with Amy.

Alice began to miss follow-up appointments with Lynn and was not returning calls. Attempts to reach the new therapist went unanswered. Only when Alice's prescriptions ran out did Lynn hear from Alice. Lynn had been seeing Alice for 3 years at this point but was now concerned that she was participating in a treatment protocol that was inadequate and that the possibility of harm existed related to Lynn's limited ability to evaluate Alice's overall health status and thus anticipate problems and provide appropriate care.

Case Discussion

This case raises several issues. First, when a referral or replacement for services is needed, the provider has a professional responsibility to try to ensure that the replacement is appropriate based on knowledge of the patient's needs and that the philosophy of care of the replacement fits in with the established team. Expectations of the collaborative relationship need to be articulated openly. All parties must understand their respective roles and reach agreement with other members. In this case, this arrangement is most likely to serve Alice's needs and permit anticipation of emerging problems. In view of the problem encountered in this case, it is probably also prudent for the team to talk about how a change of therapist will be handled by the group. Because team relationships are inevitably altered as members change, it might be prudent to have a group meeting to discuss roles and role responsibilities. At that meeting, an important aspect to be discussed is how a breakdown in communication among the members of the team will be handled. That is, in addition to serving Alice's current needs, future issues are anticipated. This kind of planning could also be called preventive ethics. *Preventive ethics* tries to anticipate future problems and put into place a structure to deal with them. Because of the seriousness of Alice's mental health issues, optimal care for her warrants egalitarian collaborative relationships where all members can expect to have their perspective heard.

However, this current situation has gone beyond the stage when preventive ethics could play a role. Now a new avenue must be explored. As an important part of the team, the AT has some crucial information that needs to be shared for Alice's health to be optimized. Alice's CNS, Lynn Arnold, is in the best position to evaluate Alice's ongoing needs. She has the knowledge and expertise to understand the interplay of physical, chemical, and psychosocial aspects of care and how disruptions in any one of these may lead to a deterioration of Alice's health. But she can plan appropriate care and therapeutics only if she has adequate information to do this. It is unclear what Lynn's relationship with Alice is, but if a rapport has been built up, then Lynn could explore with Alice the need for, or the possibility of, a group meeting to ensure that the plan of care continues to meet her needs. She could try to discover how Alice usually contacts the AT when she has to cancel appointments. A concern here might be that Lynn's frustration with her inability to contact the new therapist and uncertainty about Alice's health might cause an inadvertent break in the alliance that Alice has formed with the new therapist, which could be harmful (breaching the principle of nonmaleficence). Lynn must be careful not to communicate negative feelings about the AT, which might make Alice feel that she has to choose between the two.

Perhaps the AT prefers a mode of communication other than the telephone. One option for Lynn might be to write her concerns in a letter to the AT, describing the original arrangement, why it was deemed important, and why ongoing communication is important to Alice's health. Sending the letter by certified mail would permit verification that the letter was received. Lynn could also try to discover if others have had similar problems and how these have been resolved. Resolution of such issues depends on the nature of the problem and clinical judgment about the patient's good and what is required to further this. Keeping the focus on the patient's needs rather than one's own frustration is most likely to lead to appropriate and sound actions.

CASE STUDY 3: THE LIMITS OF RESPONSIBILITY

Megan was referred to Beverly Sweeney, APRN, BC, by her college health service during her first semester of school. Megan presented with symptoms of major depression that included difficulty concentrating, sleep disturbance, anhedonia, increased irritability, and recurring thoughts of harming herself. A treatment plan was established that included weekly individual psychotherapy sessions and medication management. Megan had a positive response to treatment and eventually saw Ms. Sweeney every 2 weeks to work on her negative cognitions and low self-esteem. Her treatment included a prescription for a daily dose of 40 mg of citalopram, an antidepressant.

As graduation approached, it was clear that Megan would be moving out of state to pursue job opportunities and thus therapy with Ms. Sweeney would need to be terminated. Ms. Sweeney encouraged Megan to use the remaining few weeks before her move to review her experiences of therapy. Megan was able to articulate her ambivalence in saying goodbye to Ms. Sweeney. This ambivalence is understood to be a normal response to the ending of a therapeutic relationship, whether this is because treatment is no longer needed or a transfer to another therapist is needed. Megan and Ms. Sweeney spent the last few sessions discussing the need for follow-up care and how to find an appropriate provider after relocating. Because Megan felt that she needed to continue on the prescribed antidepressants, a new provider who could evaluate her progress was essential.

During their last session, Ms. Sweeney gave Megan a 1-month prescription for citalopram with three refills. They agreed that this would get Megan through the initial period of getting settled in a new area. Besides the psychological impact that a relocation can have, it takes time to find a place to live, a job, new health insurance, and new healthcare providers. Thus, a 3-month supply seemed appropriate. They parted toward the end of July with the acknowledgment that the therapy had been successful but that more follow-up would benefit Megan as she went through the stress of relocating.

Toward the end of November, Ms. Sweeney received a phone message from Megan stating that she was about to run out of her citalopram and she had only three pills left. She left a pharmacy phone number along with her cell phone number and asked if Ms. Sweeney could please call in a prescription to her new pharmacy. Ms. Sweeney was alarmed at her own emotional reaction to this situation. She felt an intense irritation and wondered what the root cause of it was.

Case Discussion

This case raises several questions. It is not known if Megan is seeing a new therapist who does not have prescription privileges or if she has other reasons for not following through on the suggested interim therapy. Is this a type of boundary issue as described by Gutheil and Gabbard (1993/2006)? Is Megan is suffering from the psychological effects of withdrawal from her therapist that has been worsened by the stress of trying to adapt to new circumstances? Gutheil and Gabbard noted that "almost all patients who enter into a psychotherapeutic process struggle with the unconscious wish to view the therapist as the ideal parent" (p. 61). Thus, Megan may be acting out her insecurity by returning to a reliance on, or a demand for, the attention of Ms. Sweeney. More information is needed before an ethical course of action can be determined.

Initially, on hearing the phone message Ms. Sweeney had viewed this problem as a dilemma. Having not seen Megan in several months, and thus not being able to evaluate her mental health status on a face-to-face basis, she wondered whether she should call in a prescription or not. She felt somewhat irritated that Megan had not acted responsibly. On the other hand, she was worried that if she did not fill the prescription, Megan might suffer withdrawal symptoms. Nevertheless, she was reluctant to fill the prescription knowing that Megan was not being monitored appropriately.

On further reflection, Ms. Sweeney felt that she had explained in great detail to Megan during a couple of their therapy sessions the unpleasant and sometimes harmful effects that abrupt withdrawal from this type of drug could have and that if she decided she did not need it any more the dosage must be slowly tapered. She began to realize that in fact this current situation did not constitute a true dilemma and that several alternative options were open to her.

She could talk to Megan on the phone and discuss with Megan her status and what her options are. If it turns out that Megan has been receiving care from a therapist who does not have prescription authority, then Megan should be encouraged to talk to her current therapist about how he or she normally handles a case where pharmaceutical intervention is seen as a necessary adjunct to therapy. Most nonprescribing clinicians have collaborative relationships with prescribers. If Megan is not having therapy, does she need it? If it is apparent that she does, perhaps a contract with Megan can be made. Ms. Sweeney could help Megan identify resources in her area and give a modified (perhaps a week's supply) prescription with the understanding that she be notified when an appointment has been made. Given that Megan is probably capable of making her own decisions (has decision-making capacity) and that she is able to appreciate the implications of her actions for her own goals and values, responsibility for the current situation properly resides with her. In fact, to come to her rescue may not be therapeutic. It could be the equivalent of failing to respect her autonomy and may undermine the previous work done with her related to developing her self-esteem and confidence.

On reflecting about her own irritated reaction, Ms. Sweeney realizes that she has mixed feelings about Megan's behavior. One of her concerns is that her therapy with Megan was unsuccessful. She had hoped that Megan would take responsibility for her ongoing mental health by seeking out appropriate care. It is important that Ms. Sweeney sort out and understand the source and nature of her own reactions to formulate an ethical response to Megan's request, one that will maximize Megan's well-being and reduce the possibility of harm.

Complicating Ms. Sweeney's reaction is the issue of compensation because she does not get paid for her time or expertise unless she sees the patient in the office. This can be a boundary issue related to the therapeutic contract—that is, the issue of holding patients responsible for their agreed part of a contracted service agreement. Alternatively, it could be a system problem related to fair reimbursement by insurance companies, which depends for its resolution on health policy changes. This discussion is beyond the scope of the current chapter but is addressed in Chapters 2 and 4 and elsewhere in the text.

Case Conclusions

The nature of psychiatric–mental health advanced practice can present the clinician with a wide variety of difficult and ambiguous situations. Although a focus on professional goals, an understanding of ethical language and pertinent principles, and experienced clinical judgment is most likely to lead to a sound course of action, elements of uncertainty will often persist. In such cases, and where time permits, consultation with another professional or an ethics expert may be helpful. The following cases are posed for class exploration and discussion or for discussion with colleagues.

CASE STUDY 4: THE ANGRY SON

Mr. A., a 23-year-old single man employed full time as a city sanitation worker, seeks help for what he describes as unbearable anxiety and depression. In his words: "I can't stand the way I feel. Every morning I wake up and ask, 'Why me? What did I do to deserve this?'" He contacts a psychiatric CNS who has a private counseling practice. As is her usual practice, Ms. P. reviews with Mr. A. policies that she follows, including the fact that personal information divulged in therapy is confidential by law and that Ms. P. cannot share this information without his permission. She notes that the only exception to this would be if she has good reason to believe that he is in serious and imminent danger of hurting himself or someone else. Mr. A. has no intention or plan to kill himself at this time, and he agrees to call if his feelings change or if he feels in any danger of hurting himself. They agree on an initial treatment contract that includes meeting for four sessions to evaluate the best course of treatment, which may or may not include medication to help with his anxiety and depression.

Despite Mr. A.'s obvious discomfort and anxiety, he settles into a fairly comfortable rapport with Ms. P. and seems calmed by having made the decision to get help. His initial mental status exam offers no evidence of thought disorder, and although he had experienced past substance abuse with alcohol and cocaine, it has been more than a year since he has used either of these substances. He denies having any active problems with these substances.

During a therapy session, Mr. A. reveals that he is the youngest of five children and the only boy born to a couple of Italian descent. His mother worked as a court stenographer, and his father was a firefighter who left the family when Mr. A. was 5 years old. Mr. A. has no memory of his father being in the house when he was growing up and states that his father was an alcoholic. After his parents' divorce, Mr. A. continued to receive little attention from his father despite the fact that his father lived nearby. Mr. A.'s mother "disciplined" him by using ridicule. On many occasions, his sisters joined in the ridicule, commenting that he was "a sissy." He shares a particularly painful memory of having his older sister making fun of him for crying and calling him "a girl."

Three days after the session in which this was revealed, Mr. A. calls Ms. P. by phone and states, in a slurred voice, that he has a weapon and is going to kill his father. Ms. P. attempts to calm Mr. A., but he remains agitated, yelling into the phone, "My father should pay for running out on me and leaving me to be raised by women. . . . I feel like I am less than a man." Ms. P. manages to establish the fact that Mr. A. is in his home alone. She does not have the father's address and is convinced that Mr. A., in his intoxicated state, is a threat to his father and possibly to himself. Ms. P. tells Mr. A. that she is very concerned about him and does not want him to act on his feelings, adding that it is her job to do whatever she can to keep him safe. Mr. A. screams some unintelligible words into the phone and hangs up.

Ms. P. is very concerned both about the safety of Mr. A.'s father and the harm to Mr. A. if he acts on his impulse (jail, remorse, and so forth). She decides to inform the police, telling the dispatcher that Mr. A. is a psychotherapy patient in her private practice who is threatening to kill his father. She adds that Mr. A. has only just begun to acknowledge some painful memories and that he is primarily depressed and anxious. Although Mr. A. stated that he has a weapon, Ms. P. does not know for certain that this is the case. What prompts immediate concern is that he is very depressed, agitated, and intoxicated and thus may not be able to control his impulses as he might when sober.

Case Discussion/Questions to Consider

Using the decision-making framework from Chapter 2 and the information in this chapter, analyze this case. What ethical principles are important and why? Did Ms. P. have any alternative courses of action? Take into account the following concerns and describe the part they play in your analysis of the case.

1. Under what sorts of conditions is a breach in confidentiality warranted?
2. How might trust be reestablished after the danger has resolved?
3. What are the implications of alerting the police about Mr. A.'s threats if he has experienced failure in past treatment attempts?

CASE STUDY 5: A CHILD AT RISK

Jane Elder, a psychiatric nurse practitioner, is following Harriet Little, a 54-year-old married mother of two daughters. Her daughter Jackie is age 25 and her daughter Anna is age 28. Ms. Little has a major depressive disorder and meets with Ms. Elder for weekly supportive psychotherapy and medications. They have worked together for 3 years. Ms. Little's recent concern has been around her daughter Jackie, who has a long-standing problem with alcohol and drug abuse. Jackie has been separated from the father of her 3-year-old son Jeremy for the last year. Jackie's substance use resulted in Jeremy's father seeking and being granted full custody of Jeremy. For the past 3 months, Ms. Little's daughter Jackie has been able to have Jeremy for weekend overnights as she has documented to the court guardian that she has been in rehab and has had clean urine screens.

Jackie brought Jeremy to a recent holiday family visit and was observed to be slurring her words and getting into arguments. This renewed concerns that Jackie was again using substances. After Jackie left the gathering, Ms. Little's other daughter confirmed that Jackie was using substances while Jeremy was in her care. As Ms. Little related this in a therapy session, Ms. Elder reminded Ms. Little that as a mandated reporter Ms. Elder was legally bound to report abuse and neglect to the authorities. Ms. Little became distraught, crying "What about confidentiality?"

Case Discussion/Questions to Consider

Using the ethical decision-making framework from Chapter 2, the information in this chapter, and knowledge about your own state or country's rules for reporting potential or actual child abuse, analyze this case. What ethical principles are important and why? Pay particular attention to any potential conflicts between existing child abuse laws and the ethical actions of Jane Elder, the psychiatric APN.

1. What would be important to convey to Ms. Little in this situation?
2. What are the issues of patient confidentiality here?

Discussion Questions

1. Your patient, Mr. Benson, suffers from bipolar disorder. When he experiences a manic phase, he refuses to take his medicine. He typically goes on buying sprees and puts himself and his family (wife and one child) at economic risk. Last time this happened they were evicted for nonpayment of rent. His sister has taken them in several times when this happened but says she will not do it again. When his disorder is managed, he experiences remorse and regret about his risky behavior. As his long-term psychotherapist, you have decided to talk to him about a psychiatric advance directive. How would you go about discussing this with him?

2. In some Western countries, the use of drugs to either control behavior or enhance performance has escalated. Although the use of behavior-controlling drugs has been shown to be beneficial for some with extreme behavioral symptoms—calming behavior and permitting a child to focus on their studies—critics claim they are overused. The overuse is claimed to be fueled partly by pharmaceutical company interests and partly by demands from teachers and parents that something be done about a child's disruptive behavior.

   You are a psychiatric APN working in a child and family counseling group practice. Mr. and Ms. Witsend bring their 7-year-old child Timmy to be evaluated for what the teacher called "over exuberant behavior" in need of medications.

   What are your responsibilities related to these sorts of questions?

What sorts of knowledge will be helpful?
What ethical principles might be helpful and why?
How will you proceed?

References

American Nurses Association. (2001). *Code of ethics for nurses with interpretive statements*. Washington, DC: Author.

Atkinson, J. (2007). *Advance directives in mental health*. London, UK: Jessica Kingsley Publishers.

Benedict, S. (2003). Killing while caring: The nurses of Hadamar. *Issues in Mental Health Nursing, 24*(1), 59–79.

Buchanan, A., & Brock, D. (1989). *Deciding for others: The ethics of surrogate decision-making*. New York, NY: Cambridge University Press.

Chodoff, P. (1999). The case for involuntary hospitalization of the mentally ill. In T. Beauchamp & L. Walters (Eds.), *Contemporary issues in bioethics* (pp. 105–115). Belmont, CA: Wadsworth. Original work published in 1976, *American Journal of Psychiatry, 133*, 496–501.

Culver, C., & Gert, B. (1982). *Philosophy in medicine. Conceptual and ethical issues in medicine and psychiatry*. New York, NY: Oxford University Press.

Doris, J. M., & The Moral Psychology Research Group. (2010). *The moral psychology handbook*. New York, NY: Oxford University Press.

Eagleman, D. (2011). *Incognito: The secret lives of the brain*. New York, NY: Random House.

Fawcett, J. (1984). The metaparadigm of nursing: Present status and future refinements . . . for theory development. *Image, 16*(3), 84–87.

Grace, P. (2005). Ethical issues relevant to health promotion. In C. Edelman & C. L. Mandle (Eds.), *Health promotion throughout the lifespan* (6th ed., pp. 100–125). St. Louis, MO: Elsevier/Mosby.

Green, S., & Bloch, S. (2006). *An anthology of psychiatric ethics*. New York, NY: Oxford University Press.

Gutheil, T., & Gabbard, G. (2006). The concept of boundaries in clinical practice: Theoretical and risk-management dimensions. In S. Green & S. Bloch (Eds.), *An anthology of psychiatric ethics* (pp. 60–66). New York, NY: Oxford University Press. Original work published in 1993, *American Journal of Psychiatry, 150*, 188–196.

Gutheil, T., & Simon, R. (2003). Abandonment of patients in split treatment. *Harvard Review of Psychiatry, 11*, 175–179.

Halter, M. (2008). Perceived characteristics of psychiatric nurses: Stigma by association. *Archives of Psychiatric Nursing, 22*(1), 20–26.

Hardy, T. (2001/1874). *Far from the madding crowd*. New York, NY: Random House.

Howell, T., Diamond, J., & Wikler, D. (1982). Is there a case for voluntary commitment? In T. L. Beauchamp & L. R. Walters (Eds.), *Contemporary issues in bioethics* (2nd ed., pp. 163–168). Belmont, CA: Wadsworth.

International Council of Nurses. (2008). *Position statement: Mental health.* Geneva: Author. Retrieved from http://www.icn.ch/images/stories/documents/publications/position_statements/A09_Mental_Health.pdf

International Council of Nurses. (2012). *Code of ethics for nurses.* Geneva: Author. Retrieved from http://www.icn.ch/about-icn/code-of-ethics-for-nurses/

Kahneman, D. (2011). *Thinking, fast and slow.* New York, NY: Farrar, Straus & Giroux.

Kelves, D. (1999). Eugenics and human rights. *British Medical Journal, 319,* 435–438.

Kneisl, C., Wilson, H., & Trigoboff, E. (2004). *Contemporary psychiatric-mental health nursing.* Upper Saddle River, NJ: Pearson/Prentice Hall.

Lavin, M. (1986). Ulysses contracts. *Journal of Applied Philosophy, 3,* 89–101.

Meynen, G. (2010). Free will and mental disorder: Exploring the relationship. *Theoretical Medical Ethics, 31,* 429–443.

Orlando, I. (1961). *The dynamic nurse-patient relationship: Function, process, and principles.* New York, NY: Putnam.

Payton, S. (1992). The concept of the person in the Parens Patriae jurisdiction over previously competent persons. *Journal of Medicine and Philosophy, 17*(6), 605–645.

Peplau, H. (1952). *Interpersonal relations in nursing.* New York, NY: Putnam.

Perraud, S., Delaney, K., Carlson-Sabelli, L., Johnson, M., Shephard, R., & Paun, O. (2006). Advanced practice psychiatric mental health nursing, finding our core: The therapeutic relationship in the 21st century. *Perspectives in Psychiatric Care, 42*(4), 215–226.

Sadler, J. (2007). The psychiatric significance of the personal self. *Psychiatry, 70*(2), 113–129.

Tarasoff v. Regents of University of California. (1976, July 1). California Supreme Court 131. California Reporter, 14.

Travelbee, J. (1966). *Interpersonal aspects of nursing.* Philadelphia, PA: F. A. Davis.

Wakefield, J. (1992). The concept of mental disorder: On the boundary between biological facts and social values. *American Psychologist, 47,* 373–388.

Willis, D. G., Grace, P. J., & Roy, C. (2008). A central unifying focus for the discipline: Facilitating humanization, meaning, choice, quality of life and healing in living and dying. *Advances in Nursing Science, 31*(1), 28–40.

Winston, M., Winston, S., Appelbaum, P., & Rhoden, N. (1982). Case studies: Can a subject consent to a "Ulysses Contract"? *Hastings Center Report, 12*(4), 26–28.

CHAPTER 12

Nursing Ethics and Advanced Practice in the Anesthesia and Perioperative Period

Gregory Sheedy, John Welch, and Brian T. Sim

Don't be afraid. Remember I'm here. The noise in the street will soon disappear. When the soft eyes of mercy are blinded by the dark. I will stay with eyes open, stay here with eyes open, to watch over you and take away the sadness and the fear. I'll be here.

—THE OCTOBER PROJECT, 1993

Introduction

In the United States, nurse anesthetists provide a significant proportion of anesthesia care. This is also true of specially trained nurses in various countries. In addition to nurse anesthetists, other advanced practice nurses (APNs) are also involved in the perioperative period. For example, clinical nurse specialists, acute care nurse practitioners, and nurse managers may all have responsibilities based on their role as defined in a given country. The authors of this chapter are all certified registered nurse anesthetists (CRNAs), the official designation in the United States for nurses who are specially educated to provide anesthesia. For this reason, the acronym CRNA is used throughout the chapter, although as evidenced by the existence of the International Federation of Nurse Anesthetists (2013), nurses in many other countries also practice anesthesia. Nurse anesthetists, regardless of country, are faced with complex and critical decision making as a normal part of their practice of providing anesthesia care to patients. Many of these decisions must be made before a patient enters the operating room (OR) suite, and they involve some of the most difficult life issues. For example, CRNAs may have to help patients understand that they have the right to refuse life-sustaining treatment and what that means in the context of surgery and anesthesia delivery, assist patients in deciding whether to participate in controversial procedures, determine if patients are capable of giving consent for procedures, and protect patients from incompetent or dangerous healthcare providers. *Timing* is a key concept that lends a particular urgent quality to ethical decision making in anesthesia practice.

The decision for a patient to have a surgical procedure is most often determined before the anesthesia provider is introduced to the patient. In many cases, the nurse anesthetist is asked to rapidly assess the patient and proceed to surgery with minimal delay. Some of these cases involve patients whose likelihood of survival or of sustaining a reasonable quality of life after surgery is in doubt, yet no code status has been established, nor have discussions of medical futility occurred. CRNAs are often faced with problems caused by communication failures earlier in a patient's evaluation or treatment process and by the patient's lack of knowledge about the anesthesia process or about his or her medical problems.

Production pressure and moving patients through the OR in as little time as possible are realities of current-day delivery of surgical services, at least in the United States. Patients are sometimes treated as if they were commodities; they become products instead of being the focus of personalized surgical care. This creates an environment where any anesthesia care provider may be requested to participate in activities that conflict with personal and professional beliefs about what constitutes good care and their understood primary ethical obligations to the patient. Conflicts among the surgical care team members, colleagues, and surgeons develop as a result of different perspectives on what is the appropriate ethical treatment of patients requiring surgery.

Ethical conflicts in the context of anesthesia practice may also involve parties other than the anesthesia provider, the surgeon, and the patient. Primary care physicians, nurse practitioners, perioperative nurses, family members, legal counsel, patient proxies, legal guardians, and other consulting healthcare providers may also have a stake in a patient's operative and anesthesia course. Imagine the difficulty in resolving a disagreement between an appointed guardian of an incompetent patient who insists on surgery for his client, a primary care physician who insists that surgery is not consistent with the plan for comfort care, and a surgeon who has a small window of opportunity to perform the surgery because of a busy schedule.

The nurse anesthetist is placed under enormous pressure to fulfill the wishes of multiple parties while trying to advocate that the patient receive appropriate care.

Ethical dilemmas and problems arise with such frequency in the clinical practice of nurse anesthetists that becoming familiar with the facets of the ethical decision-making process is essential for facilitating good care of patients. Additionally, because of the everyday nature of many of the barriers to good (i.e., ethical) anesthesia care, overcoming obstacles and resolving problems are inescapable professional responsibilities of all CRNAs and cannot be left to ethics experts. Although ethics experts and resources can provide expertise in especially difficult cases, the nurse anesthetist best knows what constitutes good anesthesia practice for a given patient. For this reason, it is important for all CRNAs to develop confidence in their ethical decision making.

The subsequent sections of this chapter explore ethical issues of particular concern to CRNA and perianesthesia practice. Each section makes use of a key ethical principle and discusses the interplay of other ethical principles in relation to the main responsibility of practice, thus facilitating the patient's good. A case study is presented to illustrate an ethical dilemma, problem, or topic of particular concern in anesthesia practice, and then the case is analyzed, relevant ethical elements are discussed, and questions are raised. This method is designed both to provide practice in ethical analysis and to assist the CRNA in developing confidence in his or her knowledge and abilities related to ethical issues in practice.

Do-Not-Resuscitate Orders During Surgery

DNRs and the Principle of Autonomy

Do-not-resuscitate orders, or DNR orders as they are commonly called, are an apparatus by which patients are spared unwanted heroic measures in the event of a cardiac or cardiopulmonary arrest (Margolis, McGrath, Kussin, & Schwinn, 1995). Anecdotally, many healthcare providers still seem to assume that a patient's DNR directive is not valid or applicable when a patient is having surgery. Many of the anesthesia processes commonly used in surgery affect the respiratory and circulatory systems, requiring respiratory and circulatory support—the very interventions that a DNR exists to prevent. Although there is increasing awareness that DNR orders can cause problems of interpretation in the OR, and that patients have rights to make their own decisions about what medical care they will or will not accept, much confusion remains about this particular issue. Anesthesia providers often do not understand what their role should be in advising patients, and patients often do not have an appropriate understanding of what is at stake. The ethical principle of autonomy is at the forefront of ethical discussions and policy formation around the topic of honoring DNR orders during surgery and anesthesia. The ethical content of this frequently encountered issue is a conflict between the obligation to honor a patient's self-determination (i.e., autonomy) and the obligation to prevent harm (i.e., nonmaleficence) to the patient and provide beneficial care. The main questions are: What is beneficial care in each case? What is the relationship of beneficial care to a patient's autonomous choice of action?

The ethical principle of autonomy essentially argues that a patient should be free to make his or her own decisions according to his or her own will and without undue influence from others (Beauchamp & Childress, 2012). Two conditions are almost universally agreed upon as needed for autonomous decision making: (1) a level of freedom from controlling forces and (2) the capacity to make independent choices (Beauchamp & Childress, 2012).

For individuals to make an autonomous decision, then, they must not be coerced into their decision or experience other factors that limit their liberty to make a decision, such as being imprisoned or serving in the armed forces. Additionally, a person with a severe mental handicap or a person with physical or cognitive impediments to the adequate processing of information cannot make informed decisions (because the person lacks the necessary capacity for intentional action) (Beauchamp & Childress, 2012). However, even patients who are deemed incompetent or who lack the mental capacity to make mature and meaningful decisions about complex healthcare issues are permitted to make autonomous decisions for less critical matters, such as what to eat or what to wear (Beauchamp & Childress, 2012) and may be allowed to make decisions that, even if not adequately processed, are unlikely to cause harm.

There are also people who would not be deemed incompetent and who clearly have the necessary intellect to make informed, autonomous decisions, yet who appear to lack an understanding of the implications involved in a proposed course of action, perhaps because of situational stressors affecting their ability to reason or deeply rooted ideas that are not easily amenable to change. Responsibilities for identifying and addressing this problem also fall to the CRNA charged with providing anesthesia for the patient.

DNRs and The Patient Self-Determination Act

Chapter 3 discusses the Patient Self-Determination Act (PSDA) in more detail; it is also pertinent here. The PSDA became law in the United States in 1991. It mandated that all hospitals accepting Medicare funding offer written information concerning patients' rights to make decisions concerning their health care and their right to consent to or refuse medical treatment (Smith, 2000). This act was meant to, and did, stimulate increased interest in the idea of facilitating autonomous choice in healthcare decision making. In many other countries, even where this right is not protected by legislation, it is acknowledged via the country's membership in the United Nations (UN) and acceptance of the values articulated in the UN's 1948 Declaration of Human Rights. In recent years, there has been an upsurge in the medical and nursing literature nationally and internationally of discussions concerning a patient's right to self-determination with special attention to advance directives and DNR status (Margolis et al., 1995), although many forces still work against the reality of patients' wishes being adequately informed or accounted for.

Advance directives are instructions created by an adult patient used to indicate to physicians, nurses, and healthcare workers the kind of care that the patient would want to receive in the event that he or she cannot make decisions or is unlikely to participate effectively in decision making in the future. DNR orders are a specific type of advance directive used during the event of a cardiopulmonary arrest. This section deals particularly with the advance directive of DNR orders in the patient who is receiving anesthesia.

DNRs and Policy

Professional associations are among those that have addressed this topic and formulated policy statements accordingly. Such policy statements are designed to ensure that proper attention is given to a patient's needs for information so that the patient is facilitated in making choices for care that fit his or her values and beliefs rather than those of providers. Policy statements are meant to provide guidance to professionals about acceptable standards and expectations of behavior.

The American Association of Nurse Anesthetists (AANA) adopted a policy in 1994 that rejects the notion of automatically suspending DNR orders during surgery and instead recommends that the DNR status of the patient be readdressed before proceeding to surgery (AANA, 2004). In essence, the AANA recommends that the patient, or proxy, be allowed to discuss the specific aspects of the DNR order. It advises accurate documentation in the patient's chart of all agreed-upon interventions, including those that are to be withheld, and suggests provider–patient discussions during which specific circumstances under which interventions will be performed or withheld are determined. Additionally, the point at which DNR orders are to be reinstated postoperatively is defined (AANA, 2004).

The American Society of Anesthesiologists (ASA) also has a policy for requiring that DNR orders be readdressed instead of automatically suspended when proceeding with surgery (Palmer & Jackson, 2003). The ASA offers three alternatives to the DNR order during the perioperative period: (1) full suspension of code status intraoperatively and in the immediate postoperative period, (2) only certain procedures may be carried out that are deemed essential to the success of the procedure, and (3) the anesthesia provider uses his or her judgment about what constitutes appropriate interventions during the intraoperative period while the patient is receiving anesthesia and in the postoperative period based on an informed understanding of the patient's wishes (ASA, 2001).

The Association of periOperative Registered Nurses (AORN) has issued a statement similar to the preceding ones, except that the AORN declares in its position statement that each nurse has the right to withdraw from participating in a situation where the reconsideration of DNR orders is in moral conflict with his or her beliefs. However, the responsibility of that nurse to ensure the availability of a replacement is highlighted (AORN, 2009). Furthermore, such decisions should only be made with careful consideration that "moral objections by the nurse do not include personal preference, prejudice, convenience, or arbitrariness" (American Nurses Association [ANA], 2006).

DNRs and Required Reconsideration

A term used frequently when addressing the matter of DNR orders in the OR is *required reconsideration*, which essentially means that although a DNR order is a legitimate order and must be honored as such, there are circumstances, such as undergoing a surgical procedure and anesthesia, that require a reexamination of this order to ensure that a patient's wishes about and need for care are met and that a patient's caregiver is not placed in any ethically compromising positions (Cohen & Cohen, 1991).

Despite the increased attention to the issue and the body of literature addressing DNRs during surgery, many institutions still suspend DNR orders during surgery and do not have a policy of required reconsideration or any clear strategies to ensure that a patient's right to self-determination is sustained (Fallat & Deshpande, 2004). Indeed, a dilemma almost inevitably arises in the absence of guidelines because certain types of anesthesia cause autonomic and metabolic suppression, requiring what would in nonanesthesia settings be considered resuscitative efforts. This fact of anesthetic agents is not reconcilable with an order that is created to prevent resuscitative interventions. Many patients do not understand this paradox because they do not have an adequate understanding of what is entailed in using anesthesia. It is counterintuitive to insist that someone not be resuscitated during general anesthesia when general anesthesia causes a state where a patient must be mechanically ventilated to sustain oxygenation (Margolis et al., 1995). This question of compatibility between a DNR request and the nature of traditional anesthetic practice has been a source of confusion and misunderstanding for both healthcare providers and patients who do not wish to be resuscitated but who require surgery that necessitates general anesthesia.

The principle of autonomy declares that individuals have the right to determine what will be done with their bodies and to base this determination on their own set of beliefs and values (Fry, Veatch, & Taylor, 2010). According to this principle, the nurse anesthetist is obligated to recognize the validity of any request to withhold an intervention that is life saving or life sustaining, whether or not the CRNA agrees with a patient's reasoning, given a competent adult patient or a proxy whose decision is informed by the patient's values. This reflects a modern approach to ethical standards and a movement away from a more paternalistic style, where a healthcare professional would ultimately influence the decisions made concerning a patient's health care (Roberts, Geppert, Warner, Green Hammond, & Lamberton, 2005).

Does this mean that health providers must consider every decision made by a patient as worthy of honoring simply because it was "self-determined"? How strict should the criteria be for self-determination? After all, APNs have advanced training, education, and often years of clinical experience. Using sound clinical judgment, they often make difficult clinical decisions that a layperson would lack the knowledge to make. Therefore, it might be reasonable to ask if this current trend away from paternalistic health care is warranted. Is a patient's healthcare decision-making ability comparable to that of an advanced healthcare professional? A strict believer in the principle of autonomy might be inclined to support a seemingly autonomous decision of a patient without making a concerted effort to ensure that the patient understands that the agreed-upon course of action cannot meet his or her real needs. The nurse anesthetist is therefore obligated to undertake special efforts to ensure that patients and their families understand the purpose of a DNR order and the reason that they have such an order, and must seek to clarify any misconceptions surrounding such an order. This will become salient with the discussion in the first case study presented.

This first case study presented illustrates a conflict related to honoring patient autonomy. In this case, the obligation of nonmaleficence (i.e., preventing or doing no harm) seems to be in conflict with the responsibility to provide a beneficial treatment for the patient.

CASE STUDY 1: DNR IN A HEALTHY PATIENT

Tina is a 37-year-old woman who is employed at an unspecified type of healthcare facility. She arrives at the hospital's operating department to have a gynecological procedure done laparoscopically. This procedure requires general anesthesia with an endotracheal tube. Tina's medical history is simple. She has a history of asthma as a child with no recurrences in many years, takes only oral contraceptives and multivitamins, and has never received general anesthesia before. Tina has a DNR order signed by her and her primary care doctor, which lists the prohibition of cardiopulmonary resuscitation (CPR), vasoactive drugs, and airway intubation in the event of a cardiopulmonary arrest. Tina has no known cardiac abnormalities and has never had a cardiac event. There seems to be no medical data to support her decision to be a DNR patient.

Karen is the nurse anesthetist assigned to this case and she discusses this DNR order with Tina prior to surgery. Tina requests that Karen perform some form of anesthesia other than general anesthesia with an endotracheal tube because she "under no circumstances wants to be intubated." Karen instructs Tina that general anesthesia with an endotracheal tube is the common accepted practice for delivering a safe anesthetic during a laparoscopic procedure and, although it is possible to perform the procedure under spinal or epidural anesthesia, purely regional techniques are uncommon and typically utilized only with patients who are unfit to receive general anesthesia. Tina reluctantly agrees to be intubated for her surgery but insists on not changing any of the conditions of her DNR order, stating that she does not want to spend the rest of her life "on a breathing machine." Efforts by Karen to discuss the use of resuscitative drugs and other measures during the unlikely event of a cardiopulmonary arrest are unsuccessful in persuading Tina to amend her DNR status for her surgery. Karen tries to differentiate between vasoactive medications used for treating transient hypotension during anesthesia and the drugs and doses that are used during a cardiac arrest, with the intention of being clear about what Tina's requests are for her anesthesia care. Tina insists that she sees no difference and repeats her demand that her DNR be honored as it is. Karen is unable to resolve this conflict between honoring Tina's request and her duty as a CRNA to provide safe anesthesia. Karen declines to participate in Tina's surgery, and it is ultimately canceled.

Questions to Consider

1. Is Karen justified in refusing to participate in this case?
2. Is Tina's DNR order valid, and should it be honored here?
3. How could this situation have been resolved with both Karen's and Tina's autonomy respected?
4. Do CRNAs, as a group, have a responsibility to educate primary care healthcare practitioners about how to advise their patients on issues related to DNR orders and anesthesia?

Case Discussion

Although at first glance the case seems to demonstrate a conflict between the autonomy of the patient and the judgment of the practitioner, this conception misplaces the problem. Moreover, even if we recognize that a person such as Tina has the innate right to determine her own actions, this right is constrained by the fact that individuals are at times placed in a position where they are dependent on others to carry out their wishes (Fry et al., 2010). This is especially true in healthcare settings. Patients are dependent on providers to perform procedures that patients cannot carry out themselves. If it is taken as a given that Tina needs the surgery, then the question becomes whether there is enough information to determine if Tina's request can really be considered autonomous. What criteria would it have to meet? What are Karen's responsibilities here? What alternatives or strategies might resolve the situation?

Tina has a right to expect that her best interests would be the primary concern of the CRNA. It is assumed that Tina does need the laparoscopy.

However, she may not need it urgently, which would give Karen time to work with her further. There is no obvious reason to believe, given Tina's health history, that a general anesthetic would be directly harmful to her. However, there seems to be more to this story than meets the eye. Is Karen violating her obligation to "do good" here by refusing to administer her anesthesia?

Clearly Karen is not comfortable performing a solely regional anesthesia technique (spinal or epidural) for Tina, even though regional anesthesia has been used successfully in patients having laparoscopic gallbladder surgery (Imbelloni, Sant'Anna, Fornasari, & Fiahlo, 2011). The likely reason is that Tina is a healthy patient with no pulmonary disease, and Karen sees no clear indication for performing an anesthesia technique typically reserved for patients who are unfit for general anesthesia (Gramatica et al., 2002).

Perhaps Karen is focusing primarily on "avoiding harm" by refusing to be an agent of a possible, however unlikely, morbid outcome while being constrained by an order not to intervene in a proper manner. But the direct result is that the surgery is not performed, whether because of a shortage of willing anesthesia personnel or because of a busy OR schedule, and Tina will either have to reconsider her DNR status during surgery or find a willing participant to accept her conditions as they are. Alternatively, a plan could be devised to discover what Tina's fears are. However, it is unlikely that these could be addressed in the short window of time available.

Tina is not the type of patient who commonly presents with a DNR order. Usually, DNR orders are written for patients with a terminal illness or a health status tenuous enough that heroic measures of any kind could result in irreversible limitations to a patient's quality of living. However, in either case, when a patient makes a decision concerning his or her own health care, including anesthesia care, that appears to be based on fear, bias, or a deficit in medical knowledge, even though he or she may otherwise be considered competent, the nurse anesthetist is faced with making a judgment about the validity and efficacy of the decision and what to do next.

Clear communication with the patient and consideration of all the ethical elements of such situations are critical before proceeding with cases like this. As mentioned previously, the CRNA is obligated to clarify misunderstandings surrounding a patient's DNR order before proceeding with surgery. Indeed, the nurse anesthetist is obligated to assist a patient or the patient's family member in understanding the DNR order, especially when it appears that some knowledge deficit resulting from a communication problem or a lack of knowledge concerning DNR orders is present. At some point, Tina's reasons for making herself a DNR patient despite her good health will have to be addressed or this issue is likely to repeat itself with no foreseeable resolution.

Indeed, many patients with DNR orders have morbidities and prognoses that are consistent with such an order. This group of patients is increasingly having surgery for palliative treatment or other procedures that are meant to improve or sustain quality of life, rather than as a curative intervention (Margolis et al., 1995). In fact, it is estimated that 15% of patients with active DNR orders undergo surgical procedures (Margolis et al., 1995). The risk of morbidity during surgery for these patients is obviously much higher than for the collective population, but the benefit of maintaining some quality of life outweighs the risk of death. The next case is an example of honoring a patient's autonomy when the risk of morbidity is high.

CASE STUDY 2: RECONSIDERATION OF A DNR ORDER IN A HIGH-RISK PATIENT

Dan is a 91-year-old man with extensive cardiac, vascular, and pulmonary disease who comes to the ambulatory surgery center to have a cataract removed from his right eye. Dan has suffered two myocardial infarctions, the last one 18 months ago, which occurred postoperatively after he had an endovascular repair of an abdominal aortic aneurysm (AAA). Presently, Dan is very limited in his activities and spends the majority of his time lying or sitting. He is able to ambulate only for short periods in his house before becoming short of breath. His most recent development is an intraluminal leak in his endovascular repair of his AAA, which has drastically increased the size of his aneurysm, and the risk of rupture has been deemed "imminent" by his vascular surgeon "if not immediately repaired."

Dan has refused surgery for his AAA and has an advance directive consisting of a DNR order in the event of a cardiac and respiratory arrest that states that he likely would not survive another surgery and that he has "had enough." Dan is consenting to have this cataract surgery because he is having trouble reading the newspaper, and his wife affirms that he "lives to read about his favorite sports teams." Dan was a coach of a high school baseball and football team for more than 40 years, and he states that he lives for sports.

The anesthesia interventions that were discussed with him during his preoperative screening are intravenous (IV) sedation in addition to a nerve block using local anesthetic that would be instilled into the retrobulbar region of his eye. The retrobulbar block is to be performed by the surgeon in this case, but in many cases the anesthesia provider actually performs it. Dan has refused to amend any of the conditions of his DNR order for surgery.

Ben is a nurse anesthetist who is being supervised by an attending anesthesiologist, Dr. Glen. Dr. Glen recommends that the anesthesia department not get involved in this case. Ben is worried because he believes that a member of the anesthesia department would be best equipped to provide support in this case. Dr. Glen contacted Dan's vascular surgeon concerning the status of his aortic aneurysm and was told by the vascular surgeon that Dan is a very high-risk patient and that an aortic rupture is very likely without treatment. Dr. Glen suggests that the surgeon performing the cataract surgery administer the local anesthetic without sedation and proceed without the assistance of anesthesia personnel. He argues that there would be limited benefit from anesthesia because the injection of even small doses of sedating medications may be an unnecessary risk compared to their benefit and that this intervention is occasionally done without any anesthesia in other settings.

Ben disagrees with Dr. Glen and believes that allaying any pain or anxiety during the injection of local anesthetic and during surgery would be beneficial to the patient and could even prevent an ischemic cardiac event. Dr. Glen elects not to participate in this case and is replaced by a different anesthesiologist, Dr. Stuart, who agrees with Ben's position. IV sedation is administered during the retrobulbar block, and Dan's requirement for further sedatives during his operation is minimal. Dan is transferred to the recovery room after his procedure, breathing room air spontaneously. He is discharged to home 1 hour later.

Questions to Consider

1. Did Ben's decision to give Dan anesthesia comply with the conditions of Dan's DNR order?
2. Under what conditions might Ben's position be justifiable/unjustifiable?
3. Was Dr. Glen justified in his decision to withdraw from the case?
4. What conditions could you change to make Dr. Glen's position justifiable/unjustifiable?

5. Would Ben be justified in administering CPR or other resuscitative drugs and measures, such as mechanical ventilation, against the expressed will of Dan in the event of an accidental overdose of sedating medication?

6. What is Ben's obligation to ensure that Dan fully understands the consequences of refusing resuscitative treatment during this procedure?

Case Discussion

Unlike the patient in Case Study 1, Dan's decision to have a DNR order written is not in question given his health status, his understanding of what would be involved, and his goals. However, Dan's risk is infinitely higher than the previous patient's. Thus, Ben's decision to participate in Dan's case is difficult because there is a greater likelihood of a morbid outcome than in the Case 1 example. However, a focus on Dan's considered goals and the professional goals of nurse anesthesia practice (facilitating Dan's good) in this case justifies Ben's participation and could even be considered a moral responsibility of good practice.

All went well with the case, but even if it had not, Ben's decision is justified because Dan understands the risks and is willing to assume them to get a better quality of life. Ben's clinical judgment is that he could provide a *beneficial* intervention that would lower the risk that an increased cardiac output, caused by the pain and anxiety of the procedure, would cause cardiac ischemia, infarction, or rupture of the aneurysm.

What is Dr. Glen's professional responsibility? Is he acting unethically in refusing to take part? Interestingly, whereas the American Medical Association's (2001) code of medical ethics provision VI states, "A physician shall, in the provision of appropriate patient care, except in emergencies, be free to choose whom to serve, with whom to associate, and the environment in which to provide medical care," the ANA's code of ethics does not support a nurse's freedom to choose whom to serve.

Alternatively, perhaps Dr. Glen's refusal is based on a conscientious objection (discussed in detail in Chapter 3) to causing physical harm. Would this be warranted in Dan's case? Is Dr. Glen unjustified in suggesting that the patient should not receive any additional anesthesia after the surgeon provides the retrobulbar block? Dr. Glen seems to be trying to avoid harm to Dan by withholding an intervention that poses some physical risk, which in this case is IV sedation. However, Dr. Glen may be more concerned with his own well-being than the patient's. He might be fearful of being "linked" to a risky procedure—retrobulbar block poses a risk of bradycardia, which can be catastrophic to a patient like Dan if not immediately treated—rather than raising a conscientious objection to it (Morgan, Mikhail, & Murray, 2002).

It could be argued that Ben's decision to proceed is careless or negligent because of the risks involved with IV sedation in an elderly patient. Because Ben is the experienced healthcare professional, his responsibility is to ascertain what Dan knows and what measures he would agree to in the event of a problem. Then, Dan's DNR order would reflect this discussion and the agreed-upon interventions should an episode of bradycardia or even apnea occur (Morgan et al., 2002).

This case is another example of the constraints in honoring a patient's right to make decisions concerning his or her own health care. Dan likely possesses little or no knowledge of the complications of a retrobulbar block, and he appears not to be interested in hearing them at the time of his surgery. However, it could be argued that poor timing is at fault. These possibilities should be introduced when the patient has time to process the information. Ben has to determine if Dan actually understood the possible complication of this surgery and anesthetic, or if Dan was simply being recalcitrant out of fear that his wishes would not be honored if he agrees to compromise his DNR order or because of a feeling that he could not trust the providers. The manner in which patients are addressed or engaged in discussion frequently makes a difference in their willingness or ability to process information and make an informed decision.

DNR Orders in Incompetent Patients

Some patients do not have the capacity to decide for themselves whether they want DNR orders to be instated and what the specifics of these orders should be. These patients are deemed to be mentally incompetent, from a chronic mental illness, an acute traumatic brain injury, a progressive mental illness, or because the patient is a child with a terminal illness. In these cases, a competent surrogate or parent must represent the patient's interests. Sometimes this can be ascertained by understanding the previous beliefs, values, and goals of the patient, although for some persons there may be no such available knowledge.

The related principles used for decision making are similar to those employed when dealing with patients who are able to make competent decisions concerning their health care, but the circumstances may make the decision-making process much more complex. Problems can arise when what the surrogate proposes conflicts with what are perceived to be the patient's likely wishes, and/or a caregiver objects to what the surrogate proposes, or the healthcare team does not feel that what is proposed is likely to benefit the patient and may cause harm. In these situations, it may be necessary to involve authorities who are not immediately involved in the issue and who have the skills to provide a balanced perspective. Institutions often have an ethics resource or committee that can be helpful. But in other cases when a resolution cannot be achieved and there is significant risk to the patient's interests, the legal system may be needed to provide advice or mediation.

DNR Orders in Pediatric Patients

The matter of DNRs in the pediatric patient deserves further mention here. The PSDA, which requires hospitals to recognize patients' rights to make their own decisions about their health care, does not address the needs of the pediatric patient (Fallat & Deshpande, 2004). A recent survey of anesthesiologists and surgeons revealed that less than half of those surveyed collectively felt that the institutions where they worked had effective policies in place for pediatric patients whose medical status requires a DNR order (Fallat & Deshpande, 2004).

The purpose of a DNR order for a pediatric patient undergoing surgery is to prevent resuscitative measures that would provide no clear benefit to the patient and possibly prolong a poor quality of life (Fallat & Deshpande, 2004). This assumes that a cardiopulmonary arrest is the direct result of a terminal illness. However, as mentioned earlier, like the surgery itself, the anesthesia process may place an additional strain on the pediatric patient, and an arrest can be precipitated in the course of anesthesia induction. Some anesthesia providers view DNR orders in a pediatric patient as a breach of the obligation of nonmaleficence (i.e., doing no harm) because it prevents intervention in the event that death occurs. Others, however, take it to be harmful to prolong a child's poor quality of life with heroic measures (Fallat & Deshpande, 2004). The basis for either perspective needs to be justified in terms of what definitions of suffering and harm are being used by the parties, and who should be the ultimate decision maker.

It is easy to see here that the sensitivity inherent in dealing with the pediatric population and their families necessitates special attention to such issues. In these situations, the DNR status, as it relates to the pediatric patient having surgery, is better addressed at the time of its activation rather than readdressed or "reconsidered" at the time of surgery. This allows more time for the family to discuss with providers what constitutes resuscitative efforts during anesthesia and surgery and to consider what treatments, if any, can reasonably be withheld during the perioperative period. This also allows a family the time to access other sources of advice or information so that they can be comfortable with their decision.

As with adults, the importance of discussing in detail the goals of the family and the patient as they relate to the patient's illness and surgery cannot be overstated. However, it may be more useful with pediatric patients to have a procedure-directed focus to avoid any ambiguity (Fallat & Deshpande, 2004). The parent or surrogate of the pediatric patient should be provided with a detailed list of interventions that are commonly utilized during anesthesia and those that are utilized during a cardiopulmonary arrest. Perhaps a good strategy is to offer booklets for parents and guardians that show some of the more common or likely anesthesia protocols. The purpose is to show the crossover of interventions between what can be considered common medical and airway techniques to achieve stable hemodynamics during anesthesia and those that are used under more emergent circumstances. Such interventions could include endotracheal intubation or reintubation, tracheostomy, vasoactive medications, chest compressions, IV fluid therapy, blood transfusions, IV colloid therapy, and electrical countershock (Waisel, Jackson, & Fine, 2003). The parent and child should also be assured that in the event of a suspension of DNR orders during surgery, such orders may be reinstated in the event of a full cardiopulmonary arrest or when it becomes clear that resuscitative efforts would be ineffective at producing any benefit to the child (Fallat & Deshpande, 2004).

The Jehovah's Witness Patient

Background

There are few more ethically challenging situations for healthcare professionals than patients who have religious beliefs that prevent them from accepting potentially lifesaving interventions such as blood and blood products. For example, the beliefs of Jehovah's Witnesses prevent them from accepting whole blood, packed red blood cells, platelets, white blood cells, and some forms of autotransfusion. It is not surprising that these beliefs can give rise to ethical and sometimes legal problems for healthcare providers. Hemostatic resuscitation for traumatic blood loss became common practice only during World War II (American Red Cross, 2013). Interestingly, Jehovah's Witness leaders proclaimed in 1945 that receiving such transfusions would prevent followers from eternal salvation (Benson, 1989). With over 7 million believers in 200 countries, APNs across settings and countries are likely to be faced with the ethical challenges of the Jehovah's Witness faith and its rules surrounding the relatively common perioperative practice of blood product transfusion. Anesthesia providers administer a large portion of these transfusions (Sheedy, 2009). A thorough understanding of the religion, the ethical implications and considerations, and the legal precedent surrounding transfusion in Jehovah's Witness patients can assist the CRNA, perianesthesia nurses, and other APNs in effectively navigating such challenges. Ultimately, increasing knowledge about a particular patient's beliefs enables the APN not only to provide good care but also to mitigate the moral distress providers sometimes experience when asked to withhold treatment they deem necessary for an individual's life.

Charles Russell began the Christian sect now known as Jehovah's Witness in the 1870s in Pennsylvania, distributing a religious journal, today called *The Watch Tower*, which covered biblical matter in a topical, sometimes literal, fashion. Early supporters of Russell's publication gathered to study his works and became known as the Zion's Watch Tower Tract Society, disputing mainstream beliefs about the immortality of the soul, the Holy Trinity, the return of Jesus in human form, and the concept of a fiery hell (Beckford, 1975). It was in this journal that a 1945 declaration banned the receipt of blood and blood products by the Witness faithful based on three Bible passages—Genesis 9:3,4; Leviticus 17:10–16; and Acts 15: 19–21—all of which condemned in one way or another the consumption of human flesh (Benson, 1989). A 1951 *Watch Tower* article expounded on the earlier proclamation, drawing links between IV fluids and IV feeding, concluding that a blood transfusion is the same as consuming blood (West, 2012). Members of the faith have since ardently followed the proviso with hopes of avoiding eternal damnation, even in cases where a transfusion could be lifesaving, frequently leading to judicial intervention, particularly in children, though early cases in adults form a legal precedent today.

As discussed in earlier chapters, "ethics" and "law" are separate concepts. Ethical reasoning often informs the law and precedes the development of regulations. But not all ethical issues reach the level of legislation. Moreover, legislation tends to address the general needs of humanity but does not always fit an individual case. Thus, while legal precedent and ethical decision making are not synonymous, one may sometimes be used to inform the other and can certainly aid the APN in understanding the underpinnings of the Jehovah's Witness transfusion debate (Sheedy, 2009). In the United States, most jurisdictions lack statutes concerning refusal of blood transfusion by Jehovah's Witnesses, but case law has provided some precedent from which modern healthcare providers can draw (Benson, 1989). Such precedent has followed a shift in U.S. healthcare ethics from the focus on paternalism—that is, beneficence over other ethical principles—toward a patient's autonomy (Grace, 2009). In the 1914 case of *Schloendorff v. Society of New York Hospital*, autonomy reigned supreme when the judge ruled that "Every human being of adult years and sound mind has a right to determine what shall be done with his own body." A later ruling in the 1965 case *United States v. George* stated that "The patient may knowingly decline treatment, but he may not demand mistreatment" (Benson, 1989). In many other countries the right to determine what treatment is acceptable and what is not is also considered a protected human right, given that the decision is "informed." With regard to children, however, the focus is on keeping them alive until they are of an age to determine for themselves what they want, as discussed later. The aforementioned and similar cases help define today's legal treatment of Jehovah's Witness patients. However, it is in the dichotomous nature of legal precedent and ethical decision making—seeking balance between autonomy, beneficence, and nonmaleficence—that has led healthcare providers to try to find a less ethically burdensome resolution to care of such patients.

Blood shortages, risks of disease transmission, cost of transfusion, patient refusal due to religious beliefs, and resolution of ethical dilemma have all led nurse anesthetists to seek alternatives to administration of blood products. Many surgeons have sought blood-sparing techniques in traditionally large blood-loss operations for the same reasons. Indeed, religious conviction may be one factor driving research to better understand the morbidity and mortality of tolerating lower hematocrit levels, leading to a more judicious approach to transfusion in all patients despite their spiritual beliefs. Blood-sparing techniques and transfusion alternatives notwith-standing, there are some cases where administration of blood products is the only option for saving a patient's life and the nurse anesthetist's ethical dilemma of autonomy over beneficence returns again to the fore.

Informed Consent

Most healthcare systems and settings in the developed world now recognize the importance of respecting patients as free individuals who, after being prudently informed, are allowed to make autonomous decisions about the care they are to receive. However, sometimes respecting a patient's autonomy can be perceived by the provider as conflicting with other ethical principles such as beneficence and nonmaleficence. It is the obligation of nurse anesthetists to obtain *informed consent* from adult patients or guardians of minor patients before administration of anesthesia. The process of informing, where pertinent, includes a discussion about the relative need for blood transfusion during a surgical procedure. In the case of Jehovah's Witness patients, obtaining informed anesthesia consent might also include a liability waiver pertaining to withholding blood and blood products (West, 2012). Consent and waiver may absolve the nurse anesthetist of medicolegal fallout, but what of his or her personal and professional ethical obligations? Ongoing evaluation of their own beliefs can help guide APNs when these situations arise.

If the nurse anesthetist anticipates large blood loss or suspects there may be a need for the use of blood products during an operation, an early and frank discussion should be had with the patient about his or her personal beliefs regarding transfusion (West, 2012). Every patient is unique and may hold individualized interpretations of his or her faith's tenets, so it is key to discuss the patient's specific commitment to the "no transfusion" stipulation. A question such as, "In the case where death is likely without a blood transfusion, do you still wish for these products to be withheld?" can help the nurse anesthetist assess the patient's specific wishes and present possible outcomes of refusing blood products. Alternatives to blood transfusion should also be presented. Some patients will accept albumin, immunoglobin, and clotting factor and may allow autotransfusion if the blood collection circuit has maintained continuity with the patient (Lindstrom & Johnstone, 2010).

Perhaps the most difficult task in the process of obtaining informed consent from a patient who is a Jehovah's Witness is how to assess for and avoid undue influence or coercion. A healthcare provider's personal bias and beliefs may infiltrate the discussion, creating a paternalistic relationship that impacts the patient's autonomous decision making. Information disseminated by the APN should be based in fact but allow the patient to express concerns, desires, and commitments (West, 2012). Bias and coercion may also come from a patient's family or community; it is important to provide privacy so that the patient can express his or her personal thoughts without influence from a spouse, parents, family, or members of his or her congregation (West, 2012). Providing the opportunity for a confidential and frank discussion may indeed save a patient's life.

CASE STUDY 3: A JEHOVAH'S WITNESS PATIENT AND DECISION MAKING IN THE FACE OF AMBIGUITY

Scott, a 20-year-old student, was transferred from a small community hospital 20 miles south of the city to a large metropolitan trauma center following a motorcycle crash. He was the helmeted driver of a motorcycle that was "t-boned" when a van ran a red light. Scott denied a loss of consciousness. He had a Glascow Coma Score of 15 when emergency medical services arrived on the scene. His evaluation at the sending hospital included head, neck, chest, abdomen, and pelvic computed tomography (CT) scans, which ruled out injury to all regions but one. The pelvic CT revealed a complex open-book fracture with bilateral trochanteric involvement. A pelvic binder was improvised with a hospital bed sheet; mild tachycardia responded to a liter bolus of lactated Ringer's solution, and pain was treated with 10 milligrams of morphine. Scott was transferred to a trauma center by helicopter for definitive treatment of the complex pelvic fracture. Having never been in a helicopter and being quite excited about it, he remained alert and oriented throughout transport, and despite remaining normotensive, he received a second liter of lactated Ringer's for a heart rate trending into the low 120s.

He was met by the trauma team, which included Jill, a nurse anesthetist. Primary and secondary trauma surveys confirmed the same findings as the referring hospital. It was clear Scott would require operative fixation of his complex pelvic fracture, and an orthopedic surgeon was consulted. On arrival, the orthopedic surgeon reviewed Scott's CT scan and alerted Jill to what he was sure would be a "long, bloody case." The plan was to attempt an interventional radiology procedure to stem the bleeding, but the surgeon was sure Scott would require open reduction and placement of an external fixation device. Scott remained alert, although his tachycardia no longer responded to fluid bolus and his systolic blood pressures were trending in the high 90s. Jill began a focused preoperative assessment before obtaining informed consent.

Jill, aware that Scott had received morphine for pain and had mild hemodynamic compromise, explained that he would require a general endotracheal anesthetic. She described the need for further IV access and explained that she would place an intra-arterial line to monitor blood pressure and laboratory values to assess oxygen delivery. As she continued, a tearful couple appeared in the doorway of the trauma suite. Smiling with relief, Scott introduced Jill to his parents. After shaking their hands, with Scott's permission to share information on his injuries, Jill explained that she was obtaining consent for anesthesia and that Scott would require immediate surgery for a complicated pelvic fracture. She expressed her concern about his hemodynamic state, explaining the degree of blood loss from a pelvic fracture of this nature and that it was very likely multiple blood products would be required to maintain hemodynamic stability and oxygen delivery. Scott's mother interjected, saying Scott was a Jehovah's Witness and that his faith precluded him from receiving blood products, stating he would sign a waiver to not receive blood products. The trauma nurse obtained the appropriate waiver paperwork, which Scott signed along with the anesthesia consent. Scott's mom asked that a notation be made on the consent as well stating "No blood products." The family did consent to albumin and autotransfusion, as long as the blood remained in a continuous circuit with Scott's body. Jill assured them this would be done but also expressed her concern that without transfusion of banked blood Scott could die. The orthopedic surgeon arrived to help escort Scott to the OR. Jill kept her eye on the vital signs, as she knew delay would lead to further hemodynamic compromise. She facilitated a quick goodbye, but not before Scott's mother, holding Jill's gaze, reminded him, "No blood, Scott."

While waiting for the elevator to the ORs, Jill prepared a dose of midazolam to help calm Scott while rapidly giving another liter of crystalloid solution. Before Jill could administer the anxiolytic, Scott said, "Please don't let me die." After some reassurance that they would take excellent care of him, Jill asked if he would be willing to receive blood products, to which Scott's only reply was, "I don't know what to do. Just don't let me die."

Questions to Consider

1. Does Scott have the capacity to sign consent and waive the use of blood products in this scenario? Why or why not?
2. What limitations does Jill face in obtaining informed consent in this case? What are the ethical principles at play in informing Scott and planning her anesthetic?
3. How would this scenario be altered if Scott had arrived to the trauma center incapacitated by head injury or medication?
4. What further ethical obligation does Jill have following her discussion with Scott at the elevator?
5. What action would Jill need to take if Scott was only 16 years old, still a minor, but otherwise presenting in the same situation?

Case Discussion

Decision-making capacity is an important component of autonomy. Indeed, a patient cannot be autonomous without the ability to decide (Van Norman, Jackson, Rosenbaum, & Palmer, 2011). Chapter 3 of this text discusses three minimal capacities for decision making, including possession of a set of values and goals, the ability to communicate and understand information, and the ability to reason and deliberate about choices. Further, it is important to assess a patient's understanding of the consequences of his or her medical decisions (Van Norman et al., 2011). Scott, since the time of his injuries, has remained conscious and coherent, with physiologic parameters that all suggest he is competent. His team contended with some mild hemo-dynamic instability, suggesting there might be some reduced oxygen-carrying capacity due to hemorrhage, which may alter Scott's mentation. Despite his hemodynamic state, Scott continues to meet the criteria described earlier and can therefore be deemed to possess appropriate decision-making capacity. Unfortunately Scott's case is not cut and dried.

Scott was involved in a very traumatic event. Apart from the crash itself, Scott was evaluated in two hospitals and transported by helicopter. He received morphine for pain and showed signs of hemodynamic compromise. While Scott may seem to be coherent in his interactions, each of these factors alters his ability to decide as he might otherwise. The trauma team did their best in the interim to improve Scott's vital signs, theoretically improving his oxygen delivery and mentation. Pain can certainly alter a patient's decision making—patients in extreme pain may decide in a way variant from their norm out of desire for pain relief. Morphine, in this case, may have altered Scott's mentation due to the known euphoric effects of mu-1 agonism by morphine, or may have put him in a state of pain relief that allows him to better focus on the decision he must make.

Jill is faced with an interesting dilemma in obtaining consent for anesthesia. Scott's parents arrived just in time for the discussion. Would Scott have disclosed the details of his family's religion had his parents not arrived? Would Jill have focused her consent on administration of blood products if Scott did not question the need for transfusion? Has Jill obtained truly informed consent if she does not mention the high possibility of death without a blood transfusion in Scott's case? These questions imply the influences of coercion, manipulation, or persuasion on Scott's consent, all of which influence Scott's autonomy. *Coercion* is the intentional and successful influence of one person over another using a threat such that the decision maker cannot resist a decision to avoid the threat (Van Norman et al., 2011). It is arguable that Scott's mother is a strong source of coercion in his choice to refuse blood products. Scott had not, in his entire course of treatment, yet mentioned his religion or concerns about transfusion. While she did not necessarily threaten Scott, his mother's preference and assumption that Scott would follow their religious doctrine were made clear, particularly with her parting reminder, which provided an unspoken threat of the consequences of his choices. *Persuasion* differs from coercion, as it is an ethically acceptable influence of one person over another using balanced information and reason to move the "other" to make a decision that is in line with that of the persuader. This type of influence is reasonable in obtaining informed consent because patients expect their healthcare providers to make recommendations about treatment, but persuasion should be resistible by the patient (Van Norman et al., 2011). In expressing her concern for Scott's condition and the possibility of death without blood transfusion, Jill was attempting to persuade Scott to change his decision on receiving blood, but Jill's recommendations were not so strong that Scott was coerced into ignoring his family's religious convictions. *Manipulation*, alternatively, attempts to alter a patient's perception of their choices by using deception, omission, or lies (Van Norman et al., 2011). Jill was certainly forthcoming with factual details about Scott's condition and the best treatment course.

The ethical and legal implications of an incapacitated patient require healthcare providers to act not just to save a patient's life but also to attempt to restore the patient's capacity to again make autonomous decisions. In

Scott's case, head injury or medicinal incapacitation would not necessarily alter Jill's actions unless an adequate surrogate decision maker were present; Scott's consent would be implied. *Implied consent* means the healthcare team assumes the patient's preference is to receive all prudent care to restore consciousness and respects that patient's desire to live. Some Jehovah's Witness patients carry wallet card information that states their refusal of blood products; however, the laws regarding the validity of these documents as legitimate healthcare directives vary from state to state and by country. Attempts should be made to locate a healthcare proxy, particularly when a patient's desires are in question as they would be if Scott carried a wallet card describing the directives of his faith. Ongoing delay in Scott's case may lead to further hemodynamic instability, such that attempting to locate a surrogate should not delay his operation. All other things being equal, Jill would not be ethically faulted by practitioners in a similar situation should she give blood products under implied consent. The pitfalls of implied consent in incapacitated patients are tied to treatments that fall outside normal procedures or treatments deemed extreme in nature; blood transfusions in the OR, particularly in an exsanguinating trauma patient, are both routine and standard of care if not expressly declined by the patient beforehand.

Scott and Jill's discussion at the elevator put a difficult twist on this scenario and creates the dichotomy that many nurse anesthetists are faced with throughout their practice. Ethical dilemmas are not, by nature, cut and dried. Jill should make all attempts to explore further Scott's wishes once the conversation can be had in private. An argument could be—and often is—made that Scott has been premedicated and that his consent thereafter is thus invalid. Van Norman and colleagues (2011), however, remind us that "Patients retain autonomy even with premedication if they are able to meet the criteria [for autonomy]. Withholding such treatment until a consent form is signed is cruel, probably coercive, and may cause such a consent to be legally invalid as well" (p. 20). The validity of this discussion, however, could be called into question considering Scott's hemodynamic status and oxygen delivery to his brain. Jill and the trauma team rendered treatment to maximize Scott's oxygen delivery to his brain and other vital organs, but it is arguable that with ongoing bleeding, his capacity to make autonomous decisions may be altered. Jill has myriad considerations in making an ethically sound decision after speaking privately with Scott. Was he being coerced by his mother, or does Scott truly wish to refuse blood products, even if this means certain death? He was clear that he did not want to die but never specifically stated that he would accept a blood transfusion. However, he also never actually spoke the words himself that he was a Jehovah's Witness. This information came to light only after Scott's family arrived. The implications of choosing against Scott's will are enormous, although it remains unclear what steps Jill should take next.

While Scott, as an adult, can make decisions about his health care that are supported through legal precedent, the same protections are not provided to minor children. The rights of Jehovah's Witness parents to decide for their children about receiving blood products vary from state to state. Thirty-nine states provide legal protection to parents of children who die from complications of withholding blood transfusions based on religious beliefs (Sheedy, 2009). Other states do not offer such protections. A 1944 U.S. Supreme Court case that originated in Massachusetts deemed that adults cannot make religious martyrs of their children, stating that children must be protected until they are of an age to make a decision for themselves (Sheedy, 2009). Indeed, young children have not yet established their religious or moral beliefs. In some states, temporary custody is given to a hospital administrator, who will sign consent for standard care in cases where parents refuse what could be lifesaving treatment. It is important for nurse anesthetists to understand their state's or country's statutes and precedent in this matter, particularly if pediatric care is not a part of their routine practice.

Truth Telling in the Operating Room: The Obligation of Veracity

Telling the truth is a basic moral precept that is part of human beings' social and moral development and is instilled during childhood. Few would question the wisdom of providing such moral lessons to a child, but as adults it is understood that what constitutes the truth is not always so easily discerned and that some truths can be unpleasant and perhaps even harmful. The truth can be very emotionally upsetting.

Nevertheless, APNs have an obligation to be honest in their discourse with patients, and their information should be accurate and presented in a way that can be easily understood and cogent for the particularities of a patient's situation. This is a responsibility of good practice, that patients are assisted to make informed decisions concerning their medical care (Hebert, Hoffmaster, Glass, & Singer, 1997). However, in doing this, APNs must understand that situations will arise where their honesty will be distressing and possibly harmful to patients and their families (Fry et al., 2010). These situations require sensitivity and clinical judgment about the boundaries of information given and the manner in which it is given. The next section deals with the implications of truth telling during the perioperative setting.

Veracity in Therapeutic Relationships

Three concepts have been advanced to support the obligation of veracity in a therapeutic relationship. These are respect for individuals, fidelity and the keeping of promises, and productive therapeutic interaction and cooperation with patients (Beauchamp & Childress, 2012).

The healthcare practitioner respects an individual by providing the most accurate information for a patient to make an informed decision and then protects the individual's control over that information (Beauchamp & Childress, 2012). The keeping of promises is seen as a central element in the fiduciary relationship between a healthcare professional and a patient. The fiduciary relationship is based on trust, and professionals have an implicit contract with patients to be honest in their discourse and faithful to their commitments (Beauchamp & Childress, 2012). Productive therapeutic relationships involve the execution of an effective therapeutic treatment plan based on an exchange with a patient of honest and accurate information and the instilling of confidence in the patient that such a care plan will be carried out (Beauchamp & Childress, 2012).

Veracity in Anesthesia Care

The therapeutic relationship between a nurse anesthetist and a patient is unique in that there is a critically short period of time in which to establish trust. This is often just a few minutes prior to surgery. It is still common practice that a surgical patient is evaluated by an anesthesia provider or a nurse practitioner in the anesthesia department to provide primary screening and address any problems or questions that a patient may have. However, this is certainly not the case for emergent or urgent cases, where there is no prescreening, and even the prescreening process is not always successful at addressing all of a patient's concerns. It is also likely that the anesthesia provider involved with the prescreening process is not the one caring for the patient on the day of surgery. Because engendering trust is vital to establishing the sort of relationship in which there is an appropriate exchange of information, a patient must be assured that any and all information that he or she receives is honest, accurate, and directed toward meeting his or her needs. Any information that is perceived as deceptive or not an honest attempt to communicate the facts undermines trust. When trust is undermined, communication becomes even more difficult.

Yet patients often ask providers difficult questions. Some questions may be very direct and stark; for example, a moribund patient asks a CRNA if he could die from receiving general anesthesia and surgery, or a parent asks for assurances that nothing bad will happen to his or her child as a result of surgery and/or anesthesia. The fact is that there are inherent risks with the performance of surgery and the delivery of anesthesia in almost all cases. However, when patients are very sick, having cardiac or respiratory conditions for example, surgery and anesthesia become even more risky to the extent that survival of surgery may be statistically problematic for some patients. Likewise, parents cannot realistically be guaranteed a perfect outcome when their child undergoes anesthesia, especially if their child has serious health issues. The CRNA needs to find a way to remain honest but supportive. Information should be provided in a way that fits the situation and is both truthful and compassionate (Krizek, 2000). Families may need to know that their ongoing concerns can be addressed.

An argument can be made that telling a moribund patient that he or she will be fine is justified. For one thing, if the patient does die, he or she will not have had to face a loss of hope and experience unnecessary suffering, and if the patient dies during surgery, the anesthetist would not be confronted by the patient with his or her dishonesty. However, a patient may not be looking for a direct answer to this question; rather, he or she may be seeking to establish some relationship by perhaps testing the veracity of the anesthetist. Thus, loss of confidence in the anesthetist's honesty may undermine a patient's confidence in the anesthetist's integrity and competence for the anesthesia delivery process, causing the patient more suffering.

The parents of the child in the preceding example may actually be looking for some reassuring words to allay their anxiety and fear, and they may receive immediate benefit from hearing the words "everything is going to be just fine." But for the same reasons mentioned earlier, if they are not convinced of the anesthetist's integrity, their confidence may be undermined. It is certainly understandable for parents to desire reassurance and for the nurse anesthetist to want to offer this promise, but the risks attendant upon violating veracity and supplying inaccurate information or in making a promise that cannot be kept are too high. One possible long-term effect is that perceptions of deception or lack of truthfulness affect the ability of patients and their families to trust healthcare professionals with whom they interact in the future. Inability to trust, then, interferes with communication and ultimately necessary information exchanges. Patients will not be forthcoming, and providers will not be able to get the information they need to plan care that is appropriate for the patient.

Anesthesia, especially general anesthesia, provides a kind of veil of secrecy and silence over a patient. A patient is made unaware of the surroundings, and there is no familial or other representation for the patient normally allowed in the OR. A patient places implicit trust in the nurse anesthetist, as well as the other care team members, to see that his or her bodily integrity is maintained during surgery. Although a patient may be wide awake during surgery, such as during spinal or epidural anesthesia, the patient is immobile and his or her vision is obstructed by surgical drapes, and reliance on trust is no less acute.

Maintaining truthfulness and integrity is also important in indirect patient care situations. The nurse anesthetist, along with allied caregivers, has professional responsibilities for truthfulness even when a particular patient is not the focus of care. CRNAs may feel pressured by colleagues, or others, to alter the details of a case, or hide certain information to protect certain parties from blame. For example, a CRNA may be asked to alter a chart to protect a fellow anesthetist who is at risk of losing his or her job as a result of having made a serious medication error or the CRNA may be asked not to report a surgeon's apparent intoxication during surgery for fear that his or her reputation would be irreparably harmed.

Even if there is no patient harm or adverse outcome in either case, not addressing such issues sensitively but honestly breaches the CRNA's fiduciary obligations to current and future patients. Examples were given earlier about how "good-natured dishonesty" may be intended to relieve anxiety or lessen the fear of unknown consequences; however, it rarely has this desired effect, and even when it does, it calls into question the integrity of the professional as this pertains to other matters. Some have noted that worries about honesty related to revealing human error have arisen in the context of a medical and media culture of blame. An Institute of Medicine (1999) report noted that systemic changes in the way healthcare institutions deal with the issue of error are warranted. A discussion of this is beyond the scope of this chapter, but it is an important topic for CRNAs to understand. Its exploration would be a good class project for enterprising CRNA students.

Further questions include the following: How honest should APNs be? How can they be honest, yet not take away a person's hope? Some would still support the idea that sometimes telling the truth can be viewed as harmful and that direct honesty can be seen as the adversary of hope (Warm & Weissman, 2000). The next case study deals with the conflict between being honest and being compassionate when bad news must be given.

CASE STUDY 4: HUSBAND'S REQUEST TO HIDE THE TRUTH

Kim is a 29-year-old healthy woman who is delivering her second child by elective cesarean section. Kim's husband, Bill, is with her in the OR and everything is thus far going well. Gail, the nurse anesthetist who initiated epidural anesthesia for Kim's C-section, is monitoring Kim's anesthesia. Dr. Ross is Kim's obstetrician and announces the delivery of a baby girl, shows the baby to Kim and Bill, and then allows the nurses in the room to take the baby for initial neonatal care.

There seems to be some increased activity in the OR near Kim's baby, and Kim asks Bill to see what's going on. Without looking in the baby's direction, Bill assures his wife that everything is just fine and the baby is doing perfectly well. Bill gestures to Gail to keep silent by placing his finger up to his lips. A pediatrician is called immediately to the room, and the nurses take Bill aside and tell him that the baby is being transferred to the neonatal intensive care unit (NICU) immediately. Bill tells his wife that the baby is going for her first bath and some normal tests and that he is required to go with her, and there's nothing to worry about. Bill whispers to Gail that she absolutely must not tell Kim about the baby's condition right now because "she will have a nervous breakdown." Bill insists that this information is "not going to help my wife right now." Gail is aware that Kim's recent medical history involves psychiatric consultation for panic disorder and anxiety attacks.

One of the surgical residents working with Dr. Ross informs Gail quietly that there is a lot of bleeding right now and she should have blood in the room available to transfuse if Kim's bleeding continues at this rate. Kim asks Gail about her baby and what all the activity was really about. Gail responds,

"I'm not sure. I need to focus on you right now, Kim." Kim becomes agitated and says, "I don't care about me. I want someone to tell me what is happening to my baby. Where's my husband?" Gail tries to calm Kim and manage her hemodynamic status during a larger than normal blood loss after a C-section. Kim's anxiety has caused her heart rate to increase and she appears distressed.

Questions to Consider

1. What should Gail tell Kim about the condition of her baby? What is her responsibility to Kim?
2. What would be the benefit of deceiving Kim? What would be the harm?
3. Does Gail have a responsibility to carry out Bill's wishes? If so, on what basis?
4. How does Kim's present condition of excessive bleeding relate to her need for information about her child's condition?
5. Under what circumstances, if any, might Gail honor Bill's request to withhold information from Kim?

Case Discussion

Bill's request that Gail deceive his wife seems rather unfair, even if he is correct that bad news would distress his wife. Gail's fiduciary obligation is to Kim, not Bill. But what if Gail simply says that the baby is "probably" fine and that babies are often taken to a specialty unit for evaluation immediately after a cesarean section? This is not really lying, as the truth is that Gail is not really sure about the nature of the baby's problem; her primary responsibility is to Kim as her patient. Reassuring Kim might be enough to relieve some of Kim's distress and will likely ensure a better outcome if it permits stabilization of Kim's vital signs.

Shopping for a right answer to a problem does not meet the requirement of veracity (complete honesty is a very tall order—what would complete honesty be?). However, clinical judgment demands that in this situation the benefits and risks of different courses of action (information exchanges are considered courses of action) be weighed to the extent that this is possible in an emergent situation. There is no universal agreement about the extent to which lying to or withholding information from a patient for the patient's perceived benefit is permissible (Beauchamp & Childress, 2012). It depends to a certain extent on knowledge of the patient and an understanding of his or her likely reactions, which is not always possible when there is limited time for interaction.

The short-term benefit of calming Kim so that her present condition is not made worse is not unimportant. There is more at stake in this case than some temporary emotional strain. However, Kim's baby could possibly require extended neonatal care, and Kim is going to have to be emotionally prepared for that in the upcoming days. If her trust in medical professionals is damaged because of a well-intentioned breach of veracity, she could possibly find it very difficult to engage in meaningful, open therapeutic relationships with members of her baby's care team. On the other hand, if her situation is critical, it may be that Gail should do what is necessary to save her life and worry about accuracy or truth telling later.

When patients belong to a vulnerable population (e.g., children, some elderly, and those with terminal illnesses), other factors may complicate the issue of veracity or truth telling. Children are developmentally immature and thus are not expected to have the emotional and mental ability to receive and interpret information in the same way as adults. Perhaps patients in their final stages of life, as well as some terminally ill patients, might be looking for an approach to information exchange that focuses on their immediate quality of life and want an emphasis on hopeful short-term goals rather than unrealistic long-term goals that, within the realities of their present condition, offer no comfort (Warm & Weissman, 2000).

Conscientious Objection in Anesthesia Practice

A Conflict of Obligation: Prioritizing Mother or Fetus?

ETHICAL OBLIGATIONS

The following are examples of another ethical quandary not uncommon in nurse anesthesia practice, that of determining the relative importance of a mother and fetus when a pregnant patient requires anesthesia for surgery or a procedure. During a preanesthesia interview, a nurse anesthetist is presented with a woman who is 28 weeks pregnant, has an acute appendicitis, and requires emergency surgery. The patient is very excited about being pregnant and refers to her fetus by name. She is, however, very anxious about the effects that anesthesia and surgery will have on her baby. How many patients are presented here? On a separate interview, a nurse anesthetist is presented with a 39-year-old female who is approximately 15 weeks pregnant and comes to the hospital to discuss her anesthesia for her elective termination of her pregnancy. How many patients are presented here?

Notice that these questions do not ask how many *lives* or how many *human entities* are presented, but specifically ask for the *number of patients*. This distinction is important in terms of the healthcare practitioner's ethical focus concerning maternal and fetal health issues.

Maternal–fetal dilemmas or considerations commonly arise in reproductive health centers, obstetric health facilities, or in other centers where pregnancy termination procedures may be common. The nurse anesthetist who objects to elective pregnancy termination on moral or religious grounds may choose not to be employed there, with the intention of avoiding moral and ethical conflicts in practice. This, however, is not so simple if a nurse anesthetist is employed at a full-service, large medical facility where a wide variety of surgical cases are performed daily, including elective abortions. The AANA's code of ethics allows a CRNA to withdraw from a case because of conflicting personal convictions, provided there is no harm to the patient or a breach of duty (AANA, 2005). In other settings, this problem has been referred to as refusal of care based on conscience. Conscience clause laws are a set of laws enacted to protect healthcare providers from having to perform functions or provide services to which they have moral or religious objections (Berlinger, 2008). Countries other than the United States may have similar or different regulations or none at all. Regardless, an ethical decision may have to be made that balances benefits and burdens of actions. Those actions that seriously compromise a provider's integrity can have negative consequences for the provider and ultimately for future patients if unaddressed. The U.S.'s conscience laws consist of both federal and individual state guidelines that were created after the deciding of the case *Roe v. Wade* in 1973; they permit physicians to abstain from having to provide abortive services as part of their practice (Berlinger, 2008).

These conscience laws are not universal in their scope and there are some differences in how they affect providers and patients from state to state. Even if a nurse anesthetist can enjoy the protection that these laws provide, there are potential conflicts and difficulties that can arise from exercising their right to refuse to participate in an abortion procedure. One such problem is in finding a replacement anesthesia provider in a timely manner so as to not delay or impede a patient's surgery, and the problem of interrupting the flow of the surgical schedule by changing anesthesia providers for other cases. A nurse anesthetist may not object to providing anesthesia for an abortion on moral or ethical grounds but may prefer not to take these kinds of cases for other reasons and may resent having to change her assignment to accommodate one of her colleague's viewpoints. The nurse anesthetist who has opted out of her surgical case may now feel strain from her colleagues because she is unwilling to perform her preassigned duties.

An objecting nurse anesthetist may also fear how his or her decisions will affect performance evaluations. They may experience reprisal from supervisors or colleagues, for example, being assigned to less desirable surgical cases because they are unwilling to participate in every surgical case.

Such practices and policies, initiated to avoid ethical conflict in anesthesia practice, have the potential to create access problems for patients who require certain services. An example of this currently in the United States occurs when some pharmacists refuse to dispense the "morning-after pill" on the grounds that it constitutes providing an abortion, to which they object (Stein, 2006). Certain populations, because of economic or logistic reasons, do not have expansive access to many healthcare services and are subject to the decisions made by a relatively small number of healthcare providers, thus creating a conflict between a patient's right to equal healthcare treatment and the right of conscience for healthcare workers (Stein, 2006).

This is a justice problem. Professional autonomy to provide or withhold services based on personal moral principles conflicts with the ethical principle of justice. Justice in this context, as discussed in Chapter 4, refers to the equal distribution of health care and the balancing of inequalities in such a way that the least well off are not unduly disadvantaged. Patients in urban areas who have insurance coverage can usually access a large or several large medical centers that offer a variety of services and have good resources in terms of provider coverage, which makes it easier for a conscientious objector to find another provider who will agree to care for the patient, whereas at smaller or rural health centers fewer practitioners are available and there may be no one to replace a provider who objects to providing a particular kind of care or service. This is an area of political concern for all providers in striving to provide good care but is of special concern to CRNAs, who provide most of the anesthesia care in many rural and semirural area institutions.

In addition to access problems, giving anesthesia in obstetrics cases can present the provider with a conflict of ethical obligations. In cases of conflict, the provider must answer the question of whose interests (maternal or fetal) prevail and under which circumstances. During a normal vaginal or cesarean delivery, the nurse anesthetist is mindful of the health and well-being of both the mother and the fetus when planning and managing an anesthetic care plan. When things go wrong, choices may need to be made, including where priorities rightly lie.

In other cases, where a woman's pregnancy has nearly come to term but complications have made a term delivery extremely dangerous to the woman's health and no realistic chance of fetal survival exists, pregnancy termination may be agreed upon by all involved as imperative for maternal survival. However, even in these seemingly less controversial cases, problems can arise. For example, what is the responsibility of the anesthesia provider if the woman asks that her fetus be given some sort of anesthetic to ensure that there is no suffering during the termination? The patient has established a tremendous maternal bond with what she thinks of as her unborn "child" and is very protective of its interests. Giving anesthesia to a late-term fetus is theoretically possible, and there is some evidence that a fetus can sense painful stimuli after 11 weeks' gestation. But no one can really say if a fetus feels pain, and fetal anesthesia in utero for abortive surgeries is not a common practice (White, 2001).

It seems that a humane approach to this problem is to further explore methods to reduce suffering in utero, even if there is only a possibility (not a certainty) that a fetus can experience pain. Is the anesthesia provider obligated to honor such a request based on the mother's autonomy to make her own decisions concerning her health care? Is this fetus now a patient, then, because the woman desires that the fetus be cared for?

These matters of maternal- and fetal-focused ethical obligations are a key characteristic of obstetric ethics and are relevant for nurse anesthesia practice, although a truly in-depth consideration of this topic is beyond the scope of this chapter. "The concept of the fetus as a patient is shaped by the interaction of the principles of beneficence and respect for autonomy for the pregnant woman and the fetus" (Chervenak, McCullough, & Birnbach, 2003, p. 1483).

An anesthesia care plan for a parturient patient is created to benefit the patient according to accepted standards of anesthesia practice. A pregnant patient's autonomy is recognized based on her belief system and her values concerning her current health status. If it is recognized that a woman has the right to autonomy based on her beliefs and values, then how is it possible to recognize the fetus's autonomy if it is not believed to possess beliefs and values because of an insufficiently developed nervous system (Chervenak et al., 2003)? The lack of justification for fetal autonomy does not diminish the practitioner's obligation of beneficence toward the fetus, but this can exist, in this example, only if the fetus is considered a patient (Chervenak et al., 2003). Two criteria are proposed for determining whether a human being should be considered a patient: (1) a human being must be presented for the purpose of medical treatment, and (2) there must be a realistic set of goals that can be achieved via an effective medical treatment plan (Chervenak et al., 2003).

Some may argue on religious grounds that a fetus is a human being at the point of conception and should be considered so despite its inability to think and reason or make autonomous decisions. Others may claim that to be awarded independent personhood, the fetus must be considered viable, meaning that it is scientifically possible for the child to exist independent of its maternal host. Viability, however, is a function of the technological setting in which it exists, and this may vary from region to region (Chervenak et al., 2003).

It comes as no surprise that "there has been no agreement on a single authoritative account of the independent moral status of the fetus" given the diverse opinions involved with this issue (Chervenak et al., 2003, p. 1483). It appears that the mother's wishes most often serve as the best guide to how her fetus should be treated, especially the previable fetus. This is because whether or not her fetus is perceived to be a patient is largely dependent upon the pregnant woman's autonomous decision to convey that status upon it.

Despite the problems of disparities in healthcare access, it is prudent for healthcare institutions to create policies that allow caregivers to decline to participate in a practice because of their moral or religious beliefs, because even the most carefully considered policy cannot eliminate moral disagreement in such a diverse cultural and religious milieu (Winkler, 2005). However, the decision to decline to participate should not be made lightly, and the provider should be convinced that a real threat to his or her personal integrity exists and seek an alternative provider for the patient. The case study for this section involves the principles of maternal beneficence and autonomy, fetal beneficence, and professional autonomy as these relate to a pregnant patient having minor surgery.

CASE STUDY 5: ELECTIVE SURGERY WITH A PREGNANT PATIENT

Sheila is a 29-year-old pregnant woman who presents to the ambulatory surgery center for repair of a large scar on her chest that occurred as a result of a poorly healed skin laceration. Tony is her nurse anesthetist and he discusses with Sheila the implications of general anesthesia, which will be necessary for this surgery. Terry, Sheila's preoperative nurse, calls Tony aside and informs him that Sheila's pregnancy test is positive. Tony asks Sheila if she is aware of the results of this test and asks her if she would mind repeating the test. Sheila admits to knowing that she is pregnant.

Sheila says, "Yes, I know. I really didn't think you guys would care. I'm having an abortion next week. I tried to get it done sooner, but next week is the earliest I could get and I have waited more than a month to get this surgery done."

Tony tells Sheila that he needs to mention this to the surgeon. Tony alerts the surgeon, who then chooses to cancel the procedure for today. The surgeon says, "Let's not mess around with this elective procedure. She can come back after her abortion." The surgeon informs Sheila that surgery cannot take place today because it violates the center's policy to perform elective surgery on a pregnant patient. Eileen is another nurse anesthetist who hears about this case and informs Tony that she would be willing to stand in for him if he objects. Tony informs Eileen that he would have chosen to withdraw on moral grounds, but the case was canceled anyway.

Questions to Consider

1. Was this procedure rightfully canceled? Which conditions would you change to make this case justifiable/unjustifiable to cancel?
2. Whose interests were met with the decision to cancel?
3. Was this a case of a patient's autonomy losing out to professional autonomy?
4. Did Tony have an obligation to Sheila's fetus?
5. If the surgeon wanted to go ahead with the case, would Tony be justified in declining for moral reasons?
6. What do you think the real reason may have been that the surgeon cancelled this case?

Case Discussion

Most anesthetic agents and sedatives that are used routinely in anesthetic practice are potentially harmful to a fetus, according to animal studies, although evidence of harm to a fetus has not been clearly established (Glosten, 2000). Aside from chemical agents, physiologic changes that can result from general or regional anesthesia such as tachycardia, bradycardia, hypotension, and hypovolemia may have deleterious effects on a fetus by impeding fetal oxygen delivery and fetal blood flow. For these reasons, pregnant women are advised to delay surgery until a time when they are no longer pregnant (Glosten, 2000).

This approach of delaying elective surgery for pregnant women could be viewed as a focus on fetal ethical obligations by avoiding the potential harmful effects of anesthesia to the fetus. Conversely, it can also be argued that this approach supports the maternal responsibility to prevent harm to the fetus as part of the woman's body, and therefore this obligation serves maternal beneficence. From a practical standpoint, it seems sensible to delay something that is not urgent until there is less risk to both the mother and her fetus.

In this case study, the woman has decided to terminate her pregnancy at a later date, so there is no explicit or implicit maternally directed obligation to prevent harm to the fetus from anesthesia. If her surgery proceeds, the obligation to provide optimal anesthesia care with concern for fetal health would be a practitioner decision because the pregnant woman is unconcerned about fetal well-being. However, this is a potentially tricky situation for the nurse anesthetist.

If the woman were to reconsider her decision to have an abortion and carried this baby to term, the anesthetist and surgeon could conceivably face legal action if the baby suffered resulting defects, but they would also be morally accountable for the use of good clinical judgment. The legal risk for the anesthetist and the surgeon lies in the fact that each would have been complicit in placing the woman's fetus at risk for a nonemergent case. There are provisions whereby a woman is directed to sign a waiver limiting the liability of the anesthesia provider for alleged harm to a fetus if a woman refuses to take a pregnancy test and her pregnancy status is unknown (Bierstein, 2006). Here the pregnancy status is known and confirmed by the patient, so freedom from either moral or legal liability cannot reasonably be claimed or expected.

Tony's decision to withdraw from this case could have been based on potential medicolegal implications, but he states that he has moral objections to giving this patient anesthesia, which probably indicates his concern about potential harm to the fetus from anesthesia. Tony's decision to withdraw could possibly have had some emotional impact on the patient, but no serious harm would have been inflicted. His withdrawal would have been much more difficult to justify, if not a breach of duty, if surgery was medically urgent and if finding someone to replace him was not possible.

The consideration of legal risk for the healthcare institution and healthcare professionals over the patient's need for this particular elective surgery was likely the true impetus for canceling the surgery in this case study. Simply put, the patient's autonomy was not permitted to place the hospital and staff in any undue medical legal jeopardy. If, hypothetically, there was no risk at all that the patient would reconsider her abortion, and there was no justification for canceling her surgery because of legal risk, then the healthcare providers involved would have to decide, based on their own interpretations of their ethical obligations, whether to proceed with this case or not.

Anesthesia and Distributive Justice

The Principle of Justice

Item 1.1 in the AANA's code of ethics states, "The CRNA renders quality anesthesia care regardless of the patient's race, religion, age, sex, nationality, disability, social or economic status" (AANA, 2005). The nurse anesthetist is obligated to provide optimal anesthesia care to everyone with medical indications for that care without regard to their ability to pay. But anesthesia care is expensive, and if anesthesia care is delivered without regard to incoming revenues or cost, then at some point it is likely that these services will no longer be possible. Politics is about who gets what and at what expense. This is a reality of societal living. Human beings rely on one another to trade goods and services fairly to exist in a functioning society. When goods become scarce or difficult to obtain, there needs to be a system for deciding fair distribution and which criteria should exist for society to determine who merits these goods.

Justice is a concept that is interpreted as fair, equitable, and appropriate treatment in light of what is owed to a person (Beauchamp & Childress, 2012). Justice is upheld, then, if someone receives something due to him or her for providing a service or producing a product or just by virtue of being human. Conversely, it is considered an injustice if something owed to a person is withheld or denied. This logical system of thought works adequately in many cases in the U.S. legal system but is more difficult to apply to the healthcare system, where defining the entitled recipient and the criteria by which that recipient receives what is due is much more complex.

Distributive Justice

The term *distributive justice* refers to fair, equitable, and appropriate distribution based on criteria that a society agrees are ethical and justifiable (Beauchamp & Childress, 2012). For distributive justice to have any relevance, society is required to devise a morally correct system for allocating its resources (Waisel & Truog, 1997). This is obviously very difficult because individuals have vastly differing abilities to obtain certain resources based on economics and opportunity. Some individuals in U.S. society cannot, or can barely, afford to pay a given copayment for a certain health service, and some could purchase entire medical centers.

Armstrong and Whitlock (1998) proposed six criteria for the justifiable distribution of resources: (1) need, (2) equity, (3) contribution, (4) ability to pay, (5) effort, and (6) merit. Although some have criticized these sorts of criteria as not addressing the needs of the oppressed, the criteria provide a useful framework for exploring the issue of resource allocation. *Need* refers to medical need and not individually determined need, such as with elective surgery, and *equity* refers to distributing the same level of service to all who are in need (Armstrong & Whitlock, 1998). *Contribution* means that an individual's entitlement is based on that person's potential contribution to society in the future, which makes sense for allocating larger resources for children, but the aged have made contributions for many years and could argue that they are entitled to the portion of the healthcare services they receive (Maddox, 1998). Allocation based on the *ability* to pay for necessary healthcare resources contradicts the code of ethics for nurse anesthetists, as well as the generally accepted principle of charitable giving of needed health services to vulnerable populations (Armstrong & Whitlock, 1998). *Effort* refers to the commitment by the patient to follow through with medical treatment and comply with prescribed healthcare routines, and *merit* implies that evidence from research or current practice supports the use of particular resources because of the benefit they supply compared to their cost (Maddox, 1998).

Examining these criteria reveals just how complicated a process it is for a society to determine where and how resources are allocated, even with a logical system of determining need. Healthcare professionals bear an enormous burden to decide when medical care for patients becomes ineffective or futile and when the allocation of expensive resources would be better directed to patients with more promising prognoses (Boudreaux, 2001). It is essential for nurse anesthetists to take a global view of this dilemma because they are so often called upon to perform anesthesia care for the purpose of improving or sustaining a patient's quality of life during that person's final stages of life, even when such services may at times prove to have little benefit (Boudreaux, 2001).

Distributive Justice in Anesthesia Practice

To examine the matter of distributive justice in everyday anesthesia practice, it is helpful to think on the level of the individual practitioner. Ethical conflicts arise when the nurse anesthetist is compelled to deliver an anesthetic regimen based on questionable criteria, such as the personal connections of the patient or a patient's perceived economic, political, or celebrity status.

A prominent anesthesia provider was asked at a clinical conference what his recommended anesthetic regime would be to prevent postoperative nausea and vomiting (PONV). His reply was, "That depends on if the patient was the wife of the CEO of this hospital because then I would use . . . and for everyone else I would use s . . ." Even though such a comment was meant to have a comedic effect, it reveals a truth about the delivery of health care: As long as there is a human element in the decision-making process determining the delivery of treatment, there is potential for inequitable care.

For example, a nurse anesthetist withholds anti-nausea medication from a patient who requires surgery after being involved in a fatal automobile collision. In the collision, a young mother was killed. The patient who is at fault for the accident was driving while under the influence of alcohol and illicit drugs. The punitive action of the anesthetist is based on personal feelings and has no basis in any justifiable criteria of resource allocation or any regard for standards of safe and effective anesthesia practice for preventing PONV. This is an unethical action that is not based on sound clinical judgment.

The next case study involves just such a problem of a nurse anesthetist making decisions of resource allocation based on her personal views of equitable delivery of anesthesia care.

CASE STUDY 6: EQUALITY IN ANESTHESIA CARE

Glen is a nurse anesthetist who is employed by a large anesthesia company that has multiple affiliations with hospitals and surgical centers throughout the city and surrounding suburban area. Today, he is working at a new ambulatory surgical facility that is housed in the city hospital and caters to an economic and culturally diverse patient population. Most of the patients who use this surgical facility live in an urban setting.

Karl is the director of anesthesia services at this facility, and he has mandated that all patients who require a general anesthetic be given rapid-acting, IV anesthetic agents only, rather than more volatile agents, because of their ability to be metabolized quickly and their effect on preventing postoperative nausea. These pharmaceutical agents are far more expensive than traditional volatile agents are when comparing total patient hours under anesthesia. Karl has declared, however, that this mandate is necessary to ensure rapid turnover times of the rooms and to prompt patient discharge, ensuring an efficient surgical facility.

Glen refuses to comply with this mandate and continues to deliver traditional volatile anesthetics in conjunction with IV agents as adjuncts as his regimen for general anesthesia for all his patients. Glen argues that he is unable to provide such expensive anesthesia for his patients in the suburban facilities where he works. In those settings, fast-acting agents are simply not available because of cost-containment measures. Glen believes that it is unfair to allocate expensive anesthesia resources for patients who, as he says, cannot pay for them or rely on "free-care" benefits to receive surgical services.

On the other hand, the patients who use the facilities in suburban locations have health insurance or pay out of pocket for their services. Glen also points out that his use of less expensive agents is in no way a breach of duty to his patients because the use of traditional techniques and agents is in full compliance with current standards of safe and effective anesthesia practice. Karl argues that the use of fast-acting anesthetic agents is necessary for the functioning of this facility and that Glen has no business making decisions based on cost of materials because such information is not salient to his practice. Glen states that all individual anesthesia providers have a responsibility to conserve medical resources and the liberal use of expensive resources is irresponsible.

Questions to Consider

1. Does Glen have a right to make such decisions?
2. Who is affected by his decision and what is the potential outcome?
3. Change the conditions to make Glen's position justifiable or unjustifiable.
4. Is Karl's mandate irresponsible in terms of use of resources?
5. Is Karl placing an unnecessary restriction on Glen's practice?
6. How can this dilemma be resolved?

Case Discussion

Glen is in direct conflict with the AANA's code of ethics in that he is making a decision to formulate a care plan based on a patient's economic status. The AANA's code of ethics uses the term *economic status*, and it can be inferred that this includes the ability to pay for anesthesia services. However, anesthesia services for certain elective cosmetic surgery cases are often legitimately denied to someone who cannot pay for such services. Denying such services is not considered discrimination because the surgery and thus the anesthesia are not medically necessary. But because Glen is not directly receiving payment from his patients for his services, he is not in a position to deny services to anyone because of an inability to pay, and, consequently, this factor is not relevant to Glen's actions.

What is interesting here is the fact that Glen is not denying his patients adequate or safe anesthesia services. There is nothing incorrect or negligent about his choices of anesthetics. He has an opportunity to use more expensive agents because of a possibly different revenue or payment structure that allows this facility to operate without such tight restrictions on the use of anesthesia drugs, but he chooses not to use them. Karl justifies the use of these more expensive products for the benefit of a more efficient facility, which may, over time, prove more cost effective than the cheaper, traditional anesthesia agents.

Glen probably makes a salient point in suggesting that all anesthesia providers have a responsibility to be conscious of cost containment and resource expenditures. It seems irresponsible to use resources as if they are on "someone else's dime." The balance possibly lies in the establishment of guidelines and policies set up for the purpose of guiding safe and effective anesthesia practice with regard to what is necessary and what may be excessive. For instance, there are medications that are routinely used by anesthesia providers and recovery room nurses to prevent, or treat, PONV. Because no healthcare provider wants his or her patient to be sick, providers are compelled to give the most effective treatment when it is available. The truth is, there are many less expensive agents that are shown to be effective in reducing the risk and incidence of PONV in some patients. Patients also have varying risk factors based on gender, age, smoking status, and history of PONV and may benefit from certain selections of medications.

Practice guidelines should take such information into account to develop effective and cost-efficient protocols for the use of antiemetic therapy during the perioperative period. Thus, clinical judgment based at least in part on knowledge of the patient is important in tailoring care. To avoid inconsistent and fragmented approaches to resource allocation, institutions, such as hospitals or other healthcare delivery facilities, are obligated to develop standards and maintain them over time to ensure that a more consistent approach is used (Winkler, 2005). Coinciding with APNs' obligation to resolve injustices they encounter in their practice is the obligation to intervene in a broader sense, such as with political action, to explore and change practices that may be unjust or result in poor care.

Glen's position, while seemingly based in logical reasoning, is not well thought out, and it is worrisome for both patients and his colleagues because it is based in a prejudicial judgment that misses the deeper question of why some people have fewer resources than others. Professional autonomy should not be used to ration care based on a patient's merit. In the case example no harm is necessarily caused, and it is not necessarily true that Glen's patients suffer, but it is troubling that Glen is using his professional power in this potentially discriminatory manner. The ability of the individual patient with ample economic resources to dictate the very details of his or her anesthesia care is not commonly recognized in our healthcare system, but it is likely a topic for future consideration in nursing and medical ethics.

Protecting Patients from Incompetent and Impaired Healthcare Providers

Fidelity and Advocacy in Anesthesia Practice

This section deals with the principle of fidelity as it pertains to the role of the nurse anesthetist as the protector or guardian of a patient's interests during anesthesia. *Fidelity* refers to being faithful to the obligation of keeping promises made in a therapeutic relationship (Beauchamp & Childress, 2012).

Keeping promises is universally recognized as vital to the nurse–patient relationship, but it has a special meaning in nurse anesthesia practice because of the increase in vulnerability created by the process of using anesthesia.

Patient advocacy and protection of a patient's welfare are hallmarks of nursing practice. The ANA's code of ethics calls for nurses to promote the health, safety, and rights of the patients in their care, and it characterizes nurses as protectors of their patients (ANA, 2001). In most clinical settings, the nurse is often the first to establish a meaningful, therapeutic relationship with a patient and spends the most time in personal contact with the patient to develop that relationship. This relationship is based on the trust that the nurse will follow through with the patient's concerns and will keep the patient's interest as a foremost concern. This includes providing mediation between the patient and other healthcare team members or family members if necessary (Schroeter, 2002). Nurses take great pride in this role and have shown remarkable leadership in promoting patient rights and developing mechanisms for ensuring quality care. The dedication to protecting a patient's rights is born from a nurse's obligation to respect a patient's autonomy, prevent harm to a patient, and promote actions for a patient's benefit, the trust formed in a therapeutic relationship, and the commitment to be faithful in that relationship (Schroeter, 2000).

This role of being the guardian of a patient's well-being is vital in the clinical setting, whether inpatient or outpatient, because of the number of different healthcare providers that a patient may come in contact with. In a large medical center, a patient is likely to have a number of different healthcare providers, all participating in different aspects of the patient's care. The nurse takes on the role of patient protector and primary advocate and attempts to ensure continuity of care for patients. Responsibilities to guard against inconsistent treatment planning, harm from incompetent professionals, and the supervision of less experienced healthcare providers are all assumed by the ethical nurse. Recent surveys of registered nurses from New England and Maryland reveal that ethical conflicts around the protection of patient rights and patient advocacy rank highest among ethical conflicts encountered in their nursing practice (Fry & Damrosch, 1994; Grace, Fry, & Schultz, 2003). A recent survey of U.S. Army CRNAs had similar findings. The most frequently encountered ethical issues involved protecting patient rights and human dignity and the personal conflict of working with incompetent or impaired colleagues (Jenkins, 2006).

The nurse anesthetist carries this role of patient guardian, protector, and advocate into the practice of anesthesia care. Advocacy has special meaning for the nurse anesthetist because it is during this period of anesthesia or deep sedation that the patient is most vulnerable (Schroeter, 2000). The need for patient advocacy during anesthesia stems from the fact that there can be no expression of autonomy or decision making by a patient who is anesthetized (Schroeter, 2002). The nurse anesthetist seeks to control the variables that can affect the patient under general anesthesia both at the time and after the anesthesia itself has dissipated. Patients are subject to noxious and possibly painful stimuli, immobility, and awkward positioning, and the physiologic depressive effects of most anesthetic agents. This commitment of being a patient guardian also applies to protecting patients from untoward actions of other health professionals in contact with patients. This obligation to advocate for patients and protect them from incompetent or impaired healthcare providers is central to the role and mission of the nurse anesthetist and is clearly stated in the AANA's code of ethics (AANA, 2005).

Incompetent and Impaired Healthcare Providers

An incompetent healthcare provider is one who engages in conduct that is unlikely to be beneficial to their patient and that may even cause harm. The incompetent behavior may include such things as being inadequately skilled in an intervention, undertaking actions that are at odds with an agreed-upon treatment plan, or not engaging in an appropriate or thorough evaluation of a patient. The behavior may range from being ill advised and unlikely to provide benefit to overtly dangerous behavior that may jeopardize the health of a patient. Examples include the photographing or recording in any way of a patient's surgery without the patient's written consent to do so, or a blatant disregard for a patient's personal integrity and assault of a patient. Although all healthcare providers should be held responsible for upholding this commitment to patients, it is the anesthesia provider who renders a patient defenseless and vulnerable by the inherent nature of CRNA practice. Thus, the obligation to defend the patient during this period of vulnerability is much more acute.

The CRNA is also a member of a collaborative care team and, in many states, practices under the supervision of a physician anesthesiologist, which necessitates an ability to work harmoniously with others for a common purpose. CRNAs may feel pressured by a supervising physician or surgeon to comply with actions that are contrary to a patient's interests. Production pressure in the OR can unwittingly drive healthcare providers to place the economic and expediency concerns of the OR over concerns of a patient. For instance, a supervising anesthesiologist may convince a patient not to have a nerve block to alleviate knee pain after total joint surgery because it may slow down the turnover in the recovery room, or a surgeon may demand unsafe positioning of a patient for surgery, risking peripheral nerve damage because diligence with proper patient positioning prolongs the time in the OR.

The abuse of narcotics and sedative drugs for personal use by anesthesia providers is a serious ongoing problem. The incidence of healthcare providers who are substance abusers is overrepresented by anesthesia providers compared to other healthcare professionals, and this number is likely an underrepresentation because of the taboo of admitting to such a problem (Booth et al., 2002). The access to rapid-acting, highly potent narcotics enables an addicted practitioner to divert these agents for his or her personal addiction; for the most part this is accomplished in complete secrecy. One of the most frightening facts concerning addicted anesthesia providers is the insidiousness of this disease, where the first signs of a problem may be overdose or death of the user (Quinlan, 1995). Because the addicted practitioner's narcotic use can go undetected, the practitioner may well be providing anesthesia care while impaired, placing patients at enormous risk (Hudson, 1998). For fellow anesthesia providers to have knowledge of such actions and do nothing is unconscionable and violates the AANA's code of ethics (2005), which states that a nurse anesthetist is obligated to protect patients from impaired healthcare providers. The code of ethics for nurse anesthetists calls for CRNAs to consider that the obligation to protect a patient's dignity and remain faithful to the delivery of safe anesthesia care pertains to all patients, not just the patients the individual CRNA is assigned to. However, confronting or reporting colleagues is no easy task.

Reporting of an impaired anesthesia provider may mean placing someone very close to the reporter in great personal turmoil and will likely lead to disciplinary action by state boards of nursing (Quinlan, 1995). The revelation of such an addiction results in an immediate life change, and the person will need counseling and rehabilitation (Quinlan, 1995). Fortunately, there is a system of anonymous reporting for persons who are suspected of practicing while impaired. The objectives of reporting are twofold: (1) protection of the patient and (2) assistance in resolving the anesthetist's problem. Successful treatment exists. The intention then is to assist the practitioner in returning to work, rather than permanently ending his or her career (Hudson, 1998). The term *impaired* as used here is not limited to the use of narcotics or alcohol (ETOH), but can also refer to emotional stress, sleep deprivation, illness, depression, and injury (Schroeter, 2002).

These personal conflicts involved with attempting to protect and advocate for patients under the nurse anesthetist's care are cited in the survey of U.S. Army CRNAs referenced earlier in this section. The survey respondents noted that encountering such issues sometimes led to decreases in morale, less job satisfaction, and "burnout" (Jenkins, 2006). The responsibility of having to expose a colleague's secret addiction, and in the process upset fellow care team members or supervisors, is daunting. Keeping a focus on promoting a patient's good and protecting him or her from harm provides the motivation for appropriate action, but it can still take an emotional toll. This is a reality of assuming a professional responsibility for the care of another human and entails placing the needs of this individual above the provider's own and others'. The next two cases involve the personal conflict and the implications of protecting patients from impaired colleagues.

CASE STUDY 7: THE NURSE ANESTHETIST WITH A NARCOTIC ADDICTION

Joe and Steve are CRNAs working at the same hospital and have been close friends for more than 2 years. Steve was on a lunch break in the staff lounge when Joe entered, looking to put something in his duffle bag. Joe and Steve began to converse when Steve tried to help Joe by putting the bag back on the shelf behind him. Several small vials of fentanyl, a short-acting narcotic used in anesthesia, fell out of the bag onto the floor. Joe acted surprised to see them there and began making excuses that he must have mistakenly placed them there, and then changed his story to say they must have fallen out of his scrub shirt pocket into his bag accidentally. Steve was not entirely shocked, however, because he had suspected Joe of diverting narcotics for some time. Joe has been acting strangely at work, taking frequent bathroom breaks, arriving to work extra early, and staying late on several occasions, despite many responsibilities at home.

Steve tells Joe that he needs to get some help and that he has a serious problem. Joe denies any illicit narcotic use initially, but as the conversation continues, he admits to Steve that he "took a few fentanyls for headaches" he's been having, "and that's all." Steve persists gently that Joe should look into treatment for substance abuse. Joe pleads with Steve not to tell anyone about this and promises that he will never do this again. Steve asks Joe if he used any today, and Joe vehemently denies doing so. Joe claims that he has to return to a case and repeats his plea to Steve to keep his confidence about this matter out of concern over losing his job and possibly his family.

Questions to Consider

1. What should Steve do next? What would you do next if you were Steve?
2. What ethical principles are involved here?
3. What is Joe obligated to do?

CASE STUDY 8: THE IMPAIRED SURGEON

The nurse in charge of the operating suite has been paging Dr. Pete for almost 3 hours with no return page. His patient, who is a 45-year-old woman who requires an appendectomy, has been waiting patiently this entire time but is beginning to get rather anxious and annoyed at the delay. Dr. Pete finally arrives, but he appears disheveled and sleep deprived. He appears confused when told his patient has been waiting for some time and that he has not returned any of his pages this evening. There does not appear to be any evidence of ETOH use, and Dr. Pete is known not to drink. He asks for the patient's chart but has difficulty reading it because he cannot find his reading glasses. His conversation with his patient is very brief; in fact, he asks her what she is here to have done and tells her that he will be ready shortly, and then leaves to change into surgical scrubs.

Denise is a nurse anesthetist and the CRNA manager of this facility, and she has also been waiting for the surgeon. The patient calls Denise over to her and asks if the surgeon always looks so ill prepared for surgery. The patient then asks if Denise thinks that Dr. Pete is "fit to do surgery this evening." Denise is tempted to make light of this issue and give excuses for his appearance, but she knows that Dr. Pete has recently experienced some turmoil in his life that seems now to be intruding into his professional life. Dr. Pete is going through a very difficult divorce and has significant financial troubles that he made known to Denise on a previous occasion.

The charge nurse confronts Denise and asks her to intervene with Dr. Pete to convince him to let someone else take care of this case. The charge nurse tells Denise that her nursing staff is concerned that Dr. Pete is not fit to perform surgery tonight because he seems too distracted and depressed. Dr. Pete is then seen coming from the changing room and without formally acknowledging Denise or the charge nurse simply says "Let's go" and makes his way toward the OR.

Questions to Consider

1. What should Denise do? What would you do?
2. What is the evidence that Dr. Pete is in any way impaired?
3. What ethical principles are involved here?
4. What are the implications for Denise if she insists that Dr. Pete not do this surgery?

Case Discussions

Steve and Denise have both been placed in very unenviable positions in which there are no easy choices. Steve's obligation is to see that Joe does not work today, or any future day, until he can resolve the matter about his bringing narcotics out of the OR, whereas Denise is obligated to protect her patient from Dr. Pete, who shows evidence of serious mental distraction resulting from an inability to successfully cope with life situations. Joe's impairment is more familiar and conceivable, because most people would agree that providing care to a patient under the influence of narcotics is unconscionable, but Dr. Pete's impairment appears to be from sleep deprivation and situational depression. Because many people in the healthcare profession sacrifice sleep to be available for their patients, some sleep deprivation is expected, and many people experience some depression from time to time as well.

If Denise and Steve act on behalf of their obligation to protect patients, whether in their care or not, their colleagues, Joe and Dr. Pete, are going to suffer some level of embarrassment, humiliation, and potential loss of finances. Joe may lose his current position, and there is no guarantee that his family will understand or sympathize with his situation. Dr. Pete will possibly face examination by hospital authorities because of his recent behavior and may be required to seek treatment and not perform surgery for a period of time. If Steve ignores this problem, a patient will be put at risk for errant practice if Joe is presently under the influence of narcotics. Ignoring this problem may also enable Joe to continue with his addiction and give him the false impression that his behavior is protected by the confidence of his colleague. If Denise does not act, she will have to give false assurance to her patient that Dr. Pete is "just fine" and she will also be negligent in keeping the promise of safely protecting her patient from harm, which is inherent in an effective nurse–patient relationship.

Nurse anesthetists need to take a global view of this commitment to protecting patients from unsafe practitioners and harmful situations while receiving anesthesia care. Patients should expect that nurse anesthetists of good moral conscience would intervene for their benefit even if there were no established nurse–patient relationship, as in the case of Steve with a patient that Joe may encounter. A patient has the right to believe that all nurse anesthetists will keep their promise of safeguarding patient interests during surgery.

Ethical Challenges During Wartime

There are many active duty military healthcare providers working in remote war zones of the world providing quality care with extremely limited resources and under circumstances unlike those faced by civilian nurses. Among this unique cadre are APNs, including CRNAs. Nurses who are also members of a country's armed forces face the unique problem of dual loyalties (Williams, 2009). "Dual loyalties are conflicts between two external accountabilities that are incompatible" (Williams, 2009, p. 8). "Dual loyalty reflects the tension between two, distinct professional obligations: the military and the medical" (Gross, 2010, p. 458). Resolving problems of dual loyalties requires a different sort of ethical decision making. The APN has to reconcile the issues of military necessity and healthcare needs. Thus the emphasis is both on maximizing possible good (i.e., beneficence) and minimizing harms (i.e., nonmaleficence). Judgments also have to be made about doing the right thing when this may be personally risky. Military needs may dictate, for example, that when there are scarce resources, these are diverted to a soldier who can return to service over an equally injured civilian. In such cases, the APN must still determine how to minimize risks to the civilian. Additionally, there is a hierarchical rule of order based on rank. The military APN is responsible for following orders, but as was learned from the problems of Abu Ghraib and other military situations, still has some responsibility to attempt to effect change when there are obvious violations of human rights (Miles, 2013). However, the bioethics community also has responsibility for highlighting disparities between military ethics and professional ethics and for conceptualizing frameworks that permit a balancing between individual and collective good and how to prioritize these dual loyalties in a given situation.

For example, a nurse anesthetist serving in the military may be tasked with distributing certain scarce medical resources while not actually being the ultimate person in charge of access and allocation. Among the limited resources in field situations are antibiotics, pain medications, and blood products. This presents a dichotomy between civilian medical ethics, in which generally adequate amounts of supplies and services are available and when they are not a just distribution is envisioned (ideally anyway), and military medical ethics, where military necessity may trump egalitarian principles. This dichotomy can be problematic for any CRNA but perhaps is especially troubling for a CRNA who mostly practices in the civilian realm but finds him- or herself deployed to military service in an area of particular scarcity as has happened recently in the United States, where reservists (people who have a civilian job but who are on standby for military service) were deployed to war zones. Consider this hypothetical situation: Karl is a CRNA with 8 years of experience. He works at a midsize community hospital. The caseload is varied; it is typically general, orthopedic, ENT, and pediatric surgical cases. Karl lives nearby with his wife of 10 years and their three young children, who are ages 6, 3, and 1.

Karl joined the Army reserves as a nurse anesthetist right out of nurse anesthesia school in order to defray some of the costs of his graduate education. Aside from his 1 weekend a month and 2 weeks a year, Karl has never been called up for active duty, until now.

With the ongoing U.S. war on terror and a resurgence of Al-Qaeda in North Africa, the U.S. Congress has authorized the use of military force. The military put combat troops on the ground to defend certain vital trade route interests from ongoing Al-Qaeda attacks. There are frequent skirmishes and roadside bombs, creating many casualties. The casualties include U.S. and allied soldiers, local inhabitants, and enemy combatants.

Karl now finds himself on active duty in a forward-operating medical facility that has limited supplies. One day he receives a report of multiple incoming heavy casualties. Weather conditions are poor, making transport of the critically wounded to better-supplied bases impossible for the next

24 hours and perhaps for longer. Among the wounded is an enemy soldier responsible for detonating a roadside bomb. He sustained multiple fractures with heavy blood loss and may need a transfusion. There is also a young marine who is currently conscious; he has sustained severe thoraco-abdominal injuries, internal bleeding, and his hematocrit is falling. Another young marine has a severe concussion; he is awake but dazed. There is also a "friendly" local denizen who has suffered multiple superficial lacerations. Karl's commanding officer, a trauma surgeon, determines that the marine with severe thoraco-abdominal trauma will require extended surgery that takes many hours and that is likely to severely deplete the reserves of available blood products. He also determines that the enemy soldier, now a non-combatant, will need to be prepped for surgery. Karl, being highly trained in pain management, is ordered to assess and implement comfort measures for the marine and then prepare the enemy soldier to anesthetize for surgery. The surgery on the enemy combatant goes smoothly, and Karl discharges his care to the recovery room staff. He then discovers that the young marine has succumbed to his injuries. Karl felt, rationally or irrationally, that more could have been done to perhaps preserve the marine's life but he was ordered to provide only palliative measures.

George Washington said, of the treatment of British soldiers during the Revolutionary War, "Treat them with humanity, and let them have no reason to complain of our copying the brutal example of the British Army in their treatment of our unfortunate brethren who have fallen into their hands" (Fischer, 2004, p. 379). In line with George Washington's ideas and as a result of historic war events, the Geneva Conventions of 1949 were instituted to protect the wounded and ensure them care. Consequently, an enemy combatant becomes a noncombatant once they are wounded and no longer pose a threat (McClain & Waisel, 2011). These enemy combatants, once rendered noncombatants, whether lawful or unlawful, shall be treated with the same rights to medical care under the Convention for the Amelioration of the Condition of the Wounded and Sick in Armed Forces in the Field, also known as the Geneva Convention (Council on Foreign Relations [CFR], 2012). "They shall be treated humanely and cared for by the Party to the conflict in whose power they may be . . . they shall not willfully be left without medical assistance and care, nor shall conditions exposing them to contagion or infection be created (CFR, 2012).

This scenario creates a situation of moral distress for Karl, as described by Fry, Harvey, Hurley, and Foley (2002). *Moral distress*, as discussed earlier in the text, is the personal disequilibrium caused by acting against what a person believes to be right. The model contains two distinct domains. The first is an initial sense of distress; the second is a reactive distress caused when the initial distress is unrelieved because the case or situation is unresolved or recurring. Moral distress has it effects on the professional and can lead to distancing from patients.

The initial domain of moral distress for military nurses has two dimensions: "(1) the psychological disequilibrium experienced when military nurses encounter a barrier to their desired moral behaviors or actions; and (2) the negative feelings . . . that accompany the experience of the psychological disequilibrium of the initial moral distress" (Fry et al., 2002, p. 382).

The reactive domain of moral distress for military nurses also contains two dimensions. The first is a continued experience of moral distress when the military nurse is unable to overcome the barrier to the moral action. The second involves, over time, the effects and consequences of the initial military moral distress. Included in these effects and consequences are "loss of sleep, crying, loss of appetite, nightmares, feelings of worthlessness, loss of confidence, heart palpitations, changes in body functions and headaches" (Fry et al., 2002, p. 383).

The goals of this model are to recognize the experience of moral distress and to begin therapeutic actions to lessen the effects for the nurse (the model is the same for all professionals; it is not particular to military nurses). Among the effects of moral distress in military nurses are burnout, withdrawal from nursing practice, and reluctance to serve in future deployments (Fry et al., 2002). These effects are ultimately problematic for the just and appropriate care of the injured. The antidote to moral distress is gaining an understanding of the ethical arguments and implications and working toward resolution, either in the moment or after the fact, and either as an individual or in concert with others. In situations such as Karl's, care is triaged (as it is in any catastrophe) according to available resources, needs, and likelihood of survival. The marine with severe thoraco-abdominal injuries needs emergency surgery and may or may not survive even under the best circumstances. The enemy soldier can be stabilized relatively quickly without utilizing a majority of limited supplies. Thus, the directed actions save a life and retain valuable supplies that can be potentially used to save others without such severe injuries. George Washington's argument was based on philosophical assumptions both about the value of any individual and the consequences for societies and their members of not treating each person with dignity. One further issue is whether the shortage of supplies is real, or due to poor planning at a higher level. Analyzing and resolving this question is certainly beyond the power of Karl in the moment, but it is worth considering if there are avenues that could be pursued later.

The dual roles of healthcare professionals who work in military settings are complicated by dual loyalties—the needs of military and the goals of the profession. Military ethics is a complex field of philosophical and political study. It is one that continues to be developed. The healthcare professional working in military settings is nevertheless obliged to carefully consider what he or she is being asked to do. Ethical decision making in such settings should be aimed at balancing benefits and harms. But even when harm is unavoidable, attempts should be made to lessen it. Mindfulness is perhaps the singular most important characteristic. Studies in cognitive psychology show that people often go along with what others in their environment are doing even when there are obvious and serious ethical violations (Doris & The Moral Psychology Research Group, 2010; Eagleman, 2011; Miles, 2013).

Summary

Ethical decision-making abilities will continue to be a vital part of the skill set of the nurse anesthetist. The healthcare environment is becoming ever more complex as advances in biomedical and electronic technology allow many persons to live longer but with chronic diseases that require ongoing care. Difficult decision-making scenarios concerning all aspects of anesthesia care including the allocation of scarce and increasingly expensive medical resources will continue to challenge the CNRA's practice. Meeting these challenges will require an understanding of the nature and origins of professional responsibilities, adequate preparation in ethical decision making, and ongoing knowledge development. Remaining up to date on current literature, sharing ethical conflicts and experiences with colleagues, participating in ethics-related policy creation and conflict resolution, and personal reflection and values clarification are all necessary ingredients for good practice.

References

American Association of Nurse Anesthetists. (2004). *Considerations for development of an anesthesia department policy on do-not-resuscitate orders.* Park Ridge, IL: Author.

American Association of Nurse Anesthetists. (2005). *Code of ethics for the certified registered nurse anesthetist.* Park Ridge, IL: Author.

American Medical Association. (2001). *Principles of medical ethics.* Retrieved from http://www .ama-assn.org/ama/pub/physician-resources/medical-ethics/code-medical-ethics /principles-medical-ethics.page

American Nurses Association. (2001). *Code of ethics for nurses with interpretive statements.* Washington, DC: Author.

American Nurses Association. (2006). *Risk and responsibility.* Retrieved from http://www .nursingworld.org/MainMenuCategories/EthicsStandards/Ethics-Position-Statements /RiskandResponsibility.pdf

American Red Cross. (2013). History of blood transfusion. Retrieved from http://www .redcrossblood.org/learn-about-blood/history-blood-transfusion

American Society of Anesthesiologists. (2001). *Ethical guidelines for the anesthesia care of patients with do-not-resuscitate orders.* Park Ridge, IL: Author.

Armstrong, C. R., & Whitlock, R. (1998). The cost of care: Two troublesome cases in health care ethics. *Physician Executive, 24*(6), 32–35.

Association of periOperative Registered Nurses. (2009). *AORN position statement: Perioperative care of patients with do-not-resuscitate or allow natural death orders.* Denver, CO: Author.

Beauchamp, T. L., & Childress, J. F. (2012). *Principles of biomedical ethics* (7th ed.). New York, NY: Oxford University Press.

Beckford, J. A. (1975). *The trumpet of prophecy: A sociological study of Jehovah's Witnesses* (p. 103). Oxford: Basil Blackwell.

Benson, K. T. (1989). The Jehovah's Witness patient: Considerations for the anesthesiologist. *Anesthesia and Analgesia, 69,* 647–656.

Berlinger, N. (2008). Conscience clauses, health care providers, and parents. In *From birth to death and bench to clinic: The Hastings Center bioethics briefing book for journalists, policymakers, and campaigns* (pp. 35–40). New York, NY: The Hastings Center.

Bierstein, K. (2006). *Preoperative pregnancy testing: Mandatory or elective?* Retrieved from http:// journals.lww.com/anesthesiology/fulltext/1996/05000/preoperative_pregnancy_ testing_in_ambulatory.32.aspx

Booth, J. V., Grossman, D., Moore, J., Lineberger, C., Reynolds, J. D., Reves, J. G., & Sheffield, D. (2002). Substance abuse among physicians: A survey of academic anesthesiology programs. *Anesthesia and Analgesia, 95,* 1024–1030.

Boudreaux, A. M. (2001). *Ethics in anesthesia practice. 52nd annual refresher course lectures: Clinical updates and basic science reviews.* Retrieved from http://scholar.google.com/scholar_ url?hl=en&q=http://folk.uio.no/ulfk/Etikk/171_Boudreaux.pdf&sa=X&scisig=AAGBf m0thUGfIg6pLF9TbyQnFf-EK-gCMw&oi=scholarr

Chervenak, F. A., McCullough, L. B., & Birnbach, D. J. (2003). Ethics: An essential dimension of clinical obstetric anesthesia. *Anesthesia and Analgesia, 96,* 1480–1485.

Cohen, C. B., & Cohen, P. J. (1991). Do not resuscitate orders in the operating room. *New England Journal of Medicine, 325,* 1879–1882.

Council on Foreign Relations. (2012, December 12). Enemy combatants memorandum. Retrieved from http://www.cfr.org/international-law/enemy-combatants/p5312

Doris, J. M., & the Moral Psychology Research Group. (2010). *The moral psychology handbook.* New York, NY: Oxford University Press.

Eagleman, D., (2011). *Incognito: The secret lives of the brain*. New York, NY: Random House.

Fallat, M. E., & Deshpande, J. K. (2004). Do not resuscitate orders for pediatric patients who require anesthesia and surgery. *Pediatrics, 114*, 1686–1692.

Fischer, D. H. (2004). *Washington's crossing*. New York, NY: Oxford University Press.

Fry, S. T., & Damrosch, S. (1994). Ethics and human rights issues in nursing practice: A survey of Maryland nurses. *The Maryland Nurse, 13*(7), 11–12.

Fry, S. T., Harvey, R. M., Hurley, A. C., & Foley, B. J. (2002). Development of a model of moral distress in military nursing. *Nursing Ethics, 9*(4), 373–387.

Fry, S. T., Veatch, R. M., & Taylor, C. (2010). *Case studies in nursing ethics* (4th ed.). Sudbury, MA: Jones & Bartlett Learning.

Glosten, B. (2000). Anesthesia for obstetrics. In *Anesthesia* (5th ed., Vol. 2, pp. 2024–2068). New York, NY: Churchill Livingstone.

Grace, P. J. (2009). *Nursing ethics and professional responsibility in advanced practice*. Sudbury, MA: Jones and Bartlett.

Grace, P. J., Fry, S. T., & Schultz, G. S. (2003). Ethics and human rights issues experienced by psychiatric-mental health and substance abuse nurses. *Journal of the American Psychiatric Nurses Association, 9*(1), 17–23.

Gramatica, L., Jr., Brasesco, O. E., Mercado, L. A., Martinessi, V., Panebianco, G., Labaque, F., ... Gramatica, L. (2002). Laparoscopic cholecystectomy performed under regional anesthesia in patients with chronic obstructive disease. *Surgical Endoscopy, 16*(3), 472–475. Retrieved from www.ncbi.nlm.nih.gov/pubmed/11928031

Gross, M. L. (2010). Teaching military medical ethics: Another look at dual loyalty and triage. *Cambridge Quarterly of Healthcare Ethics, 19*, 458–464.

Hebert, P., Hoffmaster, B., Glass, K. C., & Singer, P. A. (1997). Bioethics for clinicians: Truth telling. *Canadian Medical Association Journal, 156*(2), 225–228.

Hudson, S. (1998). Reentry using naltrexone: One anesthesia department's experience. *AANA Journal, 66*, 360–364.

Imbelloni, L. E., Sant'Anna, R., Fornasari, M., & Fiahlo, J. C. (2011). Laparoscopic cholecystectomy under spinal anesthesia: Comparative study between conventional dose and low-dose hyperbaric bupivacaine. *Local Regional Anesthesia, 4*, 41–46.

Institute of Medicine. (1999). *To err is human: Building a safer health system*. Washington, DC: National Academy Press.

International Federation of Nurse Anesthetists. (2013). About IFNA. Retrieved from http://ifna-int.org/ifna/page.php?16

Jenkins, C. L. (2006). Identifying ethical issues of the department of the army civilian and army nurse corps certified registered nurse anesthetists. *Military Medicine, 171*(8), 762–769.

Krizek, T. J. (2000). Surgical error: Ethical issues of adverse events. *Archives of Surgery, 135*(11), 1359–1366.

Lindstrom, E., & Johnstone, R. (2010). Acute normovolemic hemodilution in a Jehovah's Witness patient: A case report. *AANA Journal, 78*(4), 326–330.

Maddox, P. J. (1998). Administrative ethics and the allocation of scarce resources. Retrieved from http://www.nursingworld.org/MainMenuCategories/ANAMarketplace/ANAPeriodicals/OJIN/TableofContents/Vol31998/No3Dec1998/ScarceResources.html

Margolis, J. O., McGrath, M. J., Kussin, P. S., & Schwinn, D. A. (1995). Do not resuscitate (DNR) orders during surgery: Ethical foundations for institutional policies in the United States. *Anesthesia and Analgesia, 80,* 806–809.

McClain, C. D., & Waisel, D. B. (2011). Triage and treatment during armed conflict. In G. A. Van Norman, S. Jackson, S. H. Rosenbaum, & S. K. Palmer (Eds.), *Clinical ethics in anesthesiology: A case-based textbook* (pp. 275–279). New York, NY: Cambridge University.

Miles, S. H. (2013). The new military medical ethics: Legacies of the Gulf wars and the war on terror. *Bioethics, 27*(3), 117–123.

Morgan, G. E., Mikhail, M. S., & Murray, M. J. (2002). *Clinical anesthesiology.* New York, NY: McGraw-Hill.

Palmer, S. K., & Jackson, S. (2003). *Ethics: Hot issues in legally sensitive times.* Retrieved June 17, 2007, from http://www.asahq.org

Patient Self-Determination Act. (1992, March 6). Public Law 101–508 Federal Register 57, p. 341.

Quinlan, D. (1995). The impaired anesthesia provider: The manager's role. *AANA Journal, 63*(6), 485–491.

Roberts, L. W., Geppert, C. M. A., Warner, T. D., Green Hammond, K. A., & Lamberton, L. P. (2005). Bioethics principles, informed consent, and ethical care for special populations: Curricular needs expressed by men and women physicians-in-training. *Psychosomatics, 46,* 440–450.

Schroeter, K. (2000). Advocacy in perioperative nursing practice. *AORN Journal, 71*(6), 1207–1218.

Schroeter, K. (2002). Ethics in perioperative practice—patient advocacy. *AORN Journal, 75*(5), 11–19.

Sheedy, G. (2009). Nursing ethics and nurse anesthesia practice. In Grace, P. J. (Ed.), *Nursing ethics and professional responsibility in advanced practice* (pp. 339–381). Sudbury, MA: Jones and Bartlett.

Smith, K. A. (2000). Do-not-resuscitate orders in the operating room: Required reconsideration. *Military Medicine, 165*(7), 524–527.

Stein, R. (2006, July 16). *A medical crisis of conscience: Faith drives some to refuse patient's medication or care.* Retrieved from http://www.washingtonpost.com/wp-dyn/content/article/2006/07/15/AR2006071500846_pf.html

The October Project. (1993). The eyes of mercy – Song lyrics. Retrieved from http://www.lyricsg.com/144702/the-october-project/eyes-of-mercy-lyrics

United Nations. (1948). *The universal declaration of human rights.* Retrieved from http://www.un.org/en/documents/udhr/index.shtml

Van Norman, G. A., Jackson, S., Rosenbaum, S. H., & Palmer, S. K. (Eds.). (2011). Clinical ethics in anesthesiology: A case-based textbook. Cambridge, MA: Cambridge University Press.

Waisel, D. A., Jackson, S. B., & Fine, P. C. (2003). Should do-not-resuscitate orders be suspended for surgical cases? Ethics, economics and outcome. *Current Opinion in Anesthesiology, 16*(2), 209–213.

Waisel, D. B., & Truog, R. D. (1997). An introduction to ethics. *Anesthesiology, 87*, 411–417.

Warm, E., & Weissman, D. (2000). Fast fact and concept #21: Hope and truth telling. Retrieved from http://www.mywhatever.com/cifwriter/library/eperc/fastfact/ff21.html

West, J. (2012). Ethical issues involving Jehovah's Witness patients. In *ASA syllabus on ethics.* (pp. 81–101). Retrieved from http://education.asahq.org/sites/education.asahq.org /files/users/1392/2012-ethics-syllabus.pdf

White, R. F. (2001, October). Are we overlooking fetal pain and suffering during abortion? *American Society of Anesthesiologists Newsletter, 65.*

Williams, J. R. (2009). Dual loyalties: How to resolve ethical conflict. *South African Journal of Bioethics and Law, 2*(1), 8–11.

Winkler, E. C. (2005). The ethics of policy writing: How should hospitals deal with moral disagreement about controversial medical practices? *Journal of Medical Ethics, 31*, 559–566.

Suggested Reading

Calvin, S. (2000). Ethical challenges of maternal-fetal practice in the United States. Retrieved from http://www1.umn.edu/phrm/pp/Calvin_Tokyo2000.html

Keffer, M. J., & Keffer, M. J. (1992). Do not resuscitate in the operating room. *Anesthesia and Analgesia, 74*, 901–905.

Luck, S., & Hedrick, J. (2004). The alarming trend of substance abuse in anesthesia providers. *Journal of PeriAnesthesia Nursing, 19*(5), 308–311.

Ryan, M. A. (2004). Beyond a Western bioethics. *Theological Studies, 65*, 158–177.

CHAPTER 13

Nursing Ethics and Advanced Practice: Palliative and End-of-Life Care Across the Lifespan

Vanessa Battista, Gina Santucci, Susan DeSanto-Madeya, and Pamela J. Grace

For all the compasses in the world, there's only one direction, and time is its only measure
(ROSENCRANTZ AND GUILDENSTERN ARE DEAD. STOPPARD, 1967).

We are such stuff/ As dreams are made on, and our little life/Is rounded with a sleep.
(THE TEMPEST. WILLIAM SHAKESPEARE (2004/1611)

Introduction

This chapter addresses ethical issues that arise when caring for patients who are living with life-threatening or life-limiting illness and/or who are imminently facing the end of life. Advanced practice nurses (APNs) who are specially trained in palliative and end-of-life (EOL) care serve as important resources for other nurses, physicians, and allied health professionals, as well as for patients and their loved ones. Palliative care involves an interdisciplinary approach to assisting patients and families with the physical, psychological, social, emotional, and spiritual aspects of their illnesses (Himelstein, Hilden, Boldt, & Weissman, 2004), based on what is appropriate within their family, culture, and community.

The role of the APN in any interdisciplinary setting is to maintain nursing's perspective while collaborating with others to meet the overall healthcare needs of patients. Additionally, collaborative efforts are needed to influence movements and policies that undermine the health of certain groups or the greater society. The nursing perspective, as described in-depth elsewhere in the text and captured by Willis, Grace, and Roy (2008), is concerned with humanizing the experiences of patients and attending to their contextual as well as physical needs. The nursing actions of APNs working in palliative and EOL care can be ethically appraised in terms of their focus on providing good care that meets nursing goals, including efforts to remove barriers to good care.

A significant aspect of palliative care is helping individuals and families with decision making about the interventions and therapeutics that are acceptable in relation to their personal values, lifestyles, and goals. Ethical issues and dilemmas are inherent to the nature of the problems that palliative and EOL care addresses. Individuals, including children, and their families who are facing mortality or having to adapt to other limitations often struggle with lack of knowledge and questions of ambiguity regarding what is possible and what is not, existential meaning, and what is the right choice for them or their loved one. People may not have spent much time thinking about what they want for themselves at the end of life and even when they have (e.g., when there is an advance directive) the meaning of proposed actions and interventions may not be clear. In the case of furthering the interests of children, family or guardian decision making can be very complex. Clinical knowledge is often critical for choices about acceptable interventions, but most such decision makers do not have prior clinical knowledge and even when they do, typical decision-making scenarios are highly stressful and can interfere with rational deliberations. Patients' friends and relatives may be trying to make decisions when they are also experiencing anticipatory grief, and are responsible simultaneously for meeting ongoing care needs or have a multitude of competing responsibilities.

Decision-making tasks for a patient or family are complicated by the availability of innovations that can prolong physical life without necessarily providing qualitative benefit, that is without improving a person's quality of life. Commentators have raised concerns about the existence of a "technological imperative" (Hofmann, 2002), the subtle pressure often experienced in clinical settings to use pharmacologic and technological advances to extend life without appropriate evaluation of how this fits with patients' goals.

This chapter provides a historical overview of the emergence of palliative and EOL care as a specialty practice. Background information, strategies, and resources to assist APNs faced with difficult ethical issues in palliative care and EOL situations are provided.

End-of-Life Ethical Landmark Cases

This part of the chapter includes a history of landmark cases that presented as dilemmas, but as noted previously, not all of the ethical situations that APNs face are dilemmas; rather they may manifest as difficulties in achieving the best care possible for a patient and his or her family in the face of a variety of obstacles, such as poor or late access to palliative care services and team or family conflicts. As discussed in earlier chapters, an ethical dilemma is a situation in which the better choice for those concerned is not clear or there is no easy way to choose between options. Ethical dilemmas and the situations that invoke them are built on a rich history of diverse settings, circumstances, and situations. As the field of healthcare advances, an increasing number of therapeutic interventions can be employed to sustain life for longer periods of time. However, sustaining life is not always the most ethical option. It can prolong suffering, thereby giving rise to ethical problems for families and providers. Moreover, an emphasis on prolonging life in the absence of quality of life considerations can increase suffering.

Over the last several decades, there have been a number of pediatric and adult landmark cases that have impacted significantly the way ethical issues, inherent in palliative and EOL care, are addressed. Many of these publicized seminal cases arose in the United States but still may be resonant with global practices or changes in practice. The outcomes of these cases have shaped the laws and standards by which APNs or other healthcare clinicians practice in the United States and have informed ethics discussions both in the United States and in other countries. Because healthcare systems, as well as cultural and religious perspectives, do differ among countries, an exploration of the ethical arguments and discussions around publicized or landmark cases can be helpful in clarifying what is good for individuals or societies across countries. As a result of the first case presented, thinking about the ethical permissibility of discontinuing artificial ventilation under certain conditions changed in the United States and elsewhere.

Karen Ann Quinlan

On April 14, 1975, Karen Ann Quinlan, 21 years old, was discovered moribund and not breathing after celebrating with friends. It was later reported that she had ingested alcohol and other drugs, such as diazepam. Attempts at resuscitation were only partly successful. She was comatose on arrival at the hospital (Filene, 1998) and later determined to be in a persistent vegetative state (PVS). PVS is "a state of wakefulness accompanied by an apparent complete lack of cognitive function, experienced by some patients in an irreversible coma. Vegetative functions and brainstem reflexes are intact, but the cortex is permanently damaged" (*Mosby's Medical Dictionary*, 2012). The diffuse damage is caused by a prolonged period of inadequate oxygenation. Usually a period of several months, in addition to certain tests, is needed to validate a diagnosis of PVS. In this case, Karen was artificially ventilated, a tracheostomy was eventually performed to facilitate long-term ventilation, and a nasogastric tube was inserted to permit feeding. After a period of time, her parents realized that their daughter was not going to improve (Mahon, 2010).

A few months later, on July 31, 1975, based on the medical facts of Karen's case, the family's personal and religious preferences, and previous statements made by Karen, the Quinlans requested that all interventions including the ventilator be stopped (Filene, 1998). The Quinlan's request was initially denied by Karen's neurologist, who feared that to discontinue the ventilator would be the same as "homicide" (Filene, 1998). Consequently, Mr. Quinlan sought guardianship of Karen via the New Jersey Supreme Court in the hopes of being able to make decisions for his daughter, including that the ventilator be discontinued (as Karen was over 21 years of age, Mr. Quinlan was no longer legally considered her guardian; Mahon, 2010). The Quinlans' lawyer argued that Mr. Quinlan should be able to make decisions for Karen including that she be removed from the respirator; he based his argument on constitutional grounds of privacy and religious freedom, and asserted that keeping her alive when she would not have wanted this was tantamount to "cruel and unusual punishment" (Munson, 2008). Initially, this argument failed to convince Judge Muir because he also worried that taking her off the ventilator would result in her death and thus could be considered homicide.

During the 1976 appeal, however, the New Jersey Supreme Court reversed its decision and agreed that Joseph Quinlan could make decisions on his daughter's behalf, including the decision to discontinue artificial ventilation if an ethics committee accepted that Karen could not recover from her coma. The Quinlans had wanted the immediate removal of the ventilator; however, the process of convening an ethics committee took 6 weeks, and hospital staff remained uncomfortable with discontinuing the ventilator. Karen ended up being "weaned" from the ventilator over a period of 3 weeks and she remained in PVS, without ventilator support, for 9 more years (Mahon, 2010). Karen Quinlan's case and her parents' efforts to refuse treatment that would not cure their daughter or improve her quality of life marked the first step in the consideration that substituted judgment to discontinue even life-sustaining treatments should be permitted in certain circumstances. The substituted judgment standard permits a surrogate to refuse treatment, based on their considered judgment of what the patient would have wanted had they been capable of making a decision. Around the same time, California State Senator Barry Keene sponsored the California Natural Death Act (enacted in 1977) in response to a personal experience with a neighbor's situation. This was the first state law to specify the right to refuse life-prolonging therapies and protect physicians from being sued for failing to provide treatments at the end of life (Mahon, 2010; Munson, 2008).

The Quinlan case changed thinking about the ethical permissibility of discontinuing what, at the time, were considered "extraordinary" means of keeping people alive. That is, it slowly became seen as acceptable to remove life-supporting technology when a patient did not or would not have wanted it. Ethical argument supports the idea that in such cases the cause of a person's death is not the removal of the technology but rather the underlying condition that either cannot support life or from which the patient cannot recover. The next landmark case changed thinking about artificial nutrition and hydration regarding whether and under which conditions it was permissible to stop these interventions.

Nancy Cruzan

On January 11, 1983, 25-year-old Nancy (Davis) Cruzan was driving to her rural Missouri home when she took a curve in the road too quickly and her car overturned. She was thrown from the car and found face down, unresponsive, and presumably dead. However, paramedics eventually restored her heartbeat (Colby, 2002). She had extensive surgery and required initial ventilatory support. Within a month she was breathing on her own, yet she remained unresponsive and unable to participate in decision making (Mahon, 2010). Eventually she was moved to a rehabilitation hospital, although no one truly expected her to be able to be rehabilitated (Munson, 2008). Joe Cruzan, Nancy's father, had originally consented to the insertion of a gastrostomy tube for his daughter (Mahon, 2010). However, about 1 year later, in 1984, it became clear that Nancy would never recover, and because her husband was not consistently around, her parents sought and were granted legal guardianship. Six months later they also requested a divorce between Nancy and her husband Paul Davis, which was also granted.

In 1987, Nancy's parents recognized that she was not improving and requested that the hospital stop her tube feedings. The hospital responded by seeking a court order to "prevent the removal of the feeding tube" (Mahon, 2012, p. 351). The state trial court affirmed the family's right to refuse treatment, yet the Missouri State Supreme Court reversed this decision, asserting that the state had an interest in "the preservation of life" (Missouri State Supreme Court, 1990) and that the parents did not have the right to decide for their daughter, without "clear and convincing" evidence of what she would want. The court decided that substituted judgment was not adequate and that "explicit patient preferences" had to be clear (Mahon, 2010). The case was appealed to the U.S. Supreme Court, which "supported the right of competent patients to refuse treatment, even if that decision resulted in the patient's death" and that "discontinuation of a feeding tube is no different from refusing any other medical treatment" (Mahon, 2010, p. 351).

The Supreme Court decided that states could apply a "clear and convincing evidence standard in proceedings where a guardian seeks to discontinue nutrition and hydration of a person diagnosed to be in a persistent vegetative state" (Missouri State Supreme Court, 1990). The court thus demanded "clear and convincing evidence" that the request to remove the feeding tube represented Nancy Cruzan's own wishes" (Mahon, 2010, p. 351). Friends of Nancy testified in court, recounting times in which Nancy stated that she did not want to live "like a vegetable," and another friend remarked on Cruzan's statements about Karen Quinlan's case, in which she stated that she "wouldn't want to live like that" (Mahon, 2010). These statements met the "clear and convincing" evidence standard, and the court allowed the tube to be removed. The tube was removed and Nancy was moved to the hospice wing of the hospital and later died (Mahon, 2010).

The case of Nancy Cruzan had several important implications. Similar to Karen Quinlan's case, the case centered on a young woman in PVS; however, in Cruzan's case, which escalated to the U.S. Supreme Court, the question was regarding "the discontinuation of a technology" (i.e., the feeding tube) and whether that technology "provide[d] a benefit that Cruzan could appreciate" (Mahon, 2010, p. 352). Partly as a result of this case, the right to refuse treatment extended to the right to refuse artificial nutrition and hydration. However, the U.S. Supreme Court upheld that "Missouri did not violate the Constitution in requiring clear and convincing evidence of an incompetent patient's wishes before life-sustaining interventions may be withdrawn" (Missouri State Supreme Court, 1990). A result of the Supreme

Court's deliberation was that states would be allowed some leeway in setting standards for the strength of evidence necessary for a patient's decision to be upheld or honored. Nevertheless, where a patient's stated preference is known, decisions should be based on this preference even if the patient is no longer able to articulate their preference (Mahon, 2010). Lastly, the Cruzan case promulgated the use of advance directives (Mahon, 2010). As a reminder, advance directives permit persons to say what they would want in the way of treatment and interventions in the event of incapacity. Advance directives may be in the form of written instructions or verbal instructions conveyed through a surrogate or proxy decision maker. Many countries have recognized the importance of educating people about advance directives as a way of supporting the human right to make autonomous healthcare decisions. However, in any given country the number of persons who have completed an advance directive or assigned a surrogate decision maker remains comparatively low for a variety of reasons that will be discussed later.

Terri Schiavo

The case of Terri Schiavo is very complex. It was influenced by political motivations on the part of lawmakers, social and psychological conflicts among family members, and media opportunism. Thus the ethical aspects of the case have become distorted. The implications of this highly publicized case for APN interactions with patients and families are discussed shortly, but first a few details about the case are provided.

On February 25, 1990, at age 26, Terri Schiavo had a cardiac arrest, possibly due to hypokalemia resulting from an eating disorder. In the prior 6 years she had lost more than 100 pounds (Wolfson, 2005). This was followed by prolonged anoxia leading to brain damage, and Terri was eventually diagnosed as being in PVS. In June 1990, Michael Schiavo, Terri's husband, was appointed his wife's guardian, and from 1990 through 1993, Mr. Schiavo and Terri's parents, Bob and Mary Schindler, were "united in their pursuit of cure for Terri Schiavo" (Mahon, 2010, p. 354). The amicable relationship between husband and parents deteriorated after a malpractice award of $700,000 was put into a trust fund to cover Terri's care needs and $300,000 was awarded to Michael for the loss of his wife's companionship. The award was based on a fertility doctor's failure to note an electrolyte imbalance that was assumed to have contributed to her cardiac arrest. Around this time Michael began to understand that Terri would not recover. The Schindlers encouraged Michael to move on with his life

(Dresser, 2004). In July 1993, Terri's parents went to court to have Mr. Schiavo removed as Terri's guardian.

What followed was a 12-year struggle by the Schindlers to gain guardianship of their daughter based on fears that Michael would be successful in having her feeding tube removed, allowing her to die as she would have wished. In 1998, based on previous statements his wife had made, Mr. Schiavo advocated for Terri's percutaneous endoscopic gastrostomy (PEG) tube to be removed. Her parents were adamantly opposed. What followed was a highly publicized acrimonious series of public hearings and court proceedings. On April 24, 2001, the court ordered Terri's PEG tube removed, but then 2 days later, a circuit court judge ordered the tube reinserted. The legal battles continued, resulting in a second removal of the PEG tube on October 15, 2003. Then the government intervened, and on October 21, 2003, the PEG tube was reinserted, under a statute that became known as "Terri's Law" (Mahon, 2010). The legal arguments continued and on March 18, 2005, the PEG tube was removed for a third time. In the following 2 days, the U.S. Senate and the House passed a federal version of Terri's Law, signed by President Bush (Mahon, 2010), which was again overturned. Terri Schiavo died on March 31, 2005.

The main legal arguments that sustained the final decision were as follows: (1) Terri was in a PVS from which she would not recover; there was never any data produced to contradict this diagnosis and prognosis; and (2) that there was "clear and convincing evidence" that she would not have wanted to live in this condition. Later her parents admitted that they would have tried to keep her alive even if she had left actual written instructions saying she did not want this (Wolfson, 2005).

Terri Schiavo's case was certainly one of great debate and differed from both the Quinlan and Cruzan cases in that many of the decisions were made based on conflicting and erroneous medical information (Mahon, 2010). Terri's parents were convinced that Terri "was there" and would get better and Terri's husband felt that she was "already gone" and wanted to respect his wife's wishes. "There is a distinction between killing and letting die that rests in the understanding of the current and future state of the disease" (Mahon, 2010, p. 356), and differing from previous cases, this time, the debate centered upon others' preferences and beliefs instead of the patient's preferences (Mahon, 2010). From a nursing perspective, this case can help APNs gain insights about the need for early intervention and support for such families. APNs who work in primary care, as well as hospice and palliative care settings, have a role to play in eliciting and meeting the real needs of all involved, as discussed later in this chapter.

Helga Wanglie

This case concerns another emerging issue related to what some have called the technological imperative to keep a person physically alive when the ability to recover is questionable (Baily, 2011). Helga Wanglie was an active and well-educated 85-year-old woman who tripped on a rug and broke her hip on December 14, 1989, leading to multiple successive treatments, several cardiac arrests, and eventual PVS and life-sustaining therapies (e.g., respirator and PEG tube) (Capron, 1991). Helga's case, although commonplace in nature, quickly gained attention when Mr. Wanglie, Helga's husband, aged 87 "refused to consent to the withdrawal of her treatment" (Capron, 1991, p. 26) and her physicians requested that a judge name another guardian in his place because they believed the treatment requested was futile (Capron, 1991). The request was not granted. Mr. Wanglie remained Helga's guardian, and she died 3 days later on July 4, 1991 (Capron, 1991). The significance of the Wanglie case is that it drew wide attention to the problem of requests for treatments that are not likely to meet clinical goals. Medical futility essentially means that the treatment requested cannot be of benefit or achieve the purpose intended. One of the problems with terming an intervention or set of interventions futile is that determining futility is very difficult and ambiguous.

In the Wanglie case, the significant ethical question was whether the surrogate decision maker (in this case Mr. Wanglie) was really representing what the patient would have wanted could she have spoken for herself. Another significant question related to the principle of nonmaleficence is whether providers might actually be causing more harm than good in pursuing a given course of action. The importance of futility as it relates to the role of the APN is discussed in the following sections.

Similar to the adult-based cases, there are several landmark pediatric cases that have influenced thinking about ethical decision making in critical or EOL situations. As with any change in ethical practice, the consideration of an issue changes as each case is deliberated and the aspects are teased out and analyzed. Thus insights from these cases tend to build upon each other. Futility is discussed at length later in this chapter, but it is helpful to begin with the cases that serve as recent and significant reminders of the issues that APNs may face in providing care to patients and families in times of serious illness and at the end of life.

Baby Jane Doe

Baby Jane Doe was actually the second Baby Doe case that led to what became known as the "Baby Doe Rules" in the United States. The first Baby Doe was born in 1982 with Trisomy 21 (also known as Down syndrome) and some associated problems such as esophageal atresia and tracheoesophageal fistula. Although the esophageal problems were correctable by surgery, the parents requested no treatment and a court ruling upheld the decision. Baby Doe number one died 6 days later (Mercurio, 2009). Several of the staff members who had cared for Baby Doe were alarmed by the fact that the baby had needlessly died of starvation and dehydration; the nurses reported the baby's pitiful crying (Bannon, 1982). The case subsequently became highly publicized. The outcry was related to clinicians' testimony that with surgery, Baby Doe number one could have had a reasonable quality of life, despite cognitive deficits related to the trisomy.

This first case was followed shortly by the case of Baby Jane Doe, born on October 11, 1983, with spina bifida, hydrocephaly, and microencephaly. Her providers recommended that she have "immediate surgery to reduce the fluid in her skull and close her meningomyelocele" (Annas, 1984, p. 727), which would increase her life expectancy but not change the highly likely ultimate outcome of being profoundly retarded, epileptic, paralyzed, bed-ridden, and subject to constant urinary tract infections (Annas, 1984). Even with surgery, Baby Jane Doe's prognosis was worse than Baby Doe number one's would have been; however, providing nutrition and hydration was possible for her. Her parents ultimately refused to consent to the surgery although they did agree to other treatments such as antibiotics.

Given the political uproar over the first Baby Doe case, the case of Baby Jane Doe became what Annas termed a "test case to determine the proper role of the state in decisions to withhold surgery from handicapped newborns" (Annas, 1984, p. 727). Several "right to life" lawyers became involved, and in a sudden turn of events, a guardian ad litem (GAL) who initially told the parents he agreed with their decision reversed his position at the hearing. A GAL is a person appointed by the court with the specific task of attending to the interests of another person, in this case Baby Jane Doe. The judge "ruled the infant in need of immediate surgery to preserve her life" (Annas, 1984, p. 727) and authorized the GAL to consent to it, yet Baby Doe's parents appealed (see also Chapter 7 for implications of this case in neonatal intensive care unit settings.)

What ensued was a long and complicated series of legal proceedings in which the prominent questions became whether abstaining from providing available medical care made this a case of child abuse or neglect and whether Baby Jane Doe was being "discriminatorily denied indicated medical treatment" (Annas, 1984, p. 727) because she was handicapped. The legal question was then raised if in forgoing treatment, Section 504 of the Rehabilitation Act of 1973 would be violated (Annas, 1984). The court ultimately concluded that the hospital was not in violation of Section 504, as they did not refuse to perform the surgery because of the child's handicap, but rather because of the parents' wishes (Annas, 1984). The significance of this case was paramount, however, in that it elucidated the question of "what should the role of the government be in treatment decisions for handicapped newborns?" (Annas, 1984, p. 728). In other words, the government's role should be limited, whereas the parental role should, all things being equal, be respected.

In this case, because it was unclear what the best option for Baby Jane Doe would be, her parents had the right to opt for the most conservative treatment. The case also impacted the passing of H.R. 1904, The Child Abuse Amendments of 1984, shortly thereafter. These amendments directed the development of procedures for all persons and agencies with responsibilities related to children, including healthcare professionals, "to insure that nutrition (including fluid maintenance), medically indicated treatment, general care, and appropriate social services are provided to infants at risk with life-threatening congenital impairments" (Annas, 1984, p. 728). Another important ethical point in the Baby Doe cases has to do with whether decisions for infants should primarily be about their best interests or whether parental interests should count. The ethical concern in the first Baby Doe case was that she was denied treatment that could have saved her life merely because of a handicap, whereas another child in similar circumstances that received treatment would have had the opportunity to experience life.

For the next seminal case, that of Baby K, the ethical questions are several, including (1) what constitutes a "human" life, and (2) whether it is ever permissible to try to maintain the physical entity of an infant who will never be capable of "experiencing" life and for what purpose.

Stephanie Keene, Baby K

Stephanie Keene, also known as Baby K, was born on October 13, 1992, with anencephaly, a neurological condition resulting from the congenital absence of any cerebral cortex or cerebellum, and consequently only a "reflexive, unconscious, brainstem existence" (Doyle, 2010, p. 2). The parents had known about Baby K's condition prenatally but declined to abort the baby based on religious conviction in the sanctity of life. As a reminder, the principle of sanctity of life means that human life has absolute value (because it originates from a supreme being) apart from the ability to "experience" living. About 1,000 anencephalic infants are born in the United States each year, and although these infants do not meet the criteria for brain death, they have no possibility of consciously experiencing the world (Doyle, 2010). In most cases of anencephaly, providers and parents are in agreement that medical treatment would be futile for achieving meaningful existence. In the case of Baby K, her mother, motivated by religious conviction, was insistent that the hospital continue with advanced supportive care (primarily ventilator support). Stephanie was able to be periodically weaned from the ventilator and was cared for in an extended care nursing facility, but her respiratory status remained unstable and she required multiple hospital readmissions. At one point, the hospital petitioned the courts to permit them only to provide comfort measures in light of the prognosis of such children (Bernat, 2008). Stephanie's mother argued that "God alone should decide how long the baby should live" (Doyle, 2010, p. 3). During the following court proceedings, experts testified that the intervention of mechanical ventilation was not acceptable medical care for this condition. Moreover, the costs of providing technological and supportive care were mounting. Opposing arguments remained rooted in the idea that any human life (regardless of ability to experience) must be preserved.

The ultimate ruling from the U.S. District Court mandated that the hospital caring for Baby K mechanically ventilate her during episodes of respiratory arrest per the Emergency Medical Treatment and Active Labor Act (EMTALA), which requires that "patients who present with a medical emergency must get 'such treatment as may be required to stabilize the medical condition'" (Doyle, 2010, p. 3). The court took the stance that it is beyond "judicial function" to address moral and ethical standards regarding treatment of anencephalic infants, and as a result, Baby K was kept on mechanical ventilation and lived until the age of 2½ years (Doyle, 2010). The court's decision, however, was seen as raising problems for medical decision making and practice. Essentially it removed a physician's prerogative to act as a "moral agent" and turned the healthcare team into mere "instruments of technology" (Doyle, 2010, p. 3). This case raised several ethical questions, including: What constitutes death? What characterizes a human being? Who should be given moral standing as a human being? Is physical death always harmful? What is meant by futile treatment? And in the case of Baby K, how should we think about the costs of physical care that cannot ultimately achieve the aim of improving quality of life? It is important that APNs understand the issues and arguments to date from a historical point of view but also to take into account individual factors in a given case when providing care and support to patients and families at the end of life. For any given case, the APN may need to work collaboratively with others to determine the best solution, such as which course of action will likely produce the most good and cause the least harm for both patients and loved ones.

Emilio Gonzales

The ultimate question becomes this: When should treatment be stopped (or not started) because it cannot or is unlikely to achieve its purpose? Another case of significance in the ethical realm of (what constitutes) futility is that of Emilio Gonzales, born on November 3, 2005, with Leigh's disease, a progressive and eventually fatal neurometabolic disorder (Truog, 2007). Emilio was on life support in the intensive care unit at the Children's Hospital of Austin, Texas for 15 months and the hospital invoked The Texas Advance Directives Act (TADA). TADA was, in part, developed by members of the Baylor University Medical Center Institutional Ethics Committee and provides legal immunity to physicians who make a medical decision that treatment cannot benefit a patient (Smith, Gremillion, Slomka, & Warneke, 2007) and may even be harmful in terms of prolonged suffering. The act essentially authorizes physicians to withdraw life support if an ethics committee determines further life support is medically inappropriate. Moreover, notice must be given to the family and if the family requests, attempts must be made to transfer the patient to another facility and provider (Smith et al., 2007; Truog, 2007). In this case, Emilio's mother attempted to prevent this from happening and was successful in extending the 10-day deadline, but Emilio died on May 19, 2007, before the judge had issued a final ruling on the case (Truog, 2007).

In cases such as this, there are no clear answers. Emilio's mother and loved ones had a perspective that doing all they could to keep him alive was of utmost importance, yet the medical judgment was that "continued use of life support was causing Emilio needless suffering" and was "contributing to an undignified death" (Truog, 2007, p. 2). The American Medical

Association (AMA) and other groups have recommended that an approach based on due process of the law, thus involving an honest judicial system, is a fair method for resolving such conflicts (AMA, 1999). As such, TADA "seeks to incorporate a due-process standard by insisting that all allegations of futility go forward only after they have been reviewed and approved by the hospital ethics committee" (Truog, 2007, p. 2). This provides an opportunity to thoroughly explore the issue and make a decision that is most likely to serve the interests of the person (child or adult). Each case is different and some have questioned the ability of an ethics committee to remain both neutral and objective in considering the interests of a person especially when, as in Emilio's case, the person is a member of a minority community (Truog, 2007).

The next case, that of Ashley X, is different than previous cases, because it shifts the focus from futility to determining what physical interventions, biologic and/or surgical, that would not be sanctioned for a "normal" child, might nevertheless be ethically supportable in terms of burdens and benefits for a family providing daily care.

Ashley X

Although the case of Ashley X does not directly involve decisions regarding futility or life-sustaining treatments, it became a source of much ethical debate following the publication of a medical journal article describing "novel growth attenuation" (Kirschner, Brashler, & Savage, 2007, p. 1023), for a disabled child with a static encephalopathy of unknown origin, dependent in all activities of daily living, nonverbal, and entirely immobile. She received all nutrition via tube feedings, and her parents nicknamed her "pillow angel" because she lay on a pillow wherever they placed her (Kirschner et al., 2007). Developmentally, Ashley X was permanently equivalent to a 3-month-old child, yet at 6 years and 7 months of age, she began to show signs of puberty and grew in length rapidly, and her parents took her to an endocrinologist for evaluation. Her parents "particularly feared that continued growth would eventually make it untenable for them to care for their daughter at home, despite their strong desire to do so . . . After extensive consultation between parents and physician, a plan was devised to attenuate growth by using high-dose estrogen" (Gunther and Diekma, 2006, p. 1014). To avoid unwanted side effects of this treatment, she also underwent a hysterectomy and breast bud removal, a combination of interventions that her parents later called the "Ashley treatment." Ashley X's parents, who cared for her at home, along with her grandparents, felt that their efforts to keep their daughter small were consistent with upholding quality of life, because they could keep her mobile and allow her to continue to participate in activities outside of their home. As cited in Kirschner et al. (2007), the family also felt that "'given Ashley's mental age a nine and a half year old body is more appropriate and more dignified than a fully grown female body'" (p. 1024).

Many people in the medical community and the public did not feel the same way, however, and the case of Ashley X quickly became a source of much public attention and debate. Dr. Diekema, the chairman of the bioethics committee of the American Academy of Pediatrics, commented that most people had not even considered this a possibility, much less something that would actually be done, and that it forced people to think seriously about the reasons behind the parents' request (Coombes, 2007). The foremost concern, however, became making sure that there would not be any medical harm to Ashley; her physicians felt that there were medical benefits to the procedure such as improved circulation, digestion, muscular condition, and less bed sores (Coombes, 2007). Conversely, ethicists argued that this case brought to light the larger social issues regarding how disabled people are treated, and that "American society does not do what it should to help severely disabled children and their families" (Coombes, 2007). Several families have sought the "Ashley treatment" since this case became widely publicized, and it remains a topic of much public ethical debate. The pertinent questions for APNs that are raised by this case include the following: What sorts of palliative measures are warranted in such cases and what is the intent behind such measures? If the treatments improve parental quality of life, does this in turn improve the patient's quality of life and therefore ethically warrant the treatment? Or is the real issue related to inadequate social supports for the family? The role of APNs in such cases may include articulating the family's story and concerns, guiding them through decision making, educating others about the issues, and supporting caregivers in providing the family with care in an unbiased manner.

The next section explores the emergence of palliative care as a specialty that can provide support and resources to those who must make difficult decisions. Understanding the importance of ethical thinking in cases of EOL, futility, and ongoing highly technological care of patients and families is essential for palliative and EOL care APNs.

The Emergence of Palliative Care as a Specialty

Prior to the 1960s, healthcare provision for those with cancer was focused on attempts to cure via radiation, drugs, and surgery. Patients perceived to be in the dying process were often sent home to die because there was no longer anything an institution focused on cure could offer to them (Clark, 2007). Pain management and relief of suffering were often not attended to well (Saunders, 1978).

However, beginning in the 1950s, in both the United Kingdom and the United States, study findings shed new light on the importance of attending to the "social and clinical aspects of care for patients dying from cancer" (Clark, 2007, p. 431). Data from these studies along with the pioneering work of Dame Cicely Saunders drew attention to the particular EOL care needs of patients living with advanced malignant disease. Dame Saunders was initially a nurse who later became a physician, and she drew attention to the fact that the needs of the dying were not being met. She was particularly concerned with relieving the suffering of the dying from a holistic perspective. Influenced by her work, hospices began to develop rapidly in the 1970s (Clark, 2007). Hospices, concerned as they were with improving the quality of life of the dying and their families, were also interested in palliating suffering.

The specialty of palliative care emerged from the field of oncology with the initial goals of supporting the "physical, social, psychological, and spiritual" well-being "of patients with life-limiting illness" (Clark, 2007, p. 430) using multidisciplinary modalities. There has been some ambiguity about palliative care and its definition and goals. In 1989, the World Health Organization, with input from many sources, defined palliative care as "an approach that improves the quality of life of patients and their families facing the problems associated with life-threatening illness, through the prevention and relief of suffering by means of early identification and impeccable assessment and treatment of pain and other problems, physical, psychosocial, and spiritual" (Sepulveda, Marlin, Yoshida, & Ullrich, 2002, p. 91). The specialty of palliative care continues to gain increasing recognition and growth worldwide as it expands well beyond the world of oncology, develops further in pediatrics, and gains increasing attention from policymakers (Clark, 2007).

The Institute of Medicine's Report: *When Children Die*

The idea for the specialty of palliative care developed in response to mounting and persuasive evidence that a broad perspective was needed for the ethical care of adults who were either at the end of life or who were suffering as a result of complex illnesses and persistent applications of bio-technology. Palliative care is essential for children too; however, their needs and their families' needs differ in various ways from those of adults. In 2002, the Institute of Medicine (IOM) released a report to help palliative care professionals identify the unique needs of and care provisions for children and their families during times of illness and/or at the end of life. The report, entitled *When Children Die*, built upon two previous IOM reports, *Approaching Death: Improving Care at the End of Life* (1998) and *Improving Palliative Care for Cancer* (Foley & Gelband, 2001), and affirmed via evidence and argument the problem that "medical and other support for people with fatal or potentially fatal conditions often falls short of what is reasonably if not simply attainable" (IOM, 2002). This report paved the way for the development of pediatric palliative care as a clinical specialty facilitating the needs of children with chronic and life-threatening diseases. It elucidated the problem that children with life-limiting illnesses often fail to receive the "competent, compassionate, and consistent care that meets their physical, emotional, and spiritual needs" (IOM, 2002). The report concluded that better care is possible, but that more data and knowledge are needed to guide the effective delivery of care and to educate clinicians (IOM, 2002). There is a significant and important role for APNs trained in pediatric palliative care and who have developed the skills to work collaboratively with others in order to optimize care for this population.

The Distinction Between Palliative Care and End-of-Life Care

The terms *hospice* and *palliative care* are often erroneously used interchangeably, although hospice is now understood as a distinct part of palliative care. Both systems of care did, however, grow out of the same movement. In 1967, Dame Cicely Saunders, known as the "founding mother" of the hospice movement, was instrumental in opening the first modern-day hospice in London, St. Christopher's Hospice, which quickly became the catalyst for rapid and expansive development of hospices. Hospices were soon recognized as places where patients could go for improved pain and symptom management, as well as "psychosocial needs" and improved continuity of care (Clark, 2007). Currently, there are nearly 200 adult and pediatric hospices in existence in the United Kingdom, all of which are built on the standards first established at St. Christopher's Hospice. Hospices provide expert services to the imminently dying, based on a philosophy of striking a delicate balance between too much and too little medical treatment. Appropriate services are based on prior research evidence, clinical expertise, and inter-disciplinary support of the dying and are focused on meeting individual needs (Clark, 2007).

Although hospices function somewhat differently in the United States, in part due to differences in healthcare systems and finances, the philosophy of care is the same. Hospice care becomes an essential part of palliative care at a time when goals shift to that of comfort and away from ongoing treat-ments (Kantarjian, Wolff, & Koller, 2011). Depending on varying state laws and policies, hospice care may or may not be provided simultaneously with life-prolonging or life-sustaining treatments, may or may not include care for children, and is available on both an inpatient and an outpatient basis. Pediatric hospice care services are far less likely to be available than adult services in the United States and many other countries. The hospice model of care includes the use of trained volunteers as well as 24-hour clinical sup-port. Bereavement services are generally available for families to access for 1 year following the death of their loved one.

In the United States, adult patients are eligible for Medicare hospice ben-efits if they meet one of three criteria: (1) are over age 65 and self or spouse has previously paid into the Social Security system, (2) are under age 65 but qualify for disability, or (3) have end-stage renal disease. It is estimated that 82% of people receiving inpatient or outpatient hospice services are doing so as a result of Medicare hospice benefits (Cerminara, 2011). If the prescribing "physician" (in some state regulations the definition of physician for this purpose includes nurse practitioners) certifies that a person's prognosis is likely terminal within 6 months, the person is eligible for hospice services. Cerminara (2011) notes that there remains a great deal of confusion about who qualifies, and this has led to delayed entry into hospice for some who could benefit from hospice services earlier in their disease course. Moreover, there is confusion about how firm the criteria of having less than 6 months to live is in order to qualify. Medicare will allow certification of two 90-day periods followed by recertification as needed, as long as the patient still meets the criteria for a terminal illness. Until somewhat recently, adult U.S. patients who enrolled in hospice services were obliged to forgo curative treatments. However, the 2010 Patient Protection and Affordable Care Act contains provisions for funding some demonstration projects (15 currently) that combine disease-directed treatments with hospice services. The aim, cost-effectiveness, continues to be the same as the original impetus for Medicare coverage of hospice services (Cerminara, 2011). Nevertheless, Cerminara warns that there is a potential for this to have a contrary effect on access to hospice for persons in rural areas related to access issues.

Physicians, nurses, and APNs should remain alert to the possibility of unintended negative consequences of changes put into place by healthcare reform with the aim of improving care while reducing costs. In other countries, healthcare funding for hospice services is achieved via a variety of less cumbersome mechanisms. However, not all countries focus on hospice and palliative care, and provisions for this sort of care are sometimes nonexistent (Clark & Centeno, 2006). Elsewhere in the text it was argued that the leadership responsibilities of APNs include political activity for the purposes of meeting nursing goals. In terms of access to hospice and palliative care this is also true, along with the responsibility (of APNs) to educate others and continue to expand the nascent but rapidly growing field. APNs need to collaborate with colleagues and other healthcare providers to influence policies that negatively impact good patient care and to advocate for patients and families to receive the care that they rightfully deserve. Especially in pediatrics, hospice services may be scant, and families and providers are not always aware of this potential benefit, even when it is available. Thus, another leadership role for palliative care APNs is to help educate others about the benefits of hospice care in terms of quality of life and familial supports that hospice and palliative care can provide.

Multidisciplinary Approaches

It is widely recognized that palliative and EOL care is best delivered using a multidisciplinary approach. Palliative care APNs are professionals who have received special education and preparation in the care of patients and families living with life-threatening illness and can serve as good resources for other nurses and allied professionals. They often practice collaboratively with other palliative care team members, such as physicians, nurses, social workers, chaplains, child life specialists, and/or various therapists, as well as primary care team members, and may serve as coordinators of such interdisciplinary care, as well as act as the liaison between the patient, family, and team. By definition, "effective palliative care requires a broad multidisciplinary approach that includes the family and makes use of available community resources" and "can be successfully implemented, even if resources are limited" (Liben, Papadatou, & Wolfe, 2008, p. 852). Thus, palliative care APNs have an understanding of what the appropriate resources are and how to access them, as well as an ability to recognize ethical problems and utilize the decision-making processes that may facilitate their resolution.

International Perspectives

The specialty of palliative and EOL care is rapidly gaining popularity, not only in the United States and other Western countries, but in Eastern and developing countries as well. This is, in part, due to the spread of education and training programs for healthcare professionals, especially nurses. While the philosophy behind palliative and hospice care is universal, factors contributing to ethical dilemmas and other ethical problems for healthcare professionals, patients, and family members alike vary among countries. Examples include the high cost of care at the end of life in the United States, scarce resources in other countries, and the ever-growing number of innovations that permit the physical prolongation of life (Blank, 2011). Blank (2011) has argued that because of the "complexity of end-of-life issues, [it is] only with a thorough knowledge of what occurs across countries [that] we [can] generate the evidence necessary" (p. 204) to broaden our perspective on what is possible and what ought to be done. While it is beyond the scope of this chapter to explore each country's and culture's unique customs and practices, there are obviously distinct religious, spiritual, cultural, and familial customs and structures that affect decision making, particularly at the end of life (Blank, 2011). As discussed in earlier chapters, an important responsibility of the APN is to account for such individual and cultural influences on ethical problems in palliative and EOL care.

Ethical Decision Making: Identifying a Decision Maker

A prerequisite for ethical decision making in any population is to identify the person(s) who has the authority to make decisions. This may be the patient or someone who has appropriate knowledge of the patient's values and beliefs and thus can articulate with some degree of accuracy the patient's point of view. When the patient is a minor, parents or guardians typically serve as authorized decision makers. However, in some instances, other individuals may have decision-making authority (Kirschen & Feudtner, 2013).

For example, some children are in the legal custody of the state or may have a surrogate decision maker, such as a GAL appointed to represent that child's interests. As discussed in earlier chapters, the criteria for individuals to make their informed treatment decisions are as follows: (1) they appreciate that they have a choice; (2) they appreciate the situation and prognosis as well as risks, benefits, and consequences of treatments; (3) their decisions are stable over time and not impulsive; and (4) their decisions are consistent with their personal values and goals of care (Bernat, 2008; Lo, 1990).

This puts strong responsibilities on the healthcare provider to understand something about each patient and family and their particular needs in relation to processing information. It is necessary to consider what is needed for a patient or family member to optimally process information and to make sense of it in terms of personal goals, values, and life projects. When it comes to assisting surrogate or proxy decision makers, whose purpose is to articulate what a patient would want, healthcare providers have additional responsibilities. In such cases, the role of the APN is to help them interpret what the patient would have likely wanted, given what is known about him or her, or in pediatrics, to assist them in deciding what is in the child's best interests. This may require asking the right questions of the surrogate. For example: What do you know about Mr. or Ms. X.? What have his or her goals been? What does he or she value? But what if the patient is a child whose life goals and values are not well developed? How do APNs help a parent or guardian make the best decision for their child? Sometimes parents have difficulty realizing that their desires for their child may not actually be in the child's best interests. Additionally, parents may be anticipating the loss of their child and are under great stress. What is the responsibility of the APN in such cases? This next section explores the question in more detail.

Pediatrics

In the United States and many other countries, parents and/or legal guardians serve as medical decision makers for children. However, there may be cases where children are deemed competent to make decisions for themselves. In the United States there is a category of "mature minor." An underage child may be considered capable of making his or her own decisions for a variety of reasons. The criteria for designation as a mature minor varies, based (in the United States) on state jurisdiction, age, ability, experience, education, training, degree of maturity or judgment, and capacity to appreciate the nature of risks and consequences of procedures (Diaz et al., 2004; Hickey, 2007; Sigman & O'Connor, 1991). Children may also be deemed "emancipated" from the decisions of parents and guardians because of marital status, pregnancy, parenthood, engagement in military service, financial independence, and/or living apart from their parents (Kirschen & Feudtner, 2013). In the case of older children and adolescents who are not their own medical decision makers and who are not allowed to officially consent to treatment, it is nevertheless accepted that the child should be permitted to understand what is being suggested and why, and to assent to a course of action. There are exceptions to this ethical principle. For example, when a treatment is likely to be beneficial and it is known that the child will not assent, then a judgment has to be made about the balance of risk over benefit. It may cause more harm than good to force treatment upon a child who has been led to believe that his or her dissent will be honored.

When a child is permitted to make his or her own decisions for one of the previously stated reasons, the APN still needs to provide the support and resources the child needs. The pediatric chapter, Chapter 8, provides more in-depth discussion about how to support children who are making decisions without parental guidance or support. The American Academy of Pediatrics (AAP, 1995) has defined the concept of assent as including the following four components:

(1) an appropriate awareness of the nature of their condition
(2) knowledge of what they can expect with tests and treatments
(3) a positive clinical assessment of their understanding of the situation and the factors influencing their response; and
(4) an expression of the patient's willingness to accept care.

It is the position of the AAP that all children are entitled to comprehensible medical information and should have the opportunity to assent or dissent, and that a child's views should be given serious weight in the context of medical decision making (Kirschen & Feudtner, 2013). This can become complicated in instances when a child is able to understand information but unable to express their wishes either due to illness complications or the influence of medications (Kirschen & Feudtner, 2013). In pediatric EOL and palliative care settings, the decisions that require a child's assent can be complex and anxiety producing. A team approach that includes experts on EOL and palliative care from a variety of disciplines can result in age-appropriate, emotionally supportive environments in which a child's assent to a desired course of action is considered.

Adults and Decision Making

In the case of adults, the ethical principle of autonomy supports the right of those with decision-making capacity to accept or decline treatment or other interventions (Cerminara, 2011, p. 775). However, it is the healthcare provider's responsibility to ensure that the patient has the information needed to make an informed decision. The right to self-determination is a human right recognized by the United Nations. In the United States this right was codified in the Patient Self-Determination Act of 1991. Every state has some legally authorized form of advance directive, and guidelines exist for proxy decision makers and medical decision making. However, not all people designate a proxy decision maker, nor do they necessarily make their desires known in advance, even though efforts to educate the public about the benefits of advance directives have escalated over the past few decades.

Thus, in palliative and EOL care, the role of the APN is pivotal in providing frequent and ongoing education and guidance to patients and families as medical conditions worsen. The emphasis of the APN is on helping patients and their families focus on desired and achievable goals of care and appropriate emergency interventions (Kirschen & Feudtner, 2013). It may be that some patients are willing to accept more interventions even with the possibility of more suffering in order to achieve a goal that is meaningful to them, such as attending a child's wedding or a graduation, or it may be they do not want to accept more treatment even if there is the possibility of gaining several more months of life.

Futility at the End of Life: What Does It Mean? Who Decides?

When a patient is critically ill or at the end of life, multiple factors can influence decisions regarding care. New treatment options, advancing technology, and better outcomes have decreased morbidity and improved quality of life for many patients. Still, there are times when APNs find themselves at a crossroads. When prognosis is most certainly grim, are APNs obligated to provide a treatment that is medically feasible but clinically inappropriate? Who decides what appropriate care is? In a sense, demands for care that are inappropriate or unable to meet a person's goals or the proxy decision maker's interpretation of goals are futile. Sometimes the demand is the result of distrust of the healthcare system, and sometimes it is a problem of the decision maker's failure to separate personal needs from the best interests of their charge. Regardless of reason, the APN, along with collaborating colleagues, must try to determine what actions are needed. When a good resolution is not possible in a particular case, postcase discussions and analysis can provide insights that permit preventive ethics in future cases.

CASE STUDY: AN INFANT WITH BIRTH ANOMALIES

B.G. is 2-year-old female born with a mitochondrial disorder and multiple congenital anomalies. She has spent her entire life in the hospital, primarily in intensive care, which was necessary to address and manage her complex medical issues including hydrocephalus, seizures, and hepatic failure. Soon after birth, B.G. required a tracheotomy and gastro-jejunostomy (GJ) tube. Later, a ventricular-peritoneal (VP) shunt was placed to treat worsening hydrocephalus. At birth and during critical times when her condition deteriorated, the medical team met with the parents to discuss goals and limitations of care. The family repeatedly expressed to the healthcare team they wanted "everything done"—all medical and surgical interventions to keep their child alive and comfortable. As parents, they felt obligated to do everything possible to help their daughter. They based this decision on the hope that a miracle would occur and allow them to bring her home. During her first year of life, B.G. required seven VP shunt revisions, peritoneal dialysis, and cardiopulmonary resuscitation on multiple occasions. Her seizures were refractory to all medications.

Later, she developed multiorgan system failure, requiring continuous infusions of epinephrine and dopamine. Although B.G. never responded to painful stimuli, hydromorphone was given via a continuous intravenous infusion. Both parents repeatedly stated they would prefer their daughter to be awake as much as possible but not at the expense of having her in pain. The parents refused to attend team meetings to discuss limitations of care, nor did they want to have any discussions regarding a "do not resuscitate" (DNR) order. They insisted that the medical team continue to "do everything" — provide blood products, fluids, and all medical treatments including chest compressions, dialysis, and defibrillation if warranted. The staff felt many of the interventions the family insisted on, including providing cardiopulmonary resuscitation, were futile and only prolonged B.G.'s suffering. The case was referred to the hospital ethics committee.

Case Discussion

This case outlines several challenges in providing care when there is conflict between the medical team and family about what are considered aggressive life-sustaining interventions. The parents want everything done for their child while the medical team feels they should not be obligated to provide care deemed ineffective and futile. The family and team were in agreement about maximizing pain medications to minimize suffering, even if this meant B.G. would be heavily sedated.

What would the role of an APN with expertise both in palliative care and ethical decision making be in this situation? The goal of care for such children is to maximize the good for the child (i.e., beneficence) while minimizing harm (i.e., nonmaleficence). However, anticipating and attending to the family's needs are also an integral part of the APN's role. Early access to the expertise of a multidisciplinary palliative care team could be helpful in cohesively addressing unrealistic expectations while anticipating and attending to the psychological support needs of a family who hopes against hope that their child can be around for them to love and nurture. The knowledge base of APNs includes theories and evidence from the psychological and social literature related to the desires and needs of parents in relation to the death or impending death of a child. There are a variety of reasons why interventions that cannot meet either patient or medical goals might have been offered or might be continued. For example, the intervention might have served an initial purpose that it can no longer serve because the patient's condition and prognosis have changed. However, it is a failure of healthcare professional ethics to continue interventions that are painful when there is little hope of a quality of life. APNs who are trained in palliative care are well suited to support the healthcare team in taking ethically supportable actions in such cases.

Defining Futility

The concept of futility related to medical treatment remains complex. Ongoing biotechnological advances continue to push the barriers of what is physically possible, but that does not mean that such interventions can always meet a patient's or family's overall goals for a desired level of quality of life. Various philosophers and bioethicists have grappled with the issue of futility in the interests of assisting ethical decision making. However, the concept remains ambiguous for several reasons. Lo (2009) noted that futile medical interventions are those that would "serve no meaningful purpose, no matter how often they are repeated" (p. 69). Within the healthcare field, there has been little success in defining medical futility. One reason is that it is not clear who gets to decide whether pursuing a treatment with a 1% chance of working constitutes futility. Most clinicians will agree that the focus should instead be on how to resolve differences when families and clinicians disagree on what constitutes futile treatment (Chwang, 2009).

Schneideman, Jecker, and Johnsen (1990) asserted that the concept of futility can have both quantitative and qualitative properties, and although there is a fine distinction between the two, both refer to whether or not a treatment will produce any benefit to the patient.

Problems with Futility at the End of Life

One of the greatest challenges to nurses and others who are caring for persons at the end of life is how to manage or reconcile the distress experienced when asked to continue to provide interventions that cannot benefit the patient. Most often such interventions not only do not benefit the patient but actually cause harm in the form of increased suffering. As noted earlier in the chapter, attempts to define futility and futile interventions fail. Sometimes there is ambiguity about whether a treatment or intervention will have its desired effect. In such cases, careful deliberation with the patient's input, when possible, is most likely to reveal the best course of action. Additionally, patients or family members may change their minds about what is acceptable. When a family refuses to discontinue a medical treatment that is unwarranted, the team must attempt to understand the background story. Why was the treatment offered? What is the family hoping for? Are their needs being met? Is there a lack of trust? Are they getting conflicting information? Can providers help the family interpret what the patient would have wanted given their knowledge of him or her? It can be helpful to ask questions about the patient's previous life choices such as: Did your dad enjoy playing with the grandchildren? Did he like to be outdoors? What were his hobbies? Was mobility important to him?

Although some cases are intractable, they can still provide knowledge to change how providers approach families. Finally, when the family is acting in ways that are obviously not in a patient's best interests, it may be necessary to discuss with the legal department of an institution how to remove the proxy decision maker. The role of a proxy decision maker is to make decisions that serve the interests of the patient.

As a result of a perceived increase in demands for "futile" treatment on the part of some proxy decision makers in the United States, certain states have adopted policies that help determinations of futility to be made and in such cases permit the discontinuation of interventions that are useless (Terra, 2012; Truog, 2007). In 1999, Texas adopted The Futile Care Act, which provided physicians with a detailed approach to allow for discontinuation of life-sustaining treatment if it is considered futile by the medical team. The hospital and physician must abide by a specific course of action prior to discontinuing any treatment, including having the case reviewed by the institutional ethics committee, which allows the family's participation. If there is no consensus between the family and institution, the family may request a transfer to another hospital that is willing to provide care. If after 10 days a different provider cannot be located, the physician may unilaterally withhold or withdraw the futile therapy (Texas Health and Safety Code, 1999). One advantage of having a futility policy is that it provides a potential mechanism for solving challenging dilemmas; however, hospital-based ethics committees can be problematic because they usually consist of hospital employees, not necessarily an unbiased group of individuals (Truog, 2007). Additionally, such policies do not resolve the question of how the case developed and whether appropriate actions instituted earlier might have defused the problem.

Approaches to Help Minimize Futile Interventions

Given that medical futility is difficult to define and absolute cases of futility are rare, APNs should view cases individually to determine the benefits and burdens of each intervention. In the case of B.G., the parents' decision to continue all treatments even as their daughter's condition was rapidly deteriorating was undoubtedly shaped by multiple factors. APNs in turn make determinations based on current knowledge, prior experiences, and above all, commitment to protecting vulnerable patients. When a family asks an APN to "do everything," it is important to recognize that the family often does not know what they mean by this—they just want their loved one to be as they were previously. The APN's responsibility is to try to help them understand what the ultimate goals are and what the patient would have wanted or what is in his or her best interests. Additionally, APNs must consider how to help the family adapt to their changed or changing circumstances.

The request to "do everything" should become a mandate for open communication about genuine choices (Feudtner & Morrison, 2012) rather than a condition to back away from having candid conversations. In the case of B.G., the providers could begin by focusing on the common goals of treating pain and addressing suffering, and gradually shift the conversation to explain how certain treatments may prevent them from meeting those goals. Effective communication and insight into a complicated situation can help minimize conflict between healthcare providers, patients, and family members (Fins & Solomon, 2001; Jox, Schaider, Marckmann, & Borasio, 2012). Approaches to improve communication and minimize futility include:

1. Develop a trusting relationship
2. Allow families to express their understanding of what is occurring
3. Assure families that everything is being done
4. Ensure their loved one's comfort and dignity will always be attended to and they will not be abandoned

A provider's assertion that they can stop aggressive treatments by stating futility is often not sufficient to overrule a patient's or family's demand for more aggressive interventions (Burt, 2002). In fact, in many instances, the mention of futility alone puts a halt to legitimate conversations and consensus regarding care at the end of life.

Honoring Patient Wishes: Requests for Help with Dying

As the number of APNs who assume the overall care of persons at the end of their lives increases, there is a concomitant likelihood of encountering a request for assistance in dying. However, APNs are not the only nurses who are asked for such assistance. This may be one of the most difficult requests anyone faces in the course of a professional career, yet the person requesting is asking for help and the request must be addressed thoughtfully. In many instances, death is not the event that is feared most, but rather it is the suffering prior to and surrounding death that is the most anxiety provoking. Additionally, there is evidence to suggest that people want to have some control over their own death. Regardless of philosophical belief or emotional involvement with a patient, the APN must step back and be sure the nature and complexity of a request are understood. Additionally it is important that APNs are self-reflective about their own perspectives on death and dying.

Euthanasia is the term associated with the idea of assistance in dying. Its origins are in the Greek language. "Eu" means good or easy and "thanatos" means death (Brown, 1993); thus euthanasia means a "good death." Some philosophers have distinguished between *active euthanasia* (taking a definite action to end someone's life) and *passive euthanasia* (allowing someone to die by not intervening). There is also a distinction sometimes made among *voluntary euthanasia* (a person has asked for assistance in dying or has refused lifesaving interventions), *involuntary euthanasia* (ending a person's life against the person's wishes or without the person's knowledge), and *nonvoluntary euthanasia* (a person who is unable to make the decision is allowed to die; Munson, 2008).

In the Netherlands and Belgium, *active euthanasia* with the assistance of a physician has been legally permissible since 2002, although there are strict criteria governing the practice. Lethal injections that actually end the person's life are permitted. In the United States, active euthanasia is not permissible, although in some states such as Oregon, Washington, and Montana, physician-assisted suicide is legally permissible. Assisted suicide in these states means that after meeting criteria (including a period of deliberation), a participating physician provides the patient with life-ending medications that the patient must administer to him- or herself (Dees et al., 2013). In no country is it part of a physician's medical obligation to engage in active euthanasia or physician-assisted suicide. However, there is evidence to suggest that prior to contemporary debates about assisted suicide, voluntary and nonvoluntary euthanasia were fairly widely practiced in hospitals (Munson, 2008).

An extensive survey of U.S. physicians conducted in 1996 (Meier et al., 1998) found that incidences of euthanasia were not uncommon. The researchers surveyed physicians who were likely to encounter EOL issues. The response rate to the survey was 61% (N = 1,902). Among the results was the finding that 11% had given medicines that they knew would hasten death and 37% said they would do so if it were legal. The researchers' conclusion was that "[A] substantial proportion of physicians in the United States in the specialties surveyed report that they receive requests for physician-assisted suicide and euthanasia, and about 6% have complied with such requests at least once" (Meier et al., 1998, p. 1193). Moreover, a significant proportion of physicians had engaged in euthanasia for the purpose of relieving suffering.

The important thing to keep in mind is that although euthanasia is not legal anywhere in the United States or in many other countries, there are reasons for the intensifying public discussion about whether people have a right to the means for ending their lives in the event of unbearable suffering. Healthcare professionals hold the keys to this knowledge and to these resources. *Physician-assisted suicide* is the term used to describe the act of a physician furnishing the information, means, or medication to a patient that will help that person end his or her life. The ethical permissibility of physician-assisted suicide remains controversial even in those countries and states where legislative prohibitions do not exist. One important ethical question is whether the healthcare professional's pledge (implicit or explicit) to promote a good and at least do no harm is broken by assisting a patient to end his or her own life in the face of intractable suffering.

This issue is likely to remain polarizing in the United States because of irreconcilable belief systems. So how can the APN respond? The most important response is to elicit and validate the patient's concerns while providing appropriate resources.

It is beyond the scope of this chapter to trace the development of right-to-die legislation; however, there are numerous ethics textbooks and journal articles available that provide more information about these important topics. It is also helpful for the APN to be aware of the stance of professional nursing organizations, which mainly oppose the idea of deliberately assisting a person in ending his or her own life. The most current American Nurses Association (ANA, 1994) position statement on assisted suicide is representative of the U.S. nursing profession's voice in regard to participation in assisted suicide or active euthanasia:

> The American Nurses Association (ANA) believes that the nurse should not participate in assisted suicide. . . . Nurses, individually and collectively, have an obligation to provide comprehensive and compassionate end-of-life care which includes the promotion of comfort and the relief of pain and, at times, forgoing life-sustaining treatments. (ANA, 1994)

Currently, this position statement has been opened for revision and public comment. Of note, the expansion of legislation regarding assisted death has occurred simultaneous to the expansion of palliative care training for physicians, increased communication of patient wishes regarding life-sustaining treatment, heightened awareness of pain management techniques, and increased rates of hospice referrals and deaths occurring in homes (Quill, 2007), along with the publication of a guidebook for clinicians in 2008, *The*

Task Force to Improve the Care of Terminally-Ill Oregonians (Lachman, 2010). All of these advances allow APNs to be better equipped to address patients' and families' concerns and questions regarding these important topics. The following guidelines were developed by an interdisciplinary team to assist clinicians in responding to requests for assistance with dying:

1. Self-reflection about one's own reaction to such requests. Assume a nonjudgmental pose.
2. A genuine willingness to listen to the person's feelings and perceptions. Be alert for cues and probe for more information.
3. Evaluate possible contributing factors—What pushed the person to this point. What else is going on? What are the psychosocial and physical problems? How severe are they? Is the person coherent, delirious, depressed?
4. Ascertain whether there are issues that can be addressed or turned around. Start planning strategies with the patient as amenable.
5. Review the situation with the patient. Ask if there are other issues. Reassure the patient that his or her confidentiality will be protected to the extent reasonable given the need of other team members to know (and in the absence of serious harm to others or self).
6. Document pertinent aspects using clinical judgment. (Hudson et al., 2006)

Palliative Sedation

Palliative sedation, also known as terminal sedation, is the practice of titrating sedatives or analgesics to the point where a person no longer experiences symptoms (Davis & Ford, 2005). The goal of palliative sedation is not the cessation of life. It is a clinical decision intended to relieve intractable pain and patient awareness of suffering (Bruera, 2012; Bruinsma, Rietjens, Seymour, Anquinet, & van der Heide, 2012). Medications, specifically sedatives, are used to decrease patient consciousness when pain and suffering become intolerable (Graeff & Dean, 2007).

The Hospice and Palliative Nursing Association position paper (Hospice and Palliative Nursing Association, 2003) titled "Palliative Sedation at the End of Life" provides guidelines for advanced practice and other nurses working in palliative and hospice settings but is relevant for any nurse caring for those needing EOL care. It notes that "an array of physical and psychological symptoms and existential distress" (p. 235) may be experienced, and for the most part, they can be relieved by good care. Reports suggest that palliative sedation may be used in up to 30% of dying adult patients (Hospice and Palliative Nursing Association, 2003).

Relief of suffering is the goal of palliative sedation. Suffering includes a sense of helplessness or loss in the face of a seemingly relentless and unendurable threat to quality of life or integrity of self (Cassell, 1999). Additionally, Cherny, Coyle, and Foley (1994) proposed that consciousness, or the ability to perceive and respond to the sense of loss and hopelessness, is a condition of suffering. For the most part, it is believed that suffering can be relieved with combinations of analgesia and other therapeutics—however, sometimes it cannot.

Some commentators recommend that palliative sedation be used only when a person's death is expected within hours to a few days; other critics believe that palliative sedation can be used in other cases when intractable symptoms occur, but that the drugs should be appropriate to the symptoms and titrated only to relief of symptoms, that is, not used in ever-escalating doses (Cherny & Portnoy, 1994). General principles are that it is reserved for those who are imminently dying.

Guidelines for the use of palliative sedation have been developed by several scholars. The palliative sedation option should be discussed with patients and their families prior to the need for it (when possible). This permits patients and family members to ask questions and develop a plan. It also facilitates informed consent and thus upholds the principle of autonomy. Palliative care works best when an interdisciplinary team is available to assess the situation and collaborate both on care of the patient and support for the family. The collaborative team plans the therapeutics together (Rousseau, 2001). Team members may include a palliative care APN, the patient's physician or nurse practitioner, a pain management specialist, and allied professionals, as appropriate. Good documentation of the process and the rationale is needed.

CASE STUDY EXAMPLE: PALLIATIVE SEDATION

T.R. was a 16-year-old male who was diagnosed with rhabdomyosarcoma at the age of 6. He was treated with chemotherapy and palliative radiation to relieve pain. Soon his cancer metastasized to his lungs and spine. As T.R.'s tumors grew, his ability to participate in school and other activities gradually diminished. Throughout his diagnosis and treatment, T.R. was able to speak directly with his family and physicians regarding how and where he wanted to die. He was not afraid of dying but did share with everyone his fear of suffocating. The tumors in his lungs grew, and he required supplemental oxygen via a nasal cannula along with morphine to manage his dyspnea. T.R. and his parents met with the palliative care team; they assured him pain and dyspnea would be treated aggressively. Tumors infiltrated his abdomen, making daily activities nearly impossible. He developed a partial bowel obstruction and a nasogastric tube was placed to decompress his stomach along with medications to decrease secretions and pain.

T.R. spoke with his parents and primary oncologist and it was decided that in the event of a cardiac or respiratory arrest, he would not want to be intubated, shocked, or have chest compressions. Again, T.R. shared with them his fear of dying from suffocation and pain. T.R.'s condition deteriorated and his pain worsened along with his dyspnea. A continuous infusion of morphine was started along with a benzodiazepine to minimize anxiety. Eventually his tumors spread throughout his abdomen. His morphine infusion was increased frequently in response to worsening symptoms but without much relief. A switch to hydromorphone improved things for a short while. His pain quickly became refractory to most opioids. After discussion with his family, the decision to initiate palliative sedation was made to manage his symptoms. A continuous infusion of pentobarbital was started. T.R. died comfortably with his parents by his side.

Discussion

The preceding case demonstrates an example of justified palliative sedation. In T.R.'s case the patient, team, and family were in agreement about T.R.'s goals and how they might best be met within the constraints of ethical and legal boundaries. However, there are many reasons why intra- and/or interpersonal conflicts arise in such complex EOL situations. APNs may well be called upon to assist their peers, the patient, and family members in understanding the issues. One principle that is often relied upon to guide medical decision making about appropriate interventions and therapeutics is the rule of Double Effect.

The Rule of Double Effect

The ethical principle of double effect (Lo, 2005) is helpful in conceptualizing or rationalizing the permissibility of using high doses of drugs if necessary to alleviate a person's symptoms, even if it is known that the treatments used could shorten a person's life. "The doctrine of double effect distinguishes effects that are intended from those that are foreseen but unintended" (Lo, 2005, p. 107). Essentially, this principle asserts that the intent of an action is its most important aspect. The good effect is, of course, relief of the patient's suffering, and the unintended effect is the patient's death.

The doctrine of double effect originates within religious tradition. It is thought that when giving doses of analgesics or sedatives, focusing on the intent to alleviate suffering provides an important distinction that eradicates the concern of intending a person's death. This focus on relieving suffering permits even those with deeply held anti-euthanasia beliefs to assist in ensuring a person's comfort. It is argued that making a distinction between passive euthanasia (withholding or withdrawing life-prolonging treatments) and active euthanasia (the intentional taking of someone's life) is important and can be maintained by the doctrine of double effect. In the ethics literature, there is debate about these distinctions and their importance. Nevertheless, for many people, religious or philosophical beliefs make them uncomfortable with the idea of being involved in hastening someone's death, even if that person would prefer relief of suffering and finds the risk of death acceptable.

Autonomy in End-of-Life Decision Making

Upholding the principle of autonomy is crucially important and yet it is the most difficult to honor, especially in long-term care institutions where certain restrictions upon the personal freedom of residents are inevitable. Elders (and others) living in institutional settings are dependent to various degrees upon those who make the rules and uphold the routines. However, individuals' ability to make their own choices within the limits of the setting remains important for their well-being. Palliative and hospice care options in long-term care facilities in the United States and elsewhere remain scarce and regulations and funding complex. It will be critical to continue to develop palliative care services for such institutions.

Problems of Autonomy

Many of the ethical issues faced by APNs who care for older patients have to do with these patients' temporary or permanent loss of autonomy and how to best address this issue. Autonomy may be lost in the sense that a person has diminished decision-making ability, that is, he or she is unable to make autonomous or self-determined choices, or it may be lost in a second and more practical sense in that a person's range of choices is limited by dependence on others to meet his or her needs. The ability to carry out plans and enact choices may become limited for some older persons, which in turn affects their lifestyle options, quality of life, and even the manner of their death. For authentic choices—those that are in line with beliefs and values—to be made persons must be competent to make those choices and be relatively free to make them. The ethical principle of autonomy, as used in health care, denotes a person's capacity to determine voluntarily which choices are acceptable and unacceptable and is usually understood to be dependent upon cognitive or mental capacity. However, it is also somewhat dependent upon a person's physical ability to enact choices or resist the actions of others. For example, physical incapacities can make persons reliant on others for their daily activities, including self-care, mobility, nutrition, and other needs. As Castellucci (1998) notes, circumstances that interfere with an older adult's autonomy include "internal and external constraints" (p. 268).

Loss of Independence

When a person who previously possessed autonomy in the sense of being self-reliant and independent loses some degree of independence, as happens more frequently in the aging population than in other cohorts, a whole other set of ethical issues is presented. How can the APN assist patients in maintaining integrity and a sense of well-being when they are reliant to varying degrees upon others for their self-care needs or other services? How can older adults be protected when their well-being is threatened by a caregiver or healthcare system? What do caregivers need to help them remain healthy while being stressed as a result of caregiving activities? APNs frequently encounter all of these problems.

A person's ability to act independently can be reduced by sensory or other physical changes. Sometimes the person recognizes his or her limitations and seeks assistance from others to meet personal needs. It is not unusual, though, for a person's judgment about his or her capabilities to be in conflict with objective assessments. Thus, some people are unable or unwilling to recognize their own sensory or physical limitations. Ethical decision making in such cases may require APNs to collect data about a patient from a variety of sources, draw on colleagues and allied health professionals for assistance and resources, and educate long-term care or nursing home facilities staff about the rights and needs of residents related to palliation of symptoms and EOL care. Educating others about the role and usefulness of advance directives is an important aspect of the APN role.

Advance Directives

In Chapter 3, the need for APNs to assist people in conceptualizing what they want at the end of life was introduced. Types of advance directives were described, and important aspects of decision making were delineated. The salient idea is that there is a process involved in determining what will guide decision making at the end of life. Almost all developed countries now recognize and honor a person's right to autonomous decision making even when his or her capacity is lost. Many countries have recognized policies related to advance directives. A Swiss colleague recently informed the fourth author (Grace) that his advance directive was accessible from all over Switzerland and could be faxed elsewhere by his family if the need arose. As people develop and age, their priorities for themselves may change. The person designated as a substitute decision maker may also change for a host of reasons. Thus primary care APNs and physicians are among the first-line educators for promoting autonomy of choice even when decision-making capacity is lost. They also have an important role in keeping dialogue open with patients and making it a part of the discussion in every primary care visit.

Perhaps the single most important role of APNs related to EOL care is to help people think about what their values and goals are and to articulate these in writing. Secondly, the APN can help patients think about whom among family and acquaintances are the most likely to be able to carry out their wishes. No advance directive can address every possible scenario, but an overall picture of who the person is can inform others, including healthcare providers. In such cases where a person is socially isolated or without close family ties, assistance in identifying an appropriate legal representative or guardian is also important.

Enhancing End-of-Life Decision Making

Little has been written about the nuances of the nurse–patient relationship in relation to choices about EOL care. Clover, Browne, McErlain, and Vandenberg's (2004) small qualitative Australian study found that "patient participation is highly dependent on professionals' skill in opening up negotiation" (p. 340). When nurses were able to facilitate patients' acquisition of necessary information, patients became less passive and more able to say what they really wanted.

Additionally, providing support for the relatives or close friends of a dying patient is an important role of the APN, along with other members of the interdisciplinary team. For many people, it might be their first time encountering the death of someone close, and they must juggle personal feelings of grief with the need to make considered judgments related to the person's care. Andershed's (2006) literature review of 94 studies is revealing. Themes that emerged include the significant person (relative or friend of the dying person) as "being exposed" and experiencing "increased vulnerability" (p. 1160); they themselves were often at risk from ill health and had to find ways to cope with the tensions between "burden and capacity" (p. 1161). Not surprisingly, it was important for relatives to see that their loved one was getting good care and was "content" (p. 1162). Among the study themes that emerged from this meta-analysis was the importance of well-structured care in palliative care and hospice settings. Another very important theme in many of the studies reviewed by Andershed (2006) was the relatives' need for effective communication and information about all aspects of care. Perhaps one of the most striking insights was that relatives have different needs from the patient and desire interactions with nurses that take this into consideration. That is, nurses need to approach relatives as people in their own right with their own needs.

Withdrawing and Withholding Nutrition and Hydration

Some patients with terminal illnesses, or their family members, may question the ongoing administration of nutrition and hydration toward the end of life. Indeed, voluntary refusal of sustenance "has been proposed as an alternative to physician assisted suicide for terminally ill patients who wish to hasten death" (Ganzini et al., 2003, p. 359). It has been generally supposed that dying from dehydration is a terrible death, and thus it is worrisome when dying persons or family members request a cessation in nutrition and fluids. A study conducted by Ganzini and colleagues (2003) explored this further by surveying 102 hospice nurses working in Oregon who reported having taken care of a patient in the prior 4 years who had stopped eating or drinking a few days before that person's death. "Nurses reported that patients chose to stop eating and drinking because they were ready to die, saw continued existence as pointless, and considered their quality of life as poor" (p. 359). Eighty-five percent of the patients died within 15 days of stopping food. The nurses assigned scores for their perception of the quality of the person's death. The median score was 8 on a scale of 1 to 10, where 10 represented a highest "quality" death, given the illness suffered.

Despite such evidence, decisions to stop nutrition and hydration are certainly not without ethical implications. It is generally accepted that medical interventions can be withheld or withdrawn when competent decision makers speak on behalf of minors or patients who lack decision-making capacity (Diekema & Botkin, 2009). Interventions are deemed ethically appropriate when they meet the best interest standard, that is, "a weighing of expected burdens and benefits of that intervention" (Diekema & Botkin, 2009, p. 814). In the instance of fluid and nutrition, however, the argument is often that they are different from other medical interventions because they represent basic forms of care that can never be withdrawn, especially in children (Diekema & Botkin, 2009). The decision about whether or not to stop nutrition and hydration at the end of a person's life is a topic of ongoing debate and is wrought with personal, religious, cultural, societal, and legal implications. Many professional groups have position statements or guidelines to assist clinicians in guiding patients and families regarding these topics. For example, the AAP offers some guidelines, such as if the child is capable of eating or drinking, and shows a desire to do so, he or she should be offered food and drink, and also that decisions about whether to withhold or withdraw fluids and nutrition should be made with the same reasoning/justification as the withholding or withdrawing of any other medical treatments (Diekema & Botkin, 2009). Guidelines such as these are extensive and are available to help guide decision making, along with ethics consultations, which are strongly recommended in any situation involving ethically laden decisions, such as the withdrawal of nutrition and hydration. It is also important for the APN to examine his or her own personal beliefs, clarify where he or she stands, and refrain from projecting personal beliefs and making judgments about patients' and families' decisions.

The Role of the Advanced Practice Nurse

APNs have important roles both in providing and improving care for individuals with life-limiting or life-threatening illness and their families, including care at the end of life at any age, including infancy (as discussed in Chapter 7). The role of nursing is important because of the profession's emphasis on understanding patient experiences in response to life processes. Byock and Miles (2003) write that "quality of end-of-life care in the United States is seriously deficient" (p. 335) despite recent efforts to improve this aspect of health care. The role of the APN in palliative and EOL care can be complex as it becomes one of educator, supporter, collaborator, and consultant for other clinicians as well as patients and families. In providing such a wide array of care surrounding topics that are deeply rooted in personal, cultural, religious, and social values, ethical dilemmas abound. It is therefore also the role of the APN to recognize, contemplate, and use appropriate resources to guide such discussions and decision-making processes with patients and families.

Ethical issues that are associated with EOL situations include decision making under conditions of ambiguity, adequately informing patients and their families about treatment options, balancing quality of life against extending suffering, managing intractable suffering, and futile treatments. Decisions around EOL care and who is involved in decision making vary depending on the patient population, cultural beliefs, values, and other characteristics of the individual and setting. Other chapters in the text provide discussions related to EOL issues. For example, Chapter 7 describes the neonatal infant care unit and futility concerns, and Chapter 3 provides a discussion of advance directives and informed consent. This chapter does not repeat previous discussions but rather uses them as foundations for case exploration later. Some aspects of EOL care discussed in bioethics and applied philosophy literature provide a helpful background to discussions of futility, the ethical permissibility of withholding food and fluids at a patient's or patient surrogate's request, and the meaning and use of palliative sedation. These topics were discussed briefly in the previous subsections.

Summary

The discussion in this chapter has centered on the recognition of ethical dilemmas that arise when caring for individuals and families with life-threatening illness and/or at the end of life, and the responsibilities of APNs related to care of this population. Nursing goals and ethical principles as well as knowledge of the special needs of persons at the end of life guide the discussion about decision making. Among the responsibilities of APNs are the education and support of other nurses and allied health professionals as they provide care for this population. APNs can be influential in the education of other staff, in their collaborative relationships with interdisciplinary team members, and in formulating policies that facilitate the humane treatment of individuals and maximize their range of choices in the face of difficult decision making.

Many more issues are relevant to APN practice related to palliative and EOL care for patients and families than can be included here. Other chapters in the text provide the foundation for analyzing the issues and grasping the ethical nature of APN care in these settings. APNs have the knowledge, skills, and expertise to advocate for patients and families in the face of serious illness and to provide good care for those at the end of life.

Discussion Questions

1. Advance care planning is important in helping people think about their values and the meaning that life holds for them.
   a. What are the likely reasons that the majority of people do not explicitly make their wishes about EOL care known?
   b. What fears, including cultural and sociopolitical, might underlie this tendency?
   c. How would you go about discussing the issue of EOL care with a patient who is suspicious of healthcare providers or the healthcare system?

2. "The parents of a 12-year-old boy with terminal cancer believe they found the remedy for him to enjoy his short time left. They never told him he was dying. [They] kept their son's fatal condition from him as he battled a brain tumor pushing against his eye. Adam X was aware he had the tumor, gamely enduring bouts of chemotherapy, radiation, and steroids. But the boy remained unaware of his grim prognosis and hoped for recovery." (Dicker, 2012)
   a. What would be the issues in a case like this for an ANP with palliative care expertise?
   b. If a nurse in the oncology clinic asked for your assistance with a similar case, how would you respond?
   c. What role could preventive ethics have played in this case (preventive ethics is about recognizing the possibility of future ethical issues arising and taking preventive steps)?

References

American Academy of Pediatrics, Committee on Bioethics. (1995). Informed consent, parental permission, and assent in pediatric practice. *Pediatrics, 95*, 314–317.

American Medical Association. (1999). Medical futility in end of life care. *Journal of the American Medical Association, 281*(10), 937–941.

American Nurses Association. (1994). *Position statement on assisted suicide*. Washington, DC: Author.

Andershed, B. (2006). Relatives in end-of-life care—part 1: A systematic review of the literature the last five years, January 1999–February 2004. *Cancer and Palliative Care, 15*, 1158–1169.

Annas, G. J. (1984). The case of Baby Jane Doe: Child abuse or unlawful federal intervention? *American Journal of Public Health, 74*(7), 727–729.

Baily, M. A. (2011). Futility, autonomy and cost in end-of-life care. *Journal of Law, Medicine & Ethics, 39*(2), 172–182.

Bannon, A. (1982, Fall). The case of the Bloomington baby. *Human Life Review, 68*.

Bernat, J. L. (2008). *Ethical issues in neurology* (3rd ed). Philadelphia, PA: Wolters Kluwer/ Lippincott Williams & Wilkins.

Blank, R. H. (2011). End-of-life decision making across cultures. *Journal of Law, Medicine & Ethics, 39*(2), 201–214.

Brown, L. (Ed). (1993). *Oxford English Dictionary*. Oxford, UK: Clarendon.

Bruera, E. (2012). Palliative sedation: When and how? *Journal of Clinical Oncology, 30*(12), 1258–1259.

Bruinsma, S. M., Rietjens, J. A., Seymour, J. E., Anquinet, L., & van der Heide, A. (2012). The experiences of relatives with the practice of palliative sedation: A systematic review. *Journal of Pain and Symptom Management, 44*(3), 431–445.

Burt, R. A. (2002). The medical futility debate: Patient choice, physician obligation, and end-of-life care. *Journal of Palliative Medicine, 2*, 249–254.

Byock, I., & Miles, S. (2003). Hospice benefits and phase I cancer trials. *Annals of Internal Medicine, 138*(4), 335–337.

Capron, A. M. (1991). In re Helga Wanglie. *Hastings Center Report, 21*(5), 26–28.

Cassell, E. (1999). Diagnosing suffering: A perspective. *Annals of Internal Medicine, 131*(7), 531–534.

Castellucci, D. T. (1998). Issues for nurses regarding elder autonomy. *Nursing Clinics of North America, 33*(2), 265–274.

Cerminara, K. L. (2011). The law and its interaction with medical ethics in end-of-life decision making. *Chest, 140*(3), 775–780.

Cherny, N., Coyle, N., & Foley, K. (1994). Suffering in the advanced cancer patient: A definition and taxonomy. *Journal of Palliative Care, 102*, 57–70.

Cherny, N., & Portnoy, R. (1994). Sedation in the management of refractory symptoms: Guidelines for evaluation and treatment. *Journal of Palliative Care, 10*(2), 31–38.

Chwang, E. (2009). Futility clarified. *Journal of Law, Medicine, & Ethics 37*(3), 487–495.

Clark, D. (2007). From margins to centre: A review of the history of palliative care in cancer. *Lancet Oncology, 8*, 430–438.

Clark, D., & Centeno, C. (2006). Palliative care in Europe: An emerging approach to comparative analysis. *Clinical Medicine, 6*(2), 197–201.

Clover, A., Browne, J., McErlain, P., & Vandenberg, B. (2004). Patient approaches to clinical conversations in the palliative care settings. Issues and innovations in nursing practice. *Journal of Advanced Nursing, 48*(4), 333–341.

Colby, W. H. (2002). *Long goodbye: The deaths of Nancy Cruzan.* Carlsbad, CA: Hay House.

Coombes, R. (2007). Ashley X: A difficult moral choice. *British Medical Journal, 334,* 72–73.

Davis, M., & Ford, P. (2005). Palliative sedation: Definition, practice, outcomes. *Journal of Palliative Medicine, 8*(4), 699–701.

Dees, M. K., Vernooij-Dassen, M. J., Dekkers, W. J., Elwyn, G., Vissers, K. C., & van Weel, C. (2013). Perspectives of decision-making in requests for euthanasia: A qualitative research among patients, relatives and treating physicians in the Netherlands. *Palliative Medicine, 27*(1), 27–37.

Diaz, A., Neal, W. P., Nucci, A. T., Ludmer, P., Bitterman, J., & Edwards, S. (2004). Legal and ethical issues facing adolescent health care professionals. *Mount Sinai Journal of Medicine, 71,* 181–185.

Dicker, R. (2012, July 25). Parents didn't tell 12-year-old Adam X he was dying -- right thing to do? *The Huffington Post.* Retrieved from http://www.huffingtonpost.com/2012/07/25 /parents-didnt-12-year-old_n_1701916.html

Diekema, D. S., & Botkin, J. R. (2009). Forgoing medically provided nutrition and hydration in children. *Pediatrics, 124,* 813–822. doi: 10.1542/peds.2009-1299

Doyle, J. (2010). Baby K. A landmark case in futile medical care. *WebmedCentral Medical Ethics, 1*(10): WMC00969. Retrieved from http://www.webmedcentral.com/article_view/969

Dresser, R. (2004). Schiavo: A hard case makes questionable law. *Hastings Center Report, 34*(3), 8–9.

Feudtner, C., & Morrison, W. (2012). The darkening veil of "do everything." *Archives of Pediatrics & Adolescent Medicine, 166*(8), 694–695.

Filene, P. G. (1998). *In the arms of others: A cultural history of the right-to-die in America.* Chicago, IL: Ivan R. Dee.

Fins, J., & Solomon, M. Z. (2001). Communication in the intensive care setting: The challenges of futility disputes. *Critical Care Medicine, 29*(2), Supplement N10-15.

Foley, K. M., & Gelband, H. (2001). *Improving palliative care for cancer.* Washington, DC: National Academies Press.

Ganzini, L., Goy, E., Miller, L., Harvath, T., Jackson, A., & Delorit, M. (2003). Nurses' experiences with hospice patients who refuse food and fluids to hasten death. *New England Journal of Medicine, 349*(4), 359–365.

Graeff, A. D., & Dean, M. (2007). Palliative sedation therapy in the last weeks of life: A literature review and recommendations for standards. *Journal of Palliative Medicine, 10*(1), 67–85.

Gunther, D. F., & Diekma, D. S. (2006). Attenuating growth in children with profound developmental disability: A new approach to an old dilemma. *Archives of Pediatrics &*

Adolescent Medicine, 160(10), 1013–1017. doi:10.1001/archpedi.160.10.1013. doi:10:1001/jama.2010.920

Hickey, K. (2007). Minors' rights in medical decision making. *JONAS Healthcare Law Ethics Regulation, 9*, 100–104; quiz 105–106.

Himelstein, B. P., Hilden, J. M., Boldt, A. M., & Weissman, D. (2004). Pediatric palliative care. *New England Journal of Medicine, 350*, 1752–1762.

Hofmann, B. (2002). Is there a technological imperative in health care? *International Journal of Technology Assessment in Health Care, 18*(3), 675–689.

Hospice and Palliative Nursing Association. (2003). Palliative sedation at the end of life. *Journal of Hospice and Palliative Nursing, 5*(4), 235–237.

Hudson, P., Scholfield, P., Kelly, B., Hudson, R., Street, A., O'Connor, M., ... Aranda, S. (2006). Responding to desire to die statements form patients with advanced disease: Recommendations for health professionals. *Pallliative Medicine, 20*, 703–710.

Institute of Medicine. (1998). *Approaching death: Improving care at end of life.* Consensus Report. Retrieved from http://iom.edu/Reports/1998/Approaching-Death-Improving-Care-at-the-End-of-Life.aspx

Institute of Medicine. (2002). *When children die: Improving palliative and end-of-life care for children and their families.* Consensus report. Retrieved from http://iom.edu/Reports/2002/When-Children-Die-Improving-Palliative-and-End-of-Life-Care-for-Children-and-Their-Families.aspx

Jox, R. J., Schaider, A., Marckmann, G., & Borasio, G. N. (2012). Medical futility at the end of life: The perspectives of intensive care and palliative care clinicians. *Journal of Medical Ethics, 38*(9), 540–545.

Kantarjian, H. M., Wolff, R. A., & Koller, C. A. (Eds.). (2011). *MD Anderson Manual of Medical Oncology* (2nd ed.). Columbus, OH: McGraw-Hill.

Kirschen, M. P., & Feudtner, C. (2013). Ethical issues. In N. S. Abend & M. A. Helfaer (Eds.), *Pediatric Neurocritical Care* (pp. 485–493). New York, NY: DemosMedical.

Kirschner, K. L., Brashler, R., & Savage, T. A. (2007). Ashley X. *American Journal of Physical Medicine and Rehabilitation, 86*(12), 1023–1029.

Lachman, V. (2010). Physician-assisted suicide: Compassionate liberation or murder? *Medsurg Nursing, 19*(2), 121–125.

Liben, S., Papadatou, D., & Wolfe, J. (2008). Paediatric palliative care: Challenges and emerging ideas. *Lancet, 371*, 852–864.

Lo, B. (1990). Assessing decision-making capacity. *Journal of Law, Medicine & Ethics, 18*, 193–201.

Lo, B. (2005). *Resolving ethical dilemmas: A guide for clinicians* (3rd ed.). Philadelphia, PA: Lippincott Williams & Wilkins.

Lo, B. (2009). *Resolving ethical dilemmas: A guide for clinicians* (4th ed.). Baltimore, MD: Lippincott Williams & Wilkins.

Mahon, M. M. (2010). Clinical decision making in palliative care and end of life care. *Nursing Clinics of North America, 45*, 345–362.

Meier, D. E., Emmons, C. A., Wallenstein, S., Quill, T., Morrison, S., & Cassell, C. (1998). A national survey of physician-assisted suicide and euthanasia in the United States. *New England Journal of Medicine, 338*, 1193–1201.

Mercurio, M. R. (2009). The aftermath of Baby Doe and the evolution of newborn intensive care. *Georgia State University Law Review, 25*(4), 835–863.

Missouri State Supreme Court. (1990). *Cruzan v. Director*, Missouri Department of Health, (88-1503), 497 U.S. 261. Retrieved from http://www.law.cornell.edu/supct/html/88-1503.ZS.html

Mosby's Medical Dictionary (9th ed.). (2012). St. Louis, MO: Elsevier.

Munson, R. (2008). *Intervention and reflection: Basic issues in medical ethics*. Belmont, CA: Thompson Wadsworth.

Quill, T. E. (2007). Legal regulation of physician-assisted death—The latest report cards. *New England Journal of Medicine, 356*(19), 1911–1913.

Rousseau, P. (2001). Existential suffering and palliative sedation: A brief commentary with a proposal for clinical guidelines. *American Journal of Hospice and Palliative Care, 18*(3), 151–153.

Saunders, C. M. (1978). *The management of terminal malignant disease*. London, UK: Edward Arnold.

Schneiderman, L. J., Jecker, N. S., & Jonsen, A. R. (1990). Medical futility: Its meaning and ethical implications. *Annals of Internal Medicine, 112*(12), 949–954.

Sepulveda, C., Marlin, A., Yoshida, T., & Ullrich, A. (2002). Palliative care: The World Health Organization's global perspective. *Journal of Pain and Symptom Management, 24*, 91–96.

Shakespeare, W. (2004/1611). *The tempest*. New York, NY: Washington Square Press.

Sigman, G. S., & O'Connor, C. (1991). Exploration for physicians of the mature minor doctrine. *Journal of Pediatrics, 199*, 520–525.

Smith, M. L., Gremillion, G., Slomka, J., & Warneke, M. (2007). Texas hospitals' experience with the Texas Advance Directives Act. *Critical Care Medicine, 35*(5), 1271–1276.

Stoppard, T. (1967). *Rosencrantz and Guildenstern are dead*. London, UK: Faber and Faber.

Terra, S. P. (2012). Is determination of medical futility ethical? *Professional Case Management, 17*(3), 103–106.

Texas Health and Safety Code. (1999). Retrieved from http://www.statutes.legis.state.tx.us/Docs/HS/htm/HS.166.htm

Truog, R. D. (2007). Tackling medical futility in Texas. *New England Journal of Medicine, 357*, 1–3. doi:10.1056/NEJMp078109

Willis, D., Grace, P. J., & Roy, C. (2008). A central unifying focus for the discipline: Facilitating humanization, meaning, choice, quality of life, and healing in living and dying. *Advances in Nursing Science, 31*(1), E28–E40.

Wolfson, J. (2005). Erring on the side of Theresa Schiavo: Reflections of the special guardian ad litem. *Hastings Center Report, 35*(3), 16–19.

Supplemental Resources

General

The Ethics Committee of the American Board of Pediatrics. https://www.abp.org/abpwebsite/publicat/bioethics.pdf

Journals by Category

DECISIONS TO WITHDRAW/WITHHOLD LIFE-SUSTAINING MEDICAL INTERVENTION

American Academy of Pediatrics Committee on Bioethics. (1994). Guidelines on forgoing life-sustaining medical treatment. *Pediatrics, 93,* 532–536.

American Academy of Pediatrics Committee on Bioethics and Committee on Child Abuse and Neglect. (2000). Forgoing life-sustaining medical treatment in abused children. *Pediatrics, 106,* 1151–1153.

Carter, B. S., Hubble, C., & Weise, K. L. (2006). Palliative medicine in neonatal and pediatric intensive care. *Child & Adolescent Psychiatry Clinics of North America, 15,* 759–777.

Munson, D. (2007). Withdrawal of mechanical ventilation in pediatric and neonatal intensive care units. *Pediatric Clinics of North America, 54,* 773–785.

Paris, J. J., Graham, N., Schreiber, M. D., & Goodwin, M. (2006). Has the emphasis on autonomy gone too far? Insights from Dostoevsky on parental decision making in the NICU. *Cambridge Quarterly of Healthcare Ethics, 15,* 147–151.

Pellegrino, E. D. (2000). Decisions to withdraw life-sustaining treatment: A moral algorithm. *Journal of the American Medical Association, 283,* 1065–1067.

Reynolds, S., Cooper, A. B., & McKneally, M. (2007). Withdrawing life-sustaining treatment: Ethical considerations. *Surgical Clinics of North America, 87,* 919–936.

Sharman, M., Meert, K. L., & Sarnaik, A. P. (2005). What influences parents' decisions to limit or withdraw life support? *Pediatric Critical Care Medicine, 6,* 513–518.

Tripp, J., & McGregor, D. (2009). Withholding and withdrawing of life sustaining treatment in the newborn. *Archives of Disease in Childhood. Fetal and Neonatal Edition, 91*(1), F67– F71.

Truog, R. D., Burns, J. P., Mitchell, C., Johnson, J., & Robinson, W. (2000). Pharmacologic paralysis and withdrawal of mechanical ventilation at the end of life. *New England Journal of Medicine, 342,* 508–511.

DECISIONS TO WITHDRAW/WITHHOLD ARTIFICIAL HYDRATION/NUTRITION

Cranford, R. E. (1991). Neurologic syndromes and prolonged survival: When can artificial nutrition and hydration be forgone? *Journal of Law, Medicine & Ethics, 19,* 13–22.

Diekema, D. S., Botkin, J. R., & The American Academy of Pediatrics Committee on Bioethics. (2009). Forgoing medically provided nutrition and hydration in children. *Pediatrics, 124,* 813–822.

Nelson, L. J., Rushton, C. H., Cranford, R. E., Nelson, R. M., Glover, J. J., & Truog, R. D. (1995). Forgoing medically provided nutrition and hydration in pediatric patients. *Journal of Law, Medicine & Ethics, 23*, 33–46.

CARDIOPULMONARY RESUSCITATION AND "DO NOT RESUSCITATE" (DNR) ORDERS

American Academy of Pediatrics Committee on Bioethics & The Committee on School Health. (2010). Honoring do-not-resuscitate requests in schools. *Pediatrics, 125*, 1073–1077.

American Medical Association Council on Ethical and Judicial Affairs. (1991). Guidelines for the appropriate use of do-not-resuscitate orders. *Journal of the American Medical Association, 265*, 1868–1871.

Blackhall, L. J. (1987). Must we always use CPR? *New England Journal of Medicine, 317*, 1281–1285.

Ditillo, B. A. (2002). Should there be a choice for cardiopulmonary resuscitation when death is expected? Revisiting an old idea whose time is yet to come. *Journal of Palliative Medicine, 5*, 107–116.

Fallat, M. E., & Deshpande, J. K. (2004). Do not resuscitate orders for the pediatric patients who require anesthesia and surgery. *Pediatrics, 114*, 1686–1692.

Friedman, S. L. (2006). Parent resuscitation preferences for young people with severe developmental disabilities. *Journal of the American Medical Directors Association, 7*, 67–72.

Henderson, D. P., & Knapp, J. F. (2005). Report of the national consensus conference on family presence during pediatric cardiopulmonary resuscitation and procedures. *Pediatric Emergency Care, 21*, 787–791.

Loertscher, L., Reed, D. A., Bannon, M. P., & Mueller, P. S. (2010). Cardiopulmonary resuscitation and do-not-resuscitate orders: A guide for clinicians. *American Journal of Medicine, 123*, 4–9.

Meyer, E. C., Ritholz, M. D., Burns, J. P., & Truog, R. D. (2006). Improving the quality of end-of-life care in the pediatric intensive care unit: Parents' priorities and recommendations. *Pediatrics, 117*, 649–657.

FUTILITY

Helft, P. R., Siegler, M., & Lantos, J. (2000). The rise and fall of the futility movement. *New England Journal of Medicine, 343*, 293–295.

Moseley, K. L., Silveira, M. J., & Goold, S. D. (2005). Futility in evolution. *Clinical Geriatric Medicine, 21*(1), 211–222.

Nelson, L. J., & Nelson, R. M. (1992). Ethics and the provision of futile, harmful, or burdensome treatment to children. *Critical Care Medicine, 20*, 427–433.

Paris, J. J., & Schreiber, M. D. (1996). Physicians' refusal to provide life-prolonging medical interventions. *Clinical Perinatology, 23*, 563–571.

Schneiderman, L. J., Jecker, N. S., & Jonsen, A. R. (1990). Medical futility: Its meaning and ethical implications. *Annals of Internal Medicine, 112*, 949–954.

Tomlinson, T., & Brody, H. (1990). Futility and the ethics of resuscitation. *Journal of the American Medical Association, 264*, 1276–1280.

Truog, R. D., Brett, A. S., & Frader, J. (1992). The problem with futility. *New England Journal of Medicine, 326,* 1560–1564.

Weil, M. H., & Weil, C. J. (2000). How to respond to family demands for futile life support and cardiopulmonary resuscitation. *Critical Care Medicine, 28,* 3339–3340.

PERSISTENT/PERMANENT VEGETATIVE STATE

Ashwal, S., Bale, J. F., Jr., Coulter, D. L., Eiben, R., Garg, B. P., Hill, A., . . . Walker, R. W. (1992). The persistent vegetative state in children: Report of the Child Neurology Society Ethics Committee. *Annals of Neurology, 32,* 570–576.

Multi-Society Task Force on PVS. (1994). Medical aspects of the persistent vegetative state (Part 1). *New England Journal of Medicine, 330,* 1449–1508.

Multi-Society Task Force on PVS. (1994). Medical aspects of the persistent vegetative state (Part 2). *New England Journal of Medicine, 330,* 1572–1579.

PALLIATIVE CARE AND PAIN MANAGEMENT

American Academy of Pediatrics, Committee on Bioethics and Committee on Hospital Care. (2000). Palliative care for children. *Pediatrics, 106,* 351–357.

American Academy of Pediatrics, Committee on Fetus and Newborn and Section on Surgery; Canadian Paediatric Society Fetus and Newborn Committee, Batton, D. G., Barrington, K. J., & Wallman, C. (2006). Prevention and management of pain in the neonate: An update. *Pediatrics, 118,* 2231–2241.

Anand, K. J., & Craig, K. D. (1996). New perspectives on the definition of pain. *Pain, 67,* 3–6.

Fleischman, A. R., Nolan, K., Dubler, N. N., Epstein, M. F., Gerben, M. A., Jellinek, M. S., . . . Vaughan, C. (1994). Caring for gravely ill children. *Pediatrics, 94*(4), 433–439.

Kenny, N. P., & Frager, G. (1996). Refractory symptoms and terminal sedation of children: Ethical issues and practical management. *Journal of Palliative Care, 12,* 40–45.

Levetown, M. (1996). Ethical aspects of pediatric palliative care. *Journal of Palliative Care, 12*(3), 35–39.

Mack, J. W., & Grier, H. E. (2004). The day one talk. *Journal of Clinical Oncology, 22,* 563–566.

Steinhauser, K. E., Clipp, E. C., McNeilly, M., Christakis, N. A., McIntyre, L. M., & Tulsky, J. A. (2000). In search of a good death: Observations of patients, families, and providers. *Annals of Internal Medicine, 132,* 825–832.

Walco, G. A., Cassidy, R. C., & Schechter, N. L. (1994). Pain, hurt, and harm. The ethics of pain control in infants and children. *New England Journal of Medicine, 331,* 541–544.

Wolfe, J., Grier, H. E., Klar, N., Levin, S. B., Ellenbogen, J. M., Salem-Schatz, S., ... Weeks, J. (2000). Symptoms and suffering at the end of life in children with cancer. *New England Journal of Medicine, 342,* 326–333.

Wolfe, J., Klar, N., Grier, H. E., Duncan, J., Salem-Schatz, S., Emanuel, E. J., & Weeks, J. C. (2000). Understanding of prognosis among parents of children who died of cancer: Impact on treatment goals and integration of palliative care. *Journal of the American Medical Association, 284,* 2469–2475.

PHYSICIAN-ASSISTED SUICIDE AND EUTHANASIA

Miller, F. G., Quill, T. E., Brody, H., Fletcher, J. C., Gostin, L. O., & Meier, D. E. (1994). Regulating physician-assisted death. *New England Journal of Medicine, 331*(2), 119–123.

Verhagen, E., & Sauer, P. J. (2005). The Groningen protocol -- euthanasia in severely ill newborns. *New England Journal of Medicine, 10,* 959–962.

DECLARATION OF DEATH

1. **By neurological criteria:**

   Banasiak, K. J., & Lister, G. (2003). Brain death in children. *Current Opinions in Pediatrics, 15,* 288–293.

   Lazar, N. M., Shemie, S., Webster, G. C., & Dickens, B. M. (2001). Bioethics for clinicians: 24. Brain death. *Canadian Medical Association Journal, 164,* 833–836.

   President's Council on Bioethics. (2008). Controversies in the Determination of Death: A white paper by the President's Council on Bioethics. Retrieved from https://www.ethicshare.org/node/715643

   Truog, R. D. (2007). Brain death -- too flawed to endure, too ingrained to abandon. *Journal of Law, Medical & Ethics, 35,* 273–281.

   Wijdicks, E. F. (2001). The diagnosis of brain death. *New England Journal of Medicine, 344,* 1215–1221.

2. **By circulatory criteria:**

   Bernat, J. L. (2006). Are organ donors after cardiac death really dead? *Journal of Clinical Ethics, 17,* 122–132.

   Bernat, J. L. (2008). The boundaries of organ donation after circulatory death. *New England Journal of Medicine, 359,* 669–671.

   Truog, R. D., & Cochrane, T. I. (2006). The truth about "donation after cardiac death." *Journal of Clinical Ethics, 17,* 133–136.

Books and Book Chapters

Bluebond-Langner, M. (1980). *The private worlds of dying children.* Princeton, NJ: Princeton University Press.

Cross Cultural Health Care Program. (2000). *Death and dying in ethnic America: A research study.* Seattle, WA: Author.

Grace, P. J. (2009). Nursing ethics and advanced practice: Gerontology and end of life issues. In P. J. Grace (Ed.), *Nursing ethics and professional responsibility in advanced practice* (pp. 383–407. Sudbury, MA: Jones and Bartlett.

Levetown, M., & Carter, M. A. (1998). Child-centred care in terminal illness: An ethical framework. In D. Doyle, G. W. C. Hanks, & N. MacDonald (Eds.), *Oxford textbook of palliative medicine* (2nd ed., pp. 1107–1117). Oxford, England: Oxford University Press.

Mondragon, D. (Ed.). (1997). *Religious values of the terminally ill: A handbook for health professionals.* Las Cruces, NM: New Mexico State University Department of Health Science.

Schechter, N. L., Berde, C. B., & Yaster, M. (Eds.). (1993). Pain in infants, children, and adolescents: An overview. In *Pain in infants, children, and adolescents* (pp. 3–9). Baltimore, MD: Williams & Wilkins.

Walco, G. A., & Cassidy, R. C. (2000). The ethics of pain control in neonates and infant. In K. J. Anand, B. J. Stevens, & P. J. McGrath (Eds.), *Pain in neonates* (2nd ed., pp. 229–235). The Netherlands: Elsevier.

Wolf, S. M. (1998). Facing assisted suicide and euthanasia in children and adolescents. In L. L. Emanuel (Ed.), *Regulating how we die: The ethical, medical, and legal issues surrounding physician-assisted suicide*. Cambridge, MA: Harvard University Press.

Youngner, S. J., Arnold, R. M., & Schapiro, R. (Eds.). (1999). *The definition of death: Contemporary controversies*. Baltimore, MD: Johns Hopkins University Press.

Zucker, M. B., & Zucker, H. D. (1997). *Medical futility and the evaluation of life-sustaining interventions*. Cambridge, England: Cambridge University Press.

Online Resources

American Academy of Pediatrics
www.aap.org

American Academy of Pediatrics, Committee on Bioethics
www.aap.org/sections/bioethics/default.cfm

American Society for Bioethics and Humanities
www.asbh.org

ACT (Association for Children's Palliative Care)
www.act.org.uk

Growth House, Inc. The Yahoo of Death and Dying
www.growthhouse.orgHospice and Palliative Nurses Association
www.hpna.org

National Hospice and Palliative Care Organization
www.nhpco.org

Pediatrics Electronic Pages
www.pediatrics.org

Pediatrics Ethics Consortium
www.pediatricethics.org

Society for Adolescent Medicine
www.adolescenthealth.org

Society of Critical Care Medicine
http://www.sccm.org/Pages/default.aspx

Treuman Katz Center for Pediatric Bioethics
www.seattlechildrens.org/research/initiatives/bioethics/

Tuskegee University National Center for Bioethics in Research and Health Care
http://www.tuskegee.edu/about_us/centers_of_excellence/bioethics_center.aspx

United States Department of Health and Human Services
www.thinkculturalhealth.org

University of British Columbia Centre for Applied Ethics
www.ethics.ubc.ca/resources/biomed/

University of Buffalo Center for Clinical Ethics and Humanities in Health Care
www.wings.buffalo.edu//bioethics/ http://www.google.com/url?sa=t&rct=j&q=&esrc
=s&source=web&cd=1&cad=rja&ved=0CDEQFjAA&url=http%3A%2F%2Fwings.buf-
falo.edu%2Fbioethics%2F&ei=mnmKUdCoAdj94AOnxoHYBA&usg=AFQjCNGquaUe
fhLaDknAFRmvbHk0j927qA&bvm=bv.46226182,d.dmg

Glossary*

Accountability The responsibility of the professional for making sound clinical judgments, anticipating foreseeable harms, and being answerable for actions.

Advance directive A person's instructions that name a proxy decision maker and/or delineate acceptable interventions and that are to be used if the person's decision-making capacity is lost. The legal status of these documents varies from state to state.

Advanced practice nursing An advanced level of knowledge, skills, and experience applied to the nursing care of patients within primary care or specialty practice settings.

Aesthetics Philosophical inquiry about art or beauty.

Altruism Actions taken for or on behalf of another person that are not primarily self-serving. In the helping professions, altruism serves as a basis for ethical action along with an understanding of responsibilities incurred by assuming the professional role.

ANA Code of Ethics for Nurses with Interpretive Statements (2001) The written guidelines of the American Nurses Association that outline ethical action for all professional nurses practicing in the United States. The provisions are revised periodically as a result of societal changes and input from practicing nurses and nursing academics.

Applied ethics The application of moral philosophy and moral theory to actual situations involving human action.

---

*Prepared with assistance from my undergraduate research assistant at the time, Nora Sheehan, RN, BSN.

Assent   A child's affirmative agreement to participate in research or treatment after age- and developmentally appropriate information has been shared with and understood by the child. Failure to object to treatment or research is not the equivalent of assent.

Autonomy   An ethical principle that calls attention to a person's right to be treated with dignity and respect. It entails a right to self-determine both acceptable treatment and with whom information may be shared.

Beneficence   The ethical principle that enjoins healthcare professionals to remain focused on their professional goals in providing a good for individuals.

Care ethics   An approach to ethical decision making that focuses on the roles of relationships and contexts in achieving good for a patient. It acknowledges that relationships among patients, their families and loved ones, and their providers are important factors in decision making.

Caring   A concept that has been variously defined but that can best be described as a focused attention on and, when possible, engagement with a patient to determine that person's particular needs and the use of clinical judgment to meet those needs.

Case-based ethics or casuistry   An educational and analytic strategy whereby a landmark or epitome case (that has received some resolution or where improved understanding of nuances has occurred) is compared to and contrasted with a current problematic case or issue.

Clinical ethics residency for nurses (CERN) project   A collaborative endeavor among Massachusetts General Hospital, Boston College, and Brigham and Women's Hospital, Massachusetts. A 3-year Health Resources and Services grant funded by the U.S. Department of Health and Human Services and designed to increase the confidence of bedside and advanced practice nurses in ethical decision making and prepare them to act as unit or as department-based ethics resources.

Confidentiality   The ethical requirement for professionals, institutions, and employees of institutions to disclose information only to those who need to know for the purposes of providing care; the patient's right to say with whom his or her healthcare information may be shared.

Conflict of interest   A situation in which two or more competing interests (conscious or unconscious) exist; may result in the professional not focusing on or fulfilling professional responsibilities to patients, family members of patients, or society. For example, when a professional receives favors for promoting a good or service that is not actually the best option for a patient or when a professional is worried about losing his or her job or position because the professional does not follow the wishes of his or her employer.

Cooperation   The responsibility to collaborate with others within and outside of the profession for the purposes of achieving a good for an individual or society related to health care.

Deprofessionalization   A phenomenon in which professionals lose their ability to govern their own practice, or professions lose the rights of self-regulation. It is a problem for society because the profession is less likely to be able to meet societal expectations of the practice or service.

Descriptive ethics   Observations of what human beings take to be good actions and/or the reasons people give to justify their actions as morally good; for example, research on practice behaviors.

Dilemma   A choice that must be made between two or more actions when it is not possible to be clear about which action is preferable. In healthcare settings, a dilemma usually involves negative choices or situations where no good action is available and one must choose among equally problematic alternatives.

Distributive justice   Fair, equitable, and appropriate allocation of goods, services, and resources based on criteria that a society agrees are ethical and justifiable.

Epistemology   Philosophical inquiry about knowledge. It explores questions such as *What is knowledge?*, *What counts as knowledge and why?*, and *What are salient characteristics of human beings related to knowledge?*

Ethical practice   The use of disciplinary knowledge, skills, experience, and personal characteristics to conceptualize and act upon what is needed either at the level of the individual or of society.

Ethical principles   Rules, standards, or guidelines for action that are derived from theoretical propositions about what is good for humans.

Ethics Philosophical inquiry about the good; also called moral philosophy.

Feminist ethics An approach that takes the experience of women as a starting point by acknowledging that an individual lives in the context of societal, institutional, and interpersonal power structures. These structures give rise to injustices for women and other groups that are disadvantaged in some way.

Fidelity Refers to being faithful to the obligation of keeping promises made in a therapeutic relationship.

Fiduciary relationship An association based on trust. When there exists an inequality in knowledge, skills, or will, one party has to trust that the other—who has specialized knowledge or skills—will maintain a primary focus on meeting the first party's needs and interests.

Human rights Basic moral guarantees that a minimally good life is granted to all humans by virtue of their humanity (if granted to any), regardless of societal or political contexts. Some examples are provisions for education and health care, and protection from the effects of destitution.

Human subject A living individual about whom an investigator (whether professional or student) conducting research obtains (1) data through intervention or interaction with the individual, or (2) identifiable private information.

Implicit consent The implied permission given by the patient when entering a healthcare setting that the patient will accept certain routine evaluations and interventions, such as blood pressure measurement.

Informed consent The right of all patients—who are physically and cognitively able—to determine what is acceptable in the way of treatment and interventions. Implies that adequate information is given and is presented in a way that is comprehensible to that particular person.

Institutional review board A governmentally mandated committee charged with overseeing the protection of human subjects enrolled in research studies in an institution. The mandate for an institutional review board applies only to institutions that receive some government funding for research (almost all hospitals and research universities).

Legal rights Liberties or privileges that in democratic societies are conceived with the input of citizens and for which impingements warrant formal sanctions of some kind.

Maternal–fetal conflict   A situation in which the well-being of the mother is taken to stand in opposition to the well-being of the fetus.

Medical model   A systems model that focuses on bodily functions and disturbances.

Moral distress   The feeling of unease or discomfort experienced by healthcare providers when they cannot provide what they perceive is needed for a patient. It can be relatively transient or intractable and can lead to distancing or attrition.

Moral reasoning   The application of theoretical understandings and reasoned assumptions to determine what is good action in complex situations where the best action is at least initially unclear.

Moral residue   The persisting experience of not having acted appropriately to resolve a perceived ethical practice problem; can lead to physical as well as psychological symptoms.

Moral rights   Goods that are inherently granted to all persons in a society; these include such things as freedom to make one's own choices and freedom from state interference in personal affairs.

Moral theory   A systematic justified explanation of what good means in terms of how human beings do or should seek to live their lives.

Narrative ethics   An ethics framework that uses stories to expose and explore hidden facets of morally worrisome cases.

Negative moral right   The right to be left alone and to be free from the interference of others or from the state.

Nonmaleficence   The ethical principle that enjoins us to avoid harm in the course of providing healthcare services. The duty of the nurse is to protect the patient from any avoidable harm caused in the course of providing care.

Nontherapeutic research   Research that aims to contribute more generally to the knowledge base for benefit to others rather than benefit to the subject.

Normative ethics   Reasoned and logically explored explanations of the moral purpose of human interactions or revealed truths about good action. Prescribes which actions ought to be taken, which actions are permissible, and which actions are forbidden.

Nursing ethics (1) The study of what constitutes good nursing practice, what obstacles to good nursing practice exist, and what the responsibilities of nurses are in relation to their professional conduct; (2) how nurses act to further professional goals in the practice of individual situations.

Nursing theory Describes and explains nursing care and provides a structure or framework that facilitates practice, guides research endeavors aimed at expanding nursing's knowledge base, and underpins practitioner development and education.

Paternalism The intentional overriding of a person's preferences because these are determined by others not to be in the person's best interest.

Patient Self-Determination Act A U.S. federal law that mandates all institutions that accept Medicare (government) funding disseminate written information to all patients concerning their rights to accept or refuse medical treatment.

Political action Activities informed by nursing knowledge and clinical judgment that are undertaken by the nurse, often in collaboration with others, for the purpose of influencing necessary changes in policy at the institutional, local, or societal levels.

Positive moral right A claim that can be made against someone or some institution for assistance or for the provision of goods and services.

Practical reason A type of reasoning that acts as a constraint on emotional and instinctual drives that can result in harmful actions, on the one hand, and lack of needed action or inadequate action, on the other hand.

Practical wisdom Permits a person to understand what is a good way to live and that living a good life means habitually moderating emotional impulses by using reason.

Preventive ethics Anticipating and addressing potential problems before they arise.

Privacy The right to be free from the interference of others and the freedom to grant or withhold access to information about oneself.

Private information   Information about behavior that occurs in a context in which an individual can reasonably expect that no observation or recording is taking place, and information that has been provided for specific purposes by an individual and that the individual can reasonably expect will not be made public.

Profession   A discipline that has an extensive and specialized knowledge base, takes responsibility for developing and using its knowledge, has a practice or action orientation that is used for the good of the population served, and autonomously sets standards for and monitors the actions of its members.

Professional advocacy   Actions taken by a nurse or other professional to ensure good care at the level of the individual and at broader levels as necessary. Includes responsibilities both to address immediate situations of inadequate practice and to be active in addressing the environmental conditions that give rise to practice problems.

Professional autonomy   A profession's warrant—granted by society—to be self-governing and self-regulating.

Professional judgment   The nonlinear process of using knowledge, reasoning, tacit (experiential) knowledge, and interpersonal skills to determine—within the limits of available information—the probable best actions given the inevitable existence of some uncertainty about both the possession of adequate knowledge and the outcome of actions.

Proxy decision making   The act of deciding what healthcare actions are permissible for someone who temporarily or permanently has lost decision-making capacity, never had decision-making capacity (profound cognitive deficits), or is not yet considered sufficiently mature to make healthcare decisions (children).

Qualitative research   A form of social inquiry that is designed to understand the way people interpret and make sense of experienced phenomena.

Research   A systematic investigation—including research development, testing, and evaluation—designed to develop or contribute to generalizable knowledge.

Social contract　An agreement between an individual and society that assigns to both the individual and the society certain moral and political obligations.

Social justice　Formal systems that exist to decide who gets what in terms of social goods such as education, food, shelter, and health care.

Therapeutic research　Research that involves testing potential new treatments or therapies for a malady or condition experienced by the subject and that takes place as part of patient care.

Veracity　Truthfulness in giving patients information about their healthcare needs; facilitates autonomous choice and enhances patient decision making.

Verbal consent　The sanction given by the patient, after being educated and informed of the intended care, to be cared for by healthcare personnel, including evaluation, tests, therapeutics, and decisions about the best ways of managing chronic conditions.

Virtue ethics　In healthcare practice, the idea that a person can cultivate certain characteristics (virtues) that will predispose the person to good actions related to the profession's predetermined goals.

Virtues　Characteristics supposed to be essential for consistently good patient care and decision making. Some examples are empathy, veracity, transparency of purpose, cultural sensitivity, and motivation to act.

Written consent　The informed permission that the patient or the patient's designated proxy gives to the physician or advanced practice nurse to undertake a procedure. It consists of a signed legal document.

INDEX

Note: Page numbers followed by *b*, *f*, or *t* indicate material in boxes, figures, or tables, respectively.